SERIOUS STRENGTH TRAINING

Tudor Bompa

York University

Lorenzo Cornacchia

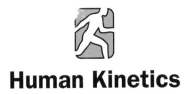

Human Kinetics

Library of Congress Cataloging-in-Publication Data

Bompa, Tudor O.
    Serious strength training / Tudor O. Bompa, Lorenzo Cornacchia.
        p.   cm.
    Includes bibliographical references and index.
    ISBN 0-88011-834-2 (paperback)
    1. Weight training.   2. Bodybuilding.   3. Muscle strength.
I. Cornacchia, Lorenzo, 1968-   .   II. Title.
GV546.B66   1998
613.7'1--dc21   98-12309
                                                              CIP

ISBN: 0-88011-834-2

Permission notices for material reprinted in this book from other sources can be found on page x.

Acquisitions Editor: Martin Barnard; **Developmental Editor**: Sydney Slobodnik; **Assistant Editors**: Katy Patterson and Jenny Simmons; **Copyeditor**: Jim Gallant; **Proofreader**: Erin Cler; **Indexer**: Gerry Lynn Messner; **Graphic Designer**: Nancy Rasmus; **Graphic Artist**: Sandra Meier; **Photo Editor**: Boyd LaFoon, **Cover Designer**: Jack Davis; **Photographer** (cover): © Quicksilver/ D.R. Goff; **Illustrator**: Denise Lowry; **Printer**: Versa

Human Kinetics books are available at special discounts for bulk purchase. Special editions or book excerpts can also be created to specification. For details, contact the Special Sales Manager at Human Kinetics.

Printed in the United States of America   10 9 8 7 6 5 4 3 2

Human Kinetics
Web site: http://www.humankinetics.com/

United States: Human Kinetics, P.O. Box 5076, Champaign, IL 61825-5076
1-800-747-4457
e-mail: humank@hkusa.com

Canada: Human Kinetics, 475 Devonshire Road, Unit 100, Windsor, ON N8Y 2L5
1-800-465-7301 (in Canada only)
e-mail: humank@hkcanada.com

Europe: Human Kinetics, P.O. Box IW14, Leeds LS16 6TR, United Kingdom
(44) 1132 781708
e-mail: humank@hkeurope.com

Australia: Human Kinetics, 57A Price Avenue, Lower Mitcham, South Australia 5062
(088) 277 1555
e-mail: humank@hkaustralia.com

New Zealand: Human Kinetics, P.O. Box 105-231, Auckland 1
(09) 523 3462
e-mail: humank@hknewz.com

CONTENTS

PREFACE

Strength training and bodybuilding are a religion, an obsession, for the many individuals whose purpose is to build and sculpt the body into a state of muscular, symmetrical perfection. It is the only sport dedicated solely to the aesthetics of the human body. The roots of strength training and bodybuilding lie in Greek and Roman antiquity. These civilizations used physical activity as a means of achieving, among other things, a perfect balance between body and mind. Sculptures from these ancient societies reflect their perceptions of the perfect human form—large, strong, well-defined muscles, all in perfect proportion, or balance.

Today, however, some bodybuilders at the professional level seem to have abandoned the ideal of the perfect human body for the novelty of a freaky body part. They seem to favor mass over symmetry, bulk over chiseled lines, bloat over definition, and quantity over quality. While mass is important, we must realize that its value does not exceed the value of symmetrical lines, well-proportioned limbs, and deeply-striated muscles. To attain the ultimate body, one must never lose sight of the balance that shapes the perfect form. Achieving this level of development requires dedication, patience, and most important, a solid understanding of the body, training principles, exercise prescription, nutrition, and planning. This book introduces a revolutionary approach to strength training and bodybuilding, that will bring the body to its perfect state, naturally, with Periodization. Read on to see how this book can help you build the ultimate physique!

Getting Bigger and Stronger!

Dr. Tudor O. Bompa developed Periodization in Romania in 1963. The Eastern Bloc countries used his unique system for years, as they achieved virtual domination of the athletic world. The system has also been published world-wide in many journals and magazines. He is also the author of several books, including *Theory and Methodology of Training: The Key to Athletic Performance* (1983, 1985, 1990, and 1994), and *Periodization of Strength: The New Wave in Strength Training* (1993). In 1988, he applied his concept of Periodization to the sport of bodybuilding, and his "Periodization of Bodybuilding" system has been published in *Ironman Magazine* as the "Ironman Training System" from 1991 to present.

Serious Strength Training is a method of organizing training to achieve optimum gains in mass, strength, and definition, without encountering the pitfalls of overtraining, stagnation, and injury. Different training phases such as anatomical adaptation, hypertrophy, maximum strength, muscle definition, and transition are manipulated according to individual training goals, to ensure peaking at appropriate times, as well as building and maintaining a splendid physique year-round. Whether you are just beginning to weight train or are a seasoned pro, Bompa has the training plan you need, complete with detailed daily training programs.

Get Lean and Ripped!

For the first time, a nutritional program has been designed to correspond with each different phase of training.

The body's needs change as training changes, so we must take nutrition into account, and not leave it to chance as in the past. The new "Periodization of Nutrition," based on Tudor Bompa's concept, gives athletes the tools needed to reach optimal levels of strength, mass, and definition.

Say good-bye to that "off season" look. Vicky Pratt's nutritional plans will help you to build the mass and strength you want, while getting and staying lean—year round. YES, it can happen to you!

Get Smart!

Cutting edge research, headed by kinesiologist and former NWA (National Wrestling Alliance) lightweight prospect, Lorenzo Cornacchia, gives you the last word on the best exercises for strength, mass, and shape. Scientific studies, using state of the art EMG (Electromyography) equipment, target the exercises that cause the greatest stimulation in the muscles and identify those exercises that might be potentially harmful. The chapter on maximum stimulation lifts ranks the exercises in order of their effectiveness, and provides pictures for each movement, to ensure proper execution.

Get Clean!

Dr. Mauro DiPasquale is the Drug Program Advisor to the WWF, and Medical Review Officer for the National Association for Stock Car Racing. Mauro is an expert in the area of ergogenic aids. He has written several books including *Drug Use and Detection in Amateur Sports* and *Beyond Anabolic Steroids*. Mauro shares his expertise on anabolic steroid side effects and other ergogenic substances.

Get Started!

For those who have been using the Periodization training system over the past few years, this plan has meant better results, with increased muscle size, tone, and definition, without the ever-present pain, strain, and exhaustion. For those about to begin using *Serious Strength Training*, don't look back. Training will never be the same again!

How to Use This Book

Part 1 gives you the background needed to plan effectively. Chapter 1 gives you an understanding of human anatomy—what happens to the body during training and why. Chapter 2 goes into detail about program design and shows you how to calculate training volume, intensity, rest intervals, number of exercises, and loading patterns. Here we introduce you to 1 rep max. Chapter 3 introduces you to short-term planning, and explains the principles and laws of bodybuilding and strength training. Here you will learn about "step-type" loading.

Part 2 shows you how to use "Periodized Workouts" to build and sculpt the ultimate physique. Chapters 4-10 take you through all of the training phases: anatomical adaptation, hypertrophy, maximum strength, mixed, muscle definition, and transition. You will also find programs for entry-level, recreational, and advanced strength trainers and bodybuilders. Yearly training programs are offered for those with special needs and interests, such as those who want to train for definition, not bulk and those who already have a strong training background. Special needs that are taken into consideration include family obligations and hectic holiday seasons that don't allow time for training.

Part 3 gives you detailed information about exercise, nutrition, and health. Chapter 11 employs scientific methods (Electromyography—EMG) to help you select the most effective exercises for maximum efficiency. Chapter 12 reviews the best information on nutrition and proposes a new approach, Periodization of Nutrition. Chapter 13 shows you techniques to use to avoid over-training and recover from fatigue and injury and chapter 14 promotes drug-free training.

ACKNOWLEDGMENTS

As our goal throughout this project has been to provide the most up-to-date and useful strength training and bodybuilding information, we called on the assistance of several noted colleagues. For their expert contributions to the completion of this book, we are grateful to the following:

Mauro Di Pasquale, BSc (Hon.), MD

Vicky Pratt, BA, Phe

Lenny Visconti, BPhe, BSc (PT), CAFC

Bill McIlroy, PhD

Roger Kelton, PhD

Louis Melo, PhD

Bruce Kripp, MSc

Teddy Temertzoglou, BScPhe

Courtney Bean, BSc (PT)

Cassandra Volpe, PhD

Jacquie Lafromboise, MSc

Shiraz Kapadia, BSc (PT)

Marni Pepper, BSc (PT)

We are equally indebted to York University for the use of its EMG research facilities and Bill McIlroy from the University of Toronto for his expertise in EMG analysis. Special thanks to Vince Scozzari, co-owner of Strictly Fitness; Steve Venet, co-owner of Pitbull Gym; Toula Reppas, owner of the Eglinton and Bayview Physiotherapy Clinic; and Joints in Motion for the use of their facilities.

We express our appreciation to several friends and close associates who have contributed either directly or indirectly to the completion of this book.

Patricia Gallacher

Bernadette Taggio

Kelly Morrell

Trevor Butler

Michael Berger

Carmela Caggianiello

Pat Caggianiello

André Elie

John Poptsis

Margaret Pratt

Douglas Adams

We would like to thank Peter Robinson (905) 336-7457 for the high professionalism demonstrated throughout the hundreds of hours necessary to take thousands of pictures (chapter 11). Our special appreciation to Sammy Wong, Sammy Wong Photography (416) 812-3692 for his exercise and nutrition pictures.

Special thanks to all the bodybuilders and fitness models who posed for the photographs.

Special thanks to Stephen Holman, Editor in Chief of *Ironman Magazine*, Tom Deters, DC, Associate Publisher of *Flex* (Weider Publications), and Robert Kennedy, editor of *Muscle Mag International*, for their many hours of kind and professional assistance.

CREDITS

Figures 1.5, 2.1, 2.2, 2.3, 2.4, 3.1, 3.2, 3.3, 3.4, 3.5, 3.6, 4.2, and 13.1 reprinted, by permission, from T.O. Bompa, 1996, *Periodization of Strength*, 4ᵗʰ ed. (Toronto: Veritas Publishing), 57, 89, 90, 91, 92, 137, 157, 158, 234.

Figures 3.7, 3.8 and 3.9 reprinted, by permission, from T.O. Bompa, 1983, *Theory and Methodology of Training*, (Dubuque, IA: Kendall/Hunt), 19, 20, 21.

Figures 13.1, 13.2, 13.3, 13.4, 13.5, 13.6, and 13.7 reprinted, by permission, from K.L. Moore, 1980, *Clinically Oriented Anatomy*, (Baltimore: Williams & Wilkins), 209, 211, 560, 571, 628, 629, 639, 812.

Tables 2.1, 2.3, 2.4, 4.1, A.1, A.2, A.3 reprinted, by permission, from T.O. Bompa, 1996, *Periodization of Strength*, 4ᵗʰ ed. (Toronto: Veritas Publishing), 64, 75, 81, 136, 261, 263-266, 267-271.

## PART 1

PLANNING A SERIOUS PROGRAM

CHAPTER 1
USING SCIENCE TO GET RESULTS

For any serious student of strength training and bodybuilding, it is important to understand muscle physiology, particularly muscle structure and the main function of muscle contraction.

The Body's Structure

The human body is constructed around a bone skeleton. Where two or more bones meet they form a *joint*, which is held together by tough bands of connective tissue called *ligaments*. The skeletal frame is covered by 656 muscles, which represent approximately 40% of the total body weight. Both ends of each muscle connect to dense connective tissue called *tendons*, which attach the muscle to the bone. All the tension developed within the muscles is directed to the bone through this tendinous linkage. The greater the tension, the stronger the pull on the tendons and bone and, consequently, the more powerful the limb's movement. The use of Periodization will increase muscle size and tone, and will also give tendons and ligaments the chance to adapt to increasing size.

Blood Supply to Muscles

All muscles contain blood vessels that branch into a fine network of tiny vessels called *capillaries* and *venules*. The capillaries are responsible for supplying oxygen-rich blood and nutrients to the tissues for energy, while the venules remove de-oxygenated blood and waste products, such as carbon dioxide, from the tissues.

The amount of blood required by a contracting skeletal muscle depends on the intensity of the exercise being performed. The blood supply needed for working muscles during a maximum strength workout may be as much as 100 times greater than the blood needed at rest.

Nerve Supply to Muscles

Muscles have two types of nerves.

- *Motor nerves* (nerves related to movement): Each motor nerve sends impulses from the *central nervous system (CNS)* to the termination point on a muscle fiber, called the *motor end plate*, resulting in a muscle contraction.

- *Sensory nerves*: These nerves relay information about pain and body orientation from the body to the CNS.

A muscle consists of special fibers, which range in length from a few inches to over three feet, and extend over the entire length of the muscle. These fibers are grouped in bundles called *fasciculi*, each separately wrapped in a sheath *(perimysium)* that holds it together.

Each muscle fiber has thread-like protein strands called *myofibrils*, which hold the contractile proteins *myosin* (thick filaments) and *actin* (thin filaments), whose actions are very important in muscle contraction (see figure 1.1). The ability of a muscle to contract and exert force is determined by its design, the cross-sectional area, the fiber length, and the number of fibers within the muscle. Genetics determines the number of fibers within the

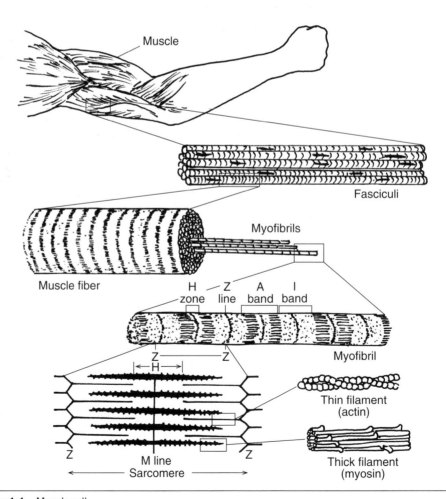

Figure 1.1 Muscle cell.

muscles, and training will not affect this, but training will have an impact on the other variables. Dedicated training increases the thickness of these muscle filaments, which increases both muscle size and force of contraction.

Mechanism of Muscular Contraction: The Sliding Filament Theory

Muscular contraction involves the two contractile proteins, actin and myosin, in a mechanical series of events called the *sliding filament theory of contraction*. Each myosin filament is surrounded by six actin filaments. The myosin filaments contain *cross-bridges*, which are tiny extensions that reach toward the actin filaments. When an impulse from the motor nerve reaches the muscle cell, it stimulates the entire fiber, creating chemical changes that allow the actin filaments to join with the myosin cross-bridges. The binding of myosin to actin via cross-bridges results in a release of energy that causes the cross-bridges to swivel, pulling or sliding the myosin filament over the actin filament. This sliding motion causes the muscle to shorten (contract), producing force. Once the stimulation ceases, the actin and myosin filaments separate, lengthening the muscle to its resting length and the contraction ceases (see figure 1.2). This cross-bridge activity explains why the muscular force generated depends upon the initial length of the muscle prior to contraction. The optimal length for muscular contraction is resting length (or slightly greater), because all of the cross-bridges can connect with the actin filaments, slowing maximal tension development.

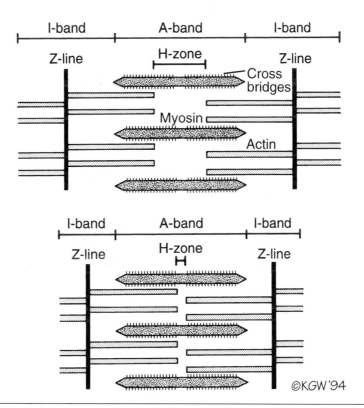

Figure 1.2   Contraction while muscle is shortened.
© K. Galasyn-Wright, Champaign, IL 1994.

The contractile force decreases when the length of the muscle prior to contraction is significantly shorter than the resting length (i.e., already partially contracted). This is due to the fact that in an already shortened muscle the actin and myosin filaments overlap to a great degree, which leaves fewer cross-bridges open to "pull" on the actin filaments. With fewer available cross-bridges less tension and force can be produced.

When the muscle lengthens too far beyond resting length the force potential will also be small, because the actin filaments are too far away from the cross-bridges to be able to join and shorten the muscle.

Contractile force diminishes as the muscle length becomes either shorter or longer than resting length. The highest force output occurs when the contraction begins at a joint angle of approximately 110-120 degrees (resting length).

The Motor Unit

Every single motor nerve entering a muscle can stimulate anywhere from one to several thousand muscle fibers. All of the muscle fibers activated by an individual motor nerve react together to its impulses, contracting and relaxing in unison. A single motor nerve together with the muscle fibers it activates creates a *motor unit* (see figure 1.3).

When a motor nerve is stimulated, the impulse sent to the muscle fibers within the motor unit either spreads completely or does not spread at all. This is the *all-or-none law*, which means that a weak impulse creates the same tension within the motor unit as a strong impulse.

This all-or-none law does not apply to the muscle as a whole. While all muscle fibers within a single motor unit respond to the stimulation of the motor nerve, not all motor units are activated during a muscular contraction. The number of motor units involved in a contraction depends on the load imposed upon the muscle, and this has a direct correlation to the force produced. For example, if the load is light, only a small number of motor units will be recruited and the strength of contraction will be low. On the other hand, if the load imposed upon the muscle is extremely heavy, then all or almost all of the motor units will be recruited resulting in a maximal force output (McDonagh and Davis, 1984). Since a muscle's motor units are recruited in sequential order, the only way to train the entire muscle is to expose it to maximum loads, so every motor unit is used for muscle contraction.

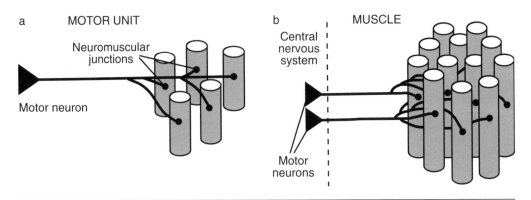

Figure 1.3   Motor unit source.
Reprinted, by permission, from Vander, Sherman, and Luciano, 1990, *Human Physiology*, 5th ed. (New York: McGraw-Hill), 296.

While the force exerted by a muscle depends upon the number of motor units recruited during a contraction, it also depends upon the number of muscle fibers within a motor unit. The number of fibers can vary between 20-500, with the average number being around 200. The more fibers in a motor unit, the higher the force output. The genetic factor that determines the number of fibers helps to explain why some people can increase muscle size and strength quite easily, while others have to fight for every small gain.

When a nerve impulse stimulates a motor unit, it responds by giving a *twitch* or a very quick contraction, followed by relaxation. If another impulse reaches the motor unit before it has time to relax, the two twitches *summate* (join forces) and produce greater tension than that produced by a single twitch.

The summation of motor units depends upon the load imposed on the muscle. (See figure 1.4.) During maximum loads (1.4c), all of the muscle's fibers summate in *synchronization* leading to maximum force output; during medium loads (1.4b), some motor units are twitching while others are relaxing, leading to medium force output. This is one of the main reasons why heavy loads lead to higher gains in maximum strength.

Muscle Fiber Types

While all motor units behave in the same way, this cannot be said for all muscle fibers. Not all muscle fibers have the same biochemical (metabolic) functions. Every muscle fiber can function under both anaerobic and aerobic conditions, although some work better under anaerobic conditions, while others work better under aerobic conditions.

The fibers that rely on and use oxygen to produce energy are aerobic, type I, red, or *slow-twitch (ST) fibers*. The fibers that do not require oxygen are anaerobic, type II, white, or *fast-twitch (FT) fibers*. ST and FT fibers exist in relatively equal proportions within the body, and this 50/50 relationship is not thought to be greatly affected by strength training and bodybuilding.

The recruitment of muscle fibers is load-dependent. During moderate and low intensity activity, ST fibers are recruited as work horses. As the load increases, a greater number of FT fibers are activated during a contraction.

The distribution of fiber types can vary, both within the same muscle and among different muscles. Usually, the arms tend to have a higher percentage of

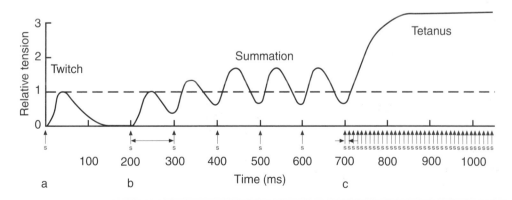

Figure 1.4   Isometric contractions produced by multiple stimuli of (b) 10 stimuli per second and (c) 100 stimuli per second, as compared with a single twitch (a).

FT fibers than the legs: biceps 55% FT, triceps 60% FT, whereas soleus (calves) 24% FT (Fox et al., 1989).

Fiber type composition (i.e., proportion of FT fibers within a muscle) plays an important role in strength training and bodybuilding. Muscles containing a high percentage of FT fibers are capable of quicker and more powerful contractions.

There are no clear differences in muscle fiber distribution between female and male athletes. An inherited propensity toward more FT fibers might indicate which individuals are genetically suited to strength training and bodybuilding. While genetics is an important factor in determining success, it is not the only one. Regardless of one's genetic endowments, every individual, through intensive training and proper nutrition, can improve his or her muscle size, tone, and definition.

Muscle Contraction

The musculoskeletal frame of the body is an arrangement of bones, attached to one another by a series of ligaments, at structures called joints. The muscles crossing these joints provide the force necessary for body movements. Skeletal muscles do not contract independently of one another. Rather, the movements performed about a joint involve several muscles, each having a different role.

Agonists or *synergists* are the muscles that work together as a team, cooperating to perform a movement.

Antagonists are the muscles that act in opposition to the agonists during a movement. In most cases, especially for skilled and experienced athletes, the antagonists are relaxed, allowing the motion to be performed with ease.

This shows that the interaction between agonist and antagonist muscle groups directly influences athletic movements. A motion that looks jerky, or is performed rigidly, might be the result of an improper interaction between the two groups. Only by concentrating on relaxing the antagonists, can one improve the flow and smoothness of a muscular contraction.

Prime movers are the muscles primarily responsible for producing a comprehensive strength movement. During a biceps curl exercise for example, the prime mover is the biceps muscle, while the triceps act as an antagonist and need to be relaxed in order to facilitate a smooth flexion.

Ronnie Coleman's muscular physique.

The *line of pull* for strength training and bodybuilding represents an imaginary line that crosses the muscle longitudinally, connecting the two extreme heads of the muscle. The highest physiological and mechanical efficiency of a muscle contraction is achieved when performed along the line of pull. An example using the biceps muscle will clarify this point. Elbow flexion can be performed with the palm held in several different positions. With the palm turned upward, the line of pull is direct, creating the highest efficiency. With the palm facing down, efficiency on contraction decreases because the tendon of the biceps muscle wraps around the bone radius. In this case, the line of pull is indirect, which wastes a large portion of the contractile force. If one is looking for maximum strength gains and optimal muscle efficiency, strength exercises must be performed along the line of pull.

Types of Muscular Contraction

Skeletal muscles are responsible for both contraction and relaxation. A muscle contracts when it is stimulated, and when the contraction stops the muscle relaxes. Bodybuilders and strength athletes use various types of contractions depending on the scope of their training phase and the equipment being used. There are three types of contractions—*isotonic*, *isometric*, and *isokinetic*.

Isotonic

Isotonic (dynamic), from the Greek "isos," meaning equal, and "tonikos," meaning tension, is the most familiar type of muscle contraction. As the term implies, during an isotonic contraction the tension should be the same throughout the entire range of motion. There are two types of isotonic contractions:

Concentric, from the Latin "com-centrum," meaning having a common center, refers to contractions in which the muscle length shortens. Concentric contractions are possible only when the resistance (i.e., weight load) starts from a position below the athlete's maximum potential. Examples of concentric contractions would include the curling action of a biceps curl, or the extending motion of a leg extension. The biceps preacher curls exercise in chapter 11 shows the curling action movement of a biceps curl—flexion.

Eccentric, or "negative" contractions, refer to the action that reverses the process of a concentric action. This simply means that eccentric contractions return the muscles to their original starting point. During a biceps curl, the eccentric component occurs when the arm extends to the starting point after the curl. During a leg extension, eccentric work is being done when the legs bend at the knee toward the starting position. During an eccentric contraction, the muscles are either yielding to the force of gravity (as in free weights), or to the force of pull of a machine. Under such conditions, the muscle lengthens as the joint angle increases, thus releasing a controlled tension. The biceps preacher curl photos also show the lowering of the barbell towards the starting stage of the biceps curl movement—extension.

Isometric

Isometric (static), from the Greek, *isos* meaning equal, and *meter* meaning unit of measurement, implies that during this type of contraction the muscle develops tension without changing its length. During an isometric contraction, the application of force against an immovable object forces the muscle to develop high tension without altering its length. The tension developed from this type of contraction is often higher than that developed during an isotonic contraction. For example, if an athlete pushes against a wall, tension is created in the muscle although it remains the same length.

Isokinetic

Isokinetic, coming from the Greek *isos* meaning equal, and *kinetic* meaning motion, describes a contraction with constant velocity over the full range of motion. Isokinetic work needs special equipment designed to allow a constant velocity of contraction regardless of the load. During the movement, both concentric and eccentric contractions are performed while the machine provides a resistance that is equal to the force generated by the athlete. The benefit of this type of training is that it allows the muscle to work maximally throughout the entire movement and eliminates the "sticking point," or weak spot, that is present in every exercise motion.

Roland Cziurlok's awesome size and strength are the result of employing maximum strength training.

Types of Strength and Their Significance in Training

Various types of strength training are needed to build and sculpt the most muscular, defined, symmetrical, and injury-free physique possible.

General strength is the foundation of the entire strength and bodybuilding program. It must be the sole focus of training during the early training phase of an experienced lifter, and during the first few years of an entry-level strength trainer or bodybuilder. A low level of general strength might be a limiting factor in overall progress. It leaves the body susceptible to injury and, potentially, even asymmetrical shape or a decreased ability to build muscle strength and size.

Maximum strength refers to the highest force that can be performed by the neuromuscular system during a maximum contraction. It reflects the heaviest load that an athlete can lift in one attempt, and is expressed as 100% of maximum, or *one repetition maximum (1RM)*. It is crucial, for training purposes, to know one's maximum strength for each exercise, since it is the basis for calculating loads for every strength phase.

Muscular endurance is defined as the muscle's ability to sustain work for a prolonged period. It is used largely in endurance training, and also plays a crucial role in bodybuilding and strength training, where it is used extensively during the "muscle definition" or "cuts" phase of training.

Muscular Adaptation to Bodybuilding and Strength Training

Systematic training results in certain structural and physiological changes, or adaptations, in the body. The size and definition of the body's muscles indicate the level of adaptation. The magnitude of these adaptations is directly proportional to the demands placed upon the body by volume (quantity) of training, frequency of training, and intensity (load) of training.

Strength cue:

> Training is beneficial to a strength trainer and bodybuilder only as long as it forces the body to adapt to the stress of physical work. In other words, if the body meets with a demand greater than that to which it is accustomed, it works to adapt to the stressor by becoming bigger and stronger. When the load is not high enough to challenge the body's *adaptation threshold*, the training effect will be nil or minimal and no adaptation will occur.

Types of Adaptation

Various body systems adapt to strength training in different ways. Muscles get bigger; bones get stronger or weaker, depending on the load; the central nervous system becomes more efficient at recruiting muscle action; and motor skills become more refined and coordinated.

Hypertrophy

One of the most visible signs of adaptation is the enlargement of muscle size—*hypertrophy*. This phenomenon is due to an increase in the cross-sectional area of individual muscle fibers. Conversely, a reduction in size resulting from inactivity is referred to as *atrophy*. Strength trainers and bodybuilders will experience two kinds of hypertrophy.

Short-term hypertrophy, as the name implies, lasts for only a few hours and is the result of the "pump" experienced during heavy training. This "pump" is largely the result of fluid accumulation (*edema*) in the muscle. Heavy lifting results in an increased amount of water being held in the intracellular spaces of the muscle, making it look even larger. When the water returns to the blood a few hours after training, the pump disappears. This is one reason why strength is not always proportional to muscle size.

Chronic hypertrophy is the result of structural changes at the muscle level. Since this is caused by an increase in either the number or size of muscle filaments, its effects are more enduring than those of short-term hypertrophy.

Individuals with a large number of fibers tend to be stronger and show more size than those with fewer fibers. The number was thought to remain constant throughout one's life because of the genetically determined number, however,

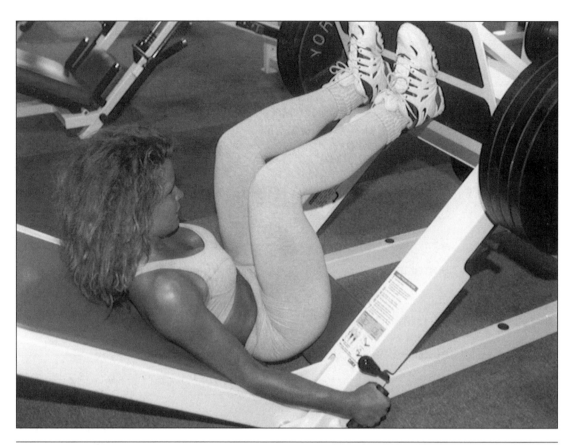

Sue Minicuccis' legs are pumped up during heavy training.

controversial theory now suggests that the heavy loads used in strength training might provoke "muscle splitting" or *hyperplasia*. If this is the case, hypertrophy might be partly induced by a possible increase in the number of muscle fibers. This theory is based on animal research and the results have not yet been duplicated in human subjects.

Strong evidence suggests that individual fiber hypertrophy accounts for most of the gains in muscle size. The increases in the muscle fiber size and number of filaments (especially the myosin filaments) have been demonstrated by many researchers (Gordon, 1967; Golber et al., 1975; MacDougall et al., 1975, 1976, 1977, and 1979; Costill et al., 1979; Dons et al., 1979; Gregory, 1981; and Fox et al., 1989). In the case of myosin, training with heavy loads increases the number of cross-bridges, leading to an increase in the cross-sectional area of the fiber and to visible gains in the force of maximum contraction.

Not all of the factors responsible for hypertrophy are fully understood. It is widely believed that growth in muscle size is stimulated mainly by a disturbance in the equilibrium between the consumption and remanufacturing of ATP (adenosine triphosphate), called the *ATP deficiency theory* (Hartman and Tünnemann, 1988). During and immediately following a heavy-load training session, protein content in the working muscles is very low, if not exhausted, due to ATP depletion. As the athlete recovers between two training sessions, the body works to replace the protein in the working muscles. During this replenishing process, the protein content in the muscles exceeds the initial levels, resulting in an increase in the size of the muscle fibers. A protein-rich diet will make this effect especially pronounced.

Another theory regarding hypertrophy suggests that the male sex hormone *testosterone* (serum androgen, a substance that has masculinizing properties) plays a role in muscle growth. The idea is that although there are no physiological differences between the muscles of women and men, male athletes usually have larger and stronger muscles. The difference is attributed to testosterone content, which is approximately ten times greater for men than for women. While testosterone seems to promote muscle growth, there is no scientific proof to indicate that it is the sole determinant of muscle size.

It is also possible that muscle hypertrophy might be attributable to a conversion of ST fibers to FT fibers. Although it is mostly speculation at this point, some research indicates that the percentage of ST fibers decreases as a result of strength training (Abernethy et al., 1990). Perhaps one reason why studies on this theory have been largely inconclusive is that research is typically conducted on subjects who are not serious strength trainers or bodybuilders. The findings might be different if a research study followed these athletes from the entry level to the professional level, instead of observing changes that occur in individuals of varying fitness levels during eight weeks of training.

Anatomical Adaptation

Research in the area of anatomical adaptation suggests that training with constant and extensive high-intensity loads might decrease the material strength of the bones (Matsuda, 1986). This means that if the load does not vary from low to maximum, the result might be a decrease in material bone strength, which might leave the athlete prone to bone injuries. The mechanical properties of bones are also affected by the mechanical demands of training. In other words, an injury-prone athlete might be one whose training exposes the bones to an intense mechanical stress without a progressive period of adaptation.

At an early age, or at the entry level, low intensity training might have a positive, stimulating effect on the length and girth of one's long bones, while high intensity, heavy-load training might permanently restrict bone growth (Matsuda, 1986) in beginners. Young and entry-level strength trainers and bodybuilders must carefully consider these facts. The most appropriate approach for these athletes is a long-term plan in which the load is progressively increased over several years. The purpose of training is to stress the body in such a way that it results in adaptation, not aggravation. A well-monitored load increment also has a positive effect for mature athletes, as it results in increased bone density, which allows the bones to better cope with the mechanical stresses of weight training.

The adaptation of tendons is of equal concern to strength training. Remember, muscles do not attach to bones directly, but rather through their extensions, called tendons. The ability of a muscle to pull forcefully against a bone and, as a result, to perform a movement, depends on the strength of the muscle's tendons. The adaptation of tendons is a long-term proposition. Tendons take a longer time to adapt to powerful contractions than muscles, therefore, muscle growth should not exceed the rate of tendon adaptation.

Nervous System Adaptation

Gains in muscle strength can also be explained by changes in both the pattern of motor unit recruitment and the synchronization of the motor units to act in

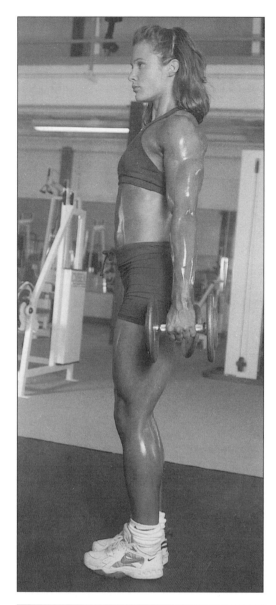

Nineteen-year-old sensation, Natalie.

unison. Let's see if we can explain this! Motor units are controlled by different nerve cells, called *neurons*, which have the capacity to produce both *excitatory* (stimulating) and *inhibitory* impulses.

Excitation is needed to initiate the contraction of a motor unit. Inhibition, on the other hand, is a mechanism that prevents the muscles from exerting more force than can be tolerated by the connective tissue (tendons) and bones. These two nervous system processes perform a sort of balancing act to ensure the safety of muscular contraction. The force outcome of a contraction depends on how many motor units will contract and how many will remain in a state of relaxation. If the number of excitatory impulses exceeds the number of inhibitory impulses, a given motor unit will be stimulated and will participate in the overall contraction and production of force. If the opposite occurs, that particular motor unit will stay relaxed. The theory is that as a result of training, inhibitory impulses can be counteracted, thus enabling the muscle to contract more powerfully. Therefore, it is fair to say that gains in strength are largely the result of an increased ability to recruit more motor units to participate in the overall force of contraction. Such an adaptive response is facilitated only by heavy and maximum loads, and is safe only after the tendons have adapted to high-intensity training.

Adaptation of Neuromuscular Coordination

Neuromuscular coordination for strength training and bodybuilding movement patterns takes time and is a function of learning. The ability to coordinate specific sequences, which involve different muscles to perform a lift, requires the precision that can only be acquired over a long period of continuous repetition. In other words, practice makes perfect. An efficient lift can be achieved only when the bodybuilder learns to relax the antagonistic muscles, so unnecessary contractions do not affect the force of the prime movers. A highly coordinated group of muscles consumes less energy during contraction, and this translates into superior performance.

It is only logical that young or entry-level strength trainers and bodybuilders are lacking in the necessary motor skills and muscle coordination. Hypertrophy, therefore, cannot be expected immediately. If young athletes are exposed to strength training, visible strength increments will be seen within the course of 4-6 weeks without a concomitant increase in muscle size. The reason for strength gain without achieving muscle hypertrophy is *neural adaptation*, which is an increase in the nervous coordination of the muscles involved. As a result of training, these entry-level athletes have learned to use their muscles effectively and economically. This motor learning effect is of major importance in the early stages of training and athletes must realize this is a necessary

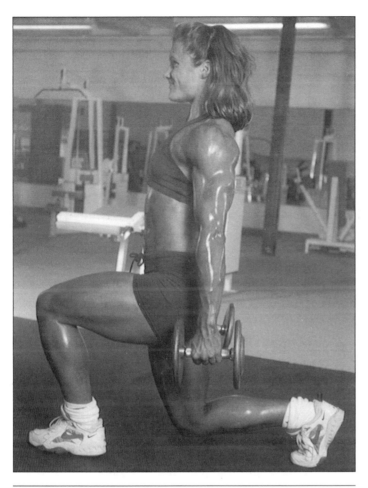

Natalie demonstrates excellent coordination and training technique.

progression. It is easy to become frustrated when improvement in size is not visibly apparent, but this will happen when the body is ready.

Principles of Strength and Bodybuilding Training

Training is a complex activity governed by principles and methodological guidelines, designed to help athletes achieve the greatest possible muscle size and definition.

Principle #1— Vary Your Training

Bodybuilding and strength training are very demanding sports that require hour after hour of dedicated training. The pressure of continually increasing training volume and intensity, along with the repetitive nature of weight lifting, can easily lead to boredom and monotony that might become obstacles to motivation and success.

The best medicine for dull, monotonous training is variety. To add variety one must be familiar with the areas of training methods and Periodization planning (see part 2), and be comfortable with a multitude of different exercises for each muscle group (see chapter 11).

Variety in training improves psychological well-being and also improves training response. The following suggestions will help you to add variety to your training.

- Choose different exercises for each specific body part instead of doing your favorite exercises each time. Mix up the order in which you perform certain exercises. Remember, both your mind and your body become bored; they both need variety.

- Incorporate variety into your loading system as suggested by the step-loading principle (discussed later in this chapter).

- Vary the type of muscular contractions done in your workouts (i.e., include concentric and eccentric work).

- Vary the speed of contraction (slow, medium, and fast).

- Vary equipment so you go from free weights to machine weights, to isokinetics, and so on.

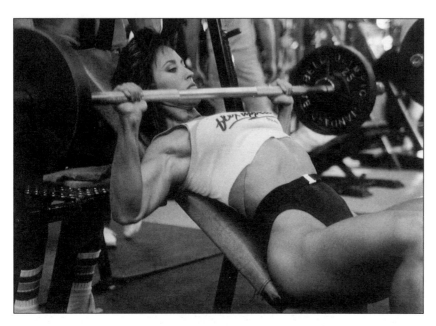

Rachel McLish takes on free weights in her workout.

Principle #2— Observe Individual Differences

No two people are alike. Rarely do two individuals come to training with exactly the same history and agenda. Everyone is different in his or her genetics, athletic background, eating habits, metabolism, training desire, and adaptation potential. For all these reasons, strength athletes and bodybuilders must have individual training programs, regardless of their level of development. Too often, entry-level athletes are seduced into following the training programs of advanced athletes. Advice given by these seasoned athletes is inappropriate for novices, no matter how well intentioned. Beginners, whose muscles, ligaments, and tendons are unaccustomed to the stresses of serious weight training, require a longer period of adjustment, or adaptation, in order to avoid injury.

Often an individual's work capacity is influenced by the following factors:

• *Training background.* The work demand should be proportional to experience, background, and age.

• *Individual capacity for work.* Not all athletes who are similar in structure and appearance have the same work tolerance. Individual work abilities must be assessed before determining the volume and intensity of work. This will increase the odds of becoming successful and remaining injury free.

• *Training load and recovery rate.* When planning and evaluating the training load, consider the factors outside training that place high demands on you. For example, heavy involvement in school, work, or family, and even the distance traveled to the gym, can affect the rate of recovery between training sessions. Destructive or negative lifestyle habits and emotional involvement should also be considered when creating a training plan.

Principle #3—Employ Step-Type Loading

The theory of progressive load increments in strength training has been known and employed since ancient times. According to Greek mythology, the first person to apply the theory was Milo of Croton, a pupil of the famous mathematician Pythagoras (580-500 BC), who was an Olympic wrestling champion himself. In his teen years, Milo decided to become the strongest man in the world, and embarked upon this mission by lifting and carrying a calf every day. As the calf grew and became heavier, Milo became stronger. Finally, when the calf had developed into a full-grown bull, Milo, thanks to a long-term progression, was able to lift the bull, and consequently became the strongest man on earth. Improvements in muscle size, tone, and definition are a direct result of the amount and quality of training performed over a long period of time. From the entry level right up to the Mr. or Ms. Olympia level, the training workload must be increased gradually in accordance with each individual's physiological and psychological abilities if gains in muscle size, tone, and definition are to continue.

The most effective technique for load patterning is the step-loading principle, because it fulfills the physiological and psychological requirements that a training load increase must be followed by a period of *unloading*. The unloading phase serves as a reprieve for the body, so it can adapt to the new, more intense stressors and regenerate itself in preparation for yet another load increase. Everyone responds differently to stress, therefore, each athlete's loading schedule must be planned according to his or her specific needs and rate of adaptation. For instance, if the load is increased too abruptly, it might exceed the body's adaptation capacity, which disrupts the physiological balance of the overload-to-adaptation cycle. Once this occurs, adaptation will be less than optimal and injuries might occur.

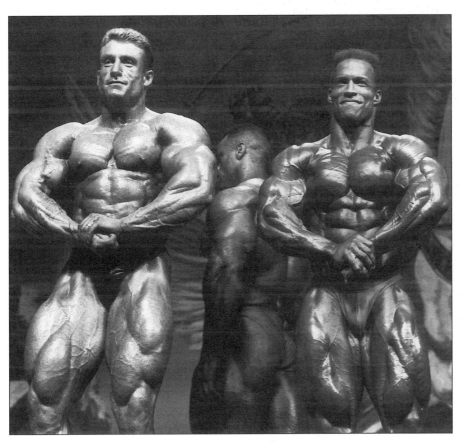

No two people are alike. Yates and Ray, both gloriously big and symmetrical, have individual looks, styles, and training needs.

The step-type approach involves the repetition of a microcycle, or a week of training (figure 1.5), in which the resistance is increased over several steps, followed by an unloading step to ensure recuperation.

Note that each step represents more than one single workout, which means that the workload is not increased at every training session. One workout provides insufficient stimulus to produce marked changes in the body. Such adaptation occurs only after repeated exposure to the same training loads. In figure 1.5, each step represents one week, each vertical line indicates a change in load, and each horizontal line represents the week over which you use and adapt to that load. The percentages indicated above each step are the suggested

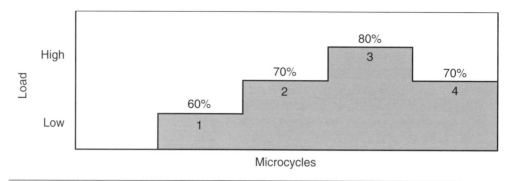

Figure 1.5   The step-type method of increasing training load.
Reprinted from Bompa 1996.

percentages of maximum load. You can see the progression for the first three weeks, as well as the decrease for the unloading phase in the fourth week.

Let's look at how your body responds to the step-loading approach. On Monday, for example, you begin a microcycle (a new step) by increasing the workload. After Monday's workout your body is in a state of fatigue—a physiological crisis—because it is unaccustomed to such stress. When the same level continues, your body will probably be comfortable with the load by Wednesday, and adapt to it in the following two days. By Friday, you should feel really good and capable of lifting even heavier loads. This illustrates that following the crisis of fatigue comes a phase of adaptation, which in turn is followed by a physiological rebound, or improvement. By the next Monday, you should feel physically and mentally comfortable, which indicates that it is time to challenge the level of adaptation once more.

Each step of the microcycle will bring improvements until you reach the unloading (regeneration) phase (step 4). This phase gives your body the time it needs to replenish its energy stores, restore a psychological balance, and rid itself of the fatigue that has accumulated over the preceding three weeks. The fourth step in this example becomes the new lowest step for another phase of load increments. Figure 1.6 illustrates how the same four microcycles (steps) shown in figure 1.5 fit into the context of a longer training cycle, where the goal is to build muscle size.

Although the load increments might seem small, it is important to remember that because you are getting stronger, your maximum weight values are increasing, which means that your percentages of maximum are increasing as well. For example, the first time you reached the high step of 80%, your 80%-of-maximum weight for a specific exercise may have been 120 lbs. Three weeks later, because of your adaptation and strength gains,

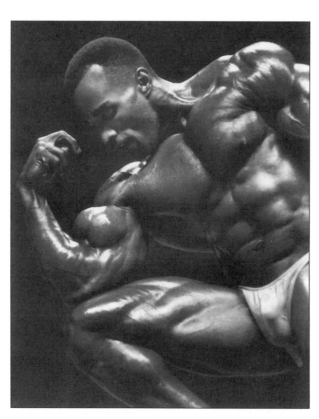

Darem Charles hits biceps pose.

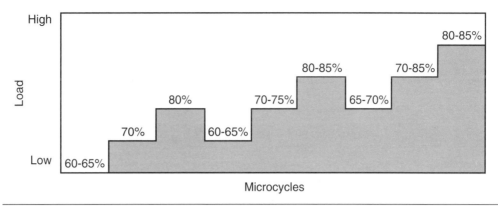

Figure 1.6   An example of how to increase the training load over a longer period of time.

your 80% may have increased to 130 lbs. Consequently, you use progressively heavier loads over the long term, despite the fact that your percentages of maximum remain the same.

Three Basic Laws of Strength and Bodybuilding Training

The training principles just discussed provide a loose guideline for general training. There are also three laws of strength training that must be adhered to if an athlete is to proceed, injury-free, to a more comprehensive, rigorous training program. Entry-level bodybuilders and strength athletes often begin training programs without being aware of the strain they will encounter, and without understanding the progression or training methodology behind the program. These are usually the people who tend to seek advice from seasoned athletes (who might not be qualified to give it), and who, consequently, find themselves out of their league and on a collision course with injury. Adherence to the following training laws will ensure the proper anatomical adaptation of a young or untrained body, before subjecting it to the rigors of strength training.

Law #1: Before Developing Muscle Strength, Develop Joint Flexibility

Most strength training exercises, especially those employing free weights, utilize the whole range of motion around major joints. In some exercises, the weight of the barbell compresses the joints to such an acute degree that if the individual does not have good flexibility, strain and pain can result. Let's take deep knee squats as an example. During a deep squat, compression of the knee joints might give an inflexible athlete a lot of pain or even injury. Also, in the deep squat position, a lack of good ankle flexibility forces the performer to stay on the balls of the feet and toes, rather than on the flat of the foot where a good base of support and balance is ensured. The development of ankle flexibility (i.e., *plantar flexion*, or bringing the toes toward the calf) is a necessity, especially for entry-level athletes.

Law #2: Before Developing Muscle Strength, Develop the Tendons

The rate of muscle strength gains always has the potential to exceed the rate at which the tendons and ligaments can adapt to higher tensions. It is crucial that the tendons and ligaments are given time to adapt in order to preserve the integrity of the bones that form the joints. Premature heavy loads and the lack of a long-term vision cause many individuals to unknowingly develop specific muscle groups without strengthening the support system. Think of it as building a house on the sand. It might look good for a little while, but at high tide the whole thing is destroyed. Build your body on a rock-solid foundation and this will not happen to you.

Tendons and ligaments are trainable and can actually increase in diameter as a result of proper anatomical adaptation training (see chapter 4), which increases their ability to withstand tension and wear. This is accomplished by following a low-load program for the first 1-2 years of training. Shortcuts are not the answer to achieving a well-developed, injury-free body. Patience will ultimately pay off.

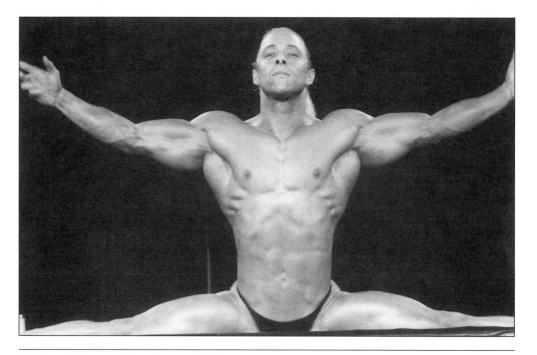

Flexibility is the cornerstone of a sound training program.

Law #3: Before Developing the Limbs, Develop the Body's Core

It is true that big arms, shoulders, and legs are impressive, and that a lot of training must be dedicated to these areas. It is also true, however, that the trunk is the link between these areas, and the limbs can only be as strong as the trunk. A poorly developed trunk represents a weak support system for the

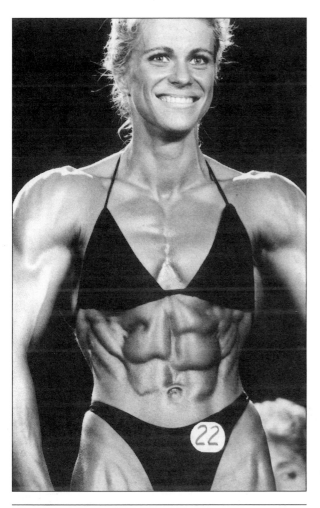

The picture of symmetry. Anja Langer knows the importance of developing the core of the body.

hard-working arms and legs. So in spite of temptation, an entry-level training program must not revolve around the legs, arms, and shoulders. The focus must first be on strengthening the "core" area of the body—the abdomen, the lower back, and the spinal column muscles.

The trunk has an abundance of abdominal and back muscles, with bundles that run in different directions surrounding the core of the body with a tight and powerful support system. All trunk muscles work as a unit to provide stabilization, or keep the trunk fixed, during movements of the arms and legs.

Back muscles consist of long and short muscles that run along the vertebral column. They work together as a unit with the rotators and diagonal muscles to perform many exercises and movements.

Abdominal muscles run lengthwise (*rectus abdominis*), crosswise (*transverse abdominis*), and diagonally (*abdominal obliques*), enabling the trunk to bend forward and sideways, rotate, and twist. The abdominal muscles play important roles in many exercises and, therefore, a weakness in this area can severely limit the effectiveness of many strength actions.

CHAPTER 2

PROGRAM DESIGN FOR MAXIMUM GAIN

Designing a training program requires athletes to understand many interconnected concepts. Awareness of how training volume, load, and intensity affect a program is important. It's also essential to understand what factors will determine loading patterns. These factors are the number of repetitions per set done, the lifting speed, and the number of sets. Rest is also a vital component of a training program. Those athletes who wish to design their own training program need to understand all of these training elements.

Training Volume

Training volume is the quantity of work performed and incorporates the following integral parts:

- The time, or duration, of training (in hours)
- The cumulative amount of weight lifted per training session or phase
- The number of exercises per training session
- The number of sets and repetitions per exercise or training session

Bodybuilders and strength trainers need to maintain training logs to correctly monitor the total volume of work performed and help plan the total volume of training for future weeks and months.

Training volume varies among individuals according to their training background, work tolerance, and biological makeup. A mature athlete with a strong strength training background will always be able to tolerate higher volumes of training. Regardless of classification, however, any dramatic or abrupt increase in training volume can be detrimental. Such increases can result in high levels of fatigue, inefficient muscular work, and greater risk of injury. This is why a well-designed, progressive plan, along with an appropriate method of monitoring load increments, is crucial to one's well-being and training success.

Training volume also changes with the type of strength training performed. For instance, high-volume training is planned during the muscle definition phase in order to burn more fat and, consequently, develop better muscle striations. Medium-volume training, on the other hand, is typical for maximum strength or power training. Muscle size and definition improve only as a result of careful and constant physiological adaptation, which depends directly upon the proper manipulation of the quantity or volume of training.

One adaptation that occurs as a result of progressively higher volumes of training is a more efficient and faster recovery time between sets and between training sessions. This makes it possible to do more work per training session, which encourages even further increases in training volume.

Training Intensity

In strength training, intensity (load) is expressed as a percentage of 1RM. Intensity is a function of the power of the nervous stimuli employed in training. The strength of a stimulus depends on the load, the speed at which a movement is performed, the variation of rest intervals between repetitions and sets, and the psychological strain that accompanies an exercise. Thus, the intensity is determined by the muscular effort involved and the CNS energy spent during strength training. Table 2.1 gives the loads employed in strength training.

Supermaximum is a load that exceeds one's maximum strength. In most cases, loads between 100 to 125% of 1RM are used by applying eccentric force, or by resisting the force of gravity. When utilizing supermaximum loads, it is advisable to have two spotters, one at each end of the barbell, to assist the performer and protect him or her from accident or injury. For example, if one employs the eccentric method in bench pressing without spotters, the barbell could fall on the performer's chest because the weight is actually heavier than he or she can lift.

During the maximum strength phase, only those athletes with a strong background or base in strength training can use supermaximum loads. Most other athletes should restrict themselves to a load of up to 100%, or 1RM.

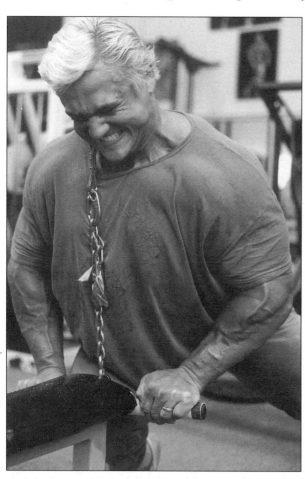

Now there's intensity. Tom Platz gives his grunting, vein-bulging, teeth-clenching best.

Table 2.1 Intensity values (loads) utilized in strength and bodybuilding training			
Intensity value	Load	% of 1RM	Type of contraction
1	Supermaximum	>105	Eccentric/isometric
2	Maximum	90–100	Concentric
3	Heavy	80–90	Concentric
4	Medium or submaximum	50–80	Concentric
5	Low	30–50	Concentric

Reprinted from Bompa 1996.

- *Maximum* load refers to a load of 90% to 100% of one's maximum.
- *Heavy* load is when one lifts 80% to 90% of maximum.
- *Medium* or *submaximum* load is a percentage 50% to 80% of maximum.
- *Low* is considered to be any load that is 30% to 50% of 1RM.

The load, however, should also relate to the type of strength being developed, as scheduled in the Periodization plan.

Number of Exercises

One of the keys to an effective training program is to have an adequate repertoire of exercises from which to choose. Athletes should build their repertoire around several key principles.

Exercises That Stimulate the Greatest Amount of Electrical Activity

The significance of this for strength and bodybuilding athletes is that the greater the electrical activity, the more muscle fibers are recruited, which results in greater increments in muscle strength and size. (See chapter 11.)

Level of Development

One of the main objectives of an entry-level strength or bodybuilding program is the development of a strong anatomical and physiological foundation. Without such a base, consistent improvement will be unlikely. Entry-level strength trainers and bodybuilders need lots of exercises (about 12 to 15) that collectively address the major muscle groups of the body. The duration of this type of training may be from one to three years, depending upon the individual's background and his or her patience to develop a progressive, solid background.

Training programs for advanced strength trainers and bodybuilders follow a completely different approach. The main training objective for these athletes is to increase muscle size, density, tone, and definition to the highest possible levels.

Individual Needs

As training progresses over the years, some strength trainers and bodybuilders might develop imbalances among different parts of the body. When this occurs, programs should be adapted to address individual specific needs by giving priority to those exercises that stress the underdeveloped parts of the body to restore symmetry.

Training Phase

As outlined by the Periodization concept, the number of exercises varies according to the phase of training. (See part 2.)

The order of exercises in bodybuilding and strength training must be *phase specific*, taking into account the scope of training for each particular phase. Just as the rest interval, volume of training, exercises, and other factors vary according to the different kinds of strength being developed, so must the order of performing exercises.

For example, in the maximum strength training phase, exercises are cycled in "vertical" sequence as they appear on the daily program sheet. Therefore, perform one set of each exercise starting from the top and moving down, repeating the cycle as often as prescribed. The advantage of this method is that it allows better recovery of each muscle group. By the time exercise #1 is repeated, enough time has elapsed to promote almost full recovery. When one is lifting 90-105% 1RM, this much rest is necessary if training is to remain at a high intensity throughout the session.

If, however, the phase of training is hypertrophy, then all of the sets for exercise #1 are performed before moving on to the next exercise. This is the "horizontal" sequence. This sequence exhausts the muscle group much faster, which leads to better increases in muscle size. Local muscle exhaustion is the main training focus of the hypertrophy phase.

Loading Patterns

There are a number of variations of distinct loading patterns that the serious training program should follow that pertain to the pyramid loading formation. These specifically include the pyramid loading pattern as well as the double, skewed, and flat pyramid loading patterns.

The Pyramid

The pyramid (figure 2.1) is one of the most popular loading patterns in strength training and bodybuilding. Notice that as the load progressively increases to maximum, the number of sets decreases proportion-

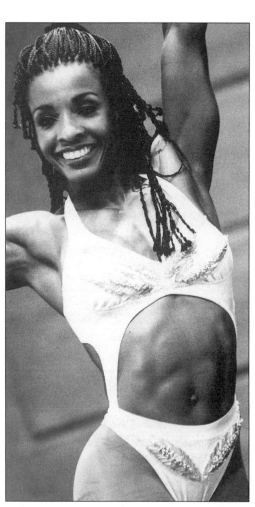

The superfit body of fitness competitor Madonna Grimes.

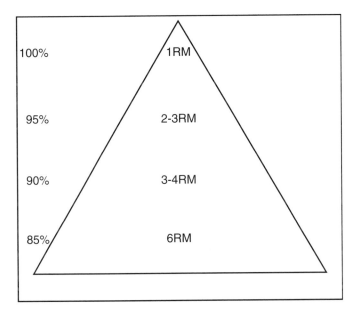

Figure 2.1   An example of the pyramid loading pattern. The number of repetitions (inside the pyramid) refers to the number per training session. Reprinted from Bompa 1996.

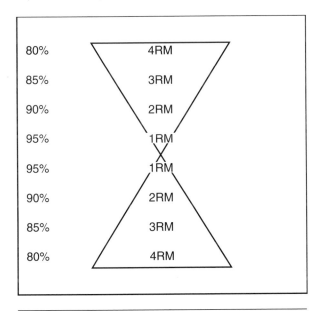

Figure 2.2   An example of the double loading pattern. Reprinted from Bompa 1996.

ately. The physiological advantage of using the pyramid is that it ensures the activation or recruitment of most, if not all, of the motor units.

The Double Pyramid

The double pyramid (figure 2.2) represents two pyramids, one mirroring the other. In this loading pattern, beginning at the bottom, the load increases progressively up to 95% 1RM and then decreases again for the last sets. Note that as the load increases, the number of repetitions, shown inside the pyramid, decreases and vice versa.

The Skewed Pyramid

The skewed pyramid (figure 2.3) proposes an improved variation of the double pyramid (Bompa, 1993). In this loading pattern, the load constantly increases throughout the session, except during the last set when it is lowered. The purpose of this last set is to provide variation and motivation, since the athlete must perform the set as quickly as possible.

The Flat Pyramid

Maximum training benefits can be achieved with the "flat pyramid" loading pattern (Bompa, 1993). A comparison between the traditional pyramids and the flat pyramid shown in figure 2.4 will explain why this is the most effective loading pattern. In the traditional pyramids, the load varies too much, often ranging between 70-100+% 1RM. Load variations of such magnitude cross over three intensity (load) borders—medium, heavy, and maximum.

In order to produce hypertrophy, the load must range between 60-80% 1RM, whereas for maximum strength the load must be between 80-100+% 1RM. The flat pyramid gives the physiological advantage of providing the best neuromuscular adaptation for a given type of strength training, because it keeps the load within one intensity level. This prevents the body from becoming confused by several different intensities.

The flat pyramid begins with a warm-up set (60% 1RM) and then the load stabilizes for the entire exercise at 70% 1RM. Another set at 60% 1RM may be performed at the end of each exercise for variety.

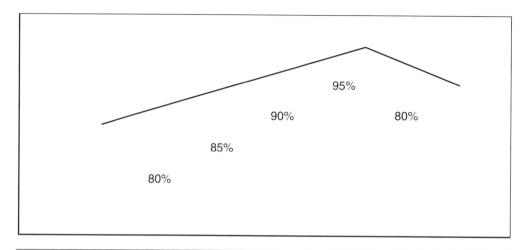

Figure 2.3 A suggested loading pattern for the skewed pyramid.
Reprinted from Bompa 1996.

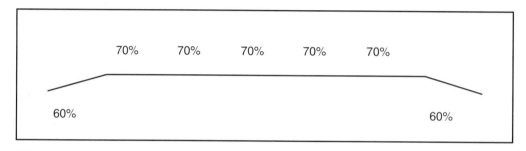

Figure 2.4 An example of the flat pyramid loading pattern.
Reprinted from Bompa 1996.

Variations of the flat pyramid are possible depending upon the phase and scope of training, as long as the load stays within the boundaries of the required intensity for a given phase:

70% - 80% - 80% - 80% - 80% - 70%

80% - 90% - 90% - 90% - 90% - 80%

85% - 95% - 95% - 95% - 95% - 85%

Repetitions Per Set

Strength trainers and bodybuilders who follow traditional thinking about the number of repetitions performed per set—those who go to the gym every day and always perform 8-12 sets—will be shocked by the numbers recommended in table 2.2. Very few people have thought of performing 150-rep sets. We will show you that this is possible, because each training phase is different and requires a separate approach to loading, rest interval, number of reps, and exercise order.

Table 2.2 Number of repetitions appropriate for each training phase		
Training phase	**Training purpose**	**Number of repetitions**
Maximum strength	Increase muscle strength or tone	1–7
Hypertrophy	Increase muscle size	6–12
Muscular endurance	Increase definition	30–150

Lifting Speed

The speed of lifting is an important component of strength and bodybuilding training. For the best results, some types of work must be executed quickly, while others must be performed at a medium pace. The speed with which one intends to lift, however, is not necessarily reflected in the appearance of the lift. For example, when lifting a heavy load that is 90% of 1RM, the performed motion might look slow, however, the force against the resistance must be applied as quickly as possible. Only under this condition will the athlete be able to synchronize and recruit all of the motor units necessary to defeat the resistance. The FT muscle fibers are recruited for action only when the application of force is fast and vigorous.

Optimum speed can usually be maintained throughout the first half of a set. Once fatigue sets in, speed often declines and a great deal of mental concentration is required to complete the intended number of repetitions.

Number of Sets

A set represents the number of exercise repetitions followed by a rest interval. The number of sets prescribed per exercise/workout depends upon several factors, including how many exercises the athlete performs in a training session, the phase of training, how many muscle groups the athlete wants to train, and how experienced the bodybuilder or strength trainer is.

Exercises in a Training Session

As the number of exercises increases, the number of sets per exercise declines. This is due to the fact that as energy and work potential decrease, the ability to perform numerous exercises and repetitions for a very high number of sets declines. As work potential improves, however, the number of sets per workout one can tolerate will improve.

Training Phase

As explained in part 2, an athlete goes through several training phases during a year of training. Each phase has a specific objective related to creating the best possible body shape. In the adaptation phase, where the scope of training is just overall adaptation, the number of sets per exercise is not high (2-3). In the hypertrophy phase, however, where the objective is to increase muscle size, it is necessary to perform the greatest number of sets one can tolerate. Please refer to the chapters on Periodization planning for details on how to incorporate these ideas into your own personal program.

Muscle Groups Trained Per Session

If training only one or two muscle groups in a given session, one is able to perform more sets per muscle group than if training three or four muscle groups.

Bodybuilder's Experience

The classification of the strength trainer or bodybuilder (i.e., entry level, recreational, advanced) also plays a part in determining the number of sets that will be included in the training session. As one becomes more experienced and achieves a high state of adaptation to weight training, one can perform more sets per body part per workout. For example, while an advanced bodybuilder might prepare for a contest by performing 20 or 30 sets for 2 or 3 muscle groups, a recreational athlete might train the same muscle groups with only 15 or 20 sets.

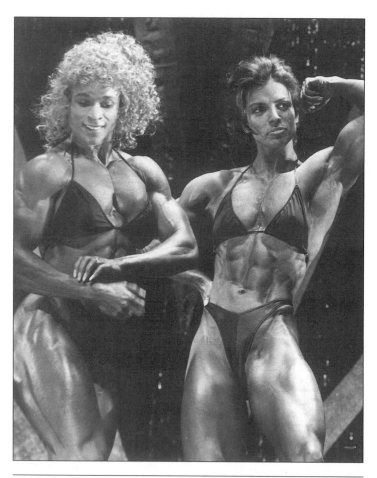

Crevalle and Bruneau strut their stuff!

Rest Interval

Energy is a crucial commodity in strength training and bodybuilding. The type of energy system used during a given workout depends upon the phase of training (i.e., hypertrophy vs. muscle definition), the load employed, and the duration of the activity. High-intensity training might tax the athlete's energy stores to such an extent that he or she becomes completely depleted. In order to complete the workout, the athlete must take a rest interval (RI) between each set to replenish the depleted fuel stores before the next set is performed.

Bodybuilders and strength trainers must realize that the RI and restoration of energy between sets and training sessions are as important as the training itself. The amount of time allowed between sets determines, to a high degree, the extent to which the energy source will be replenished prior to the next set. Careful planning of the RI is crucial if one is to avoid needless physiological and psychological stress during training.

Rest Intervals Between Sets

An inadequate RI between sets causes an increased reliance on the lactic acid (LA) system for energy. The degree to which ATP and creatine phosphate (CP), a high-energy compound stored in muscles, is replenished between sets depends on the duration of the RI. The shorter the RI, the less ATP/CP will be restored and, consequently, the less energy will be available for the next set. If the RI is too short, the energy needed for the following sets is provided by the LA system. The problem with this energy system is that its use always results in increased LA accumulation within the working muscles, leading to pain and fatigue, which impairs training ability.

It is during the RI, not during the work, that the heart pumps the highest volume of blood to the working muscles. A short RI diminishes the amount of blood reaching the working muscles, and without this supply of fuel and oxygen, the athlete will not have the energy to complete the planned training session. A longer RI is required to combat excessive LA accumulation.

Several factors influence the appropriate duration of the RI between sets, including these:

- Type of strength one is developing
- Magnitude of the load being employed
- Speed of contraction
- Number of muscle groups being worked during the session
- Level of conditioning
- Amount of rest taken between training days
- Total weight of the athlete (heavy athletes with larger muscles usually regenerate at a slower rate than lighter athletes)

See table 2.3 for guidelines on RI between sets.

Table 2.3 A guideline for RI between sets for various loads			
Load %	**Speed of performance**	**RI (minutes)**	**Applicability**
>105 (eccentric)	Slow	4–5/7	Improve maximum strength and muscle tone
80-100	Slow to medium	3–5/7	Improve maximum strength and muscle tone
60-80	Slow to medium	2	Improve muscle hypertrophy
50-80	Fast	4–5	Improve power
30-50	Slow to medium	1–2	Improve muscle definition

Reprinted from Bompa 1996.

Rest Interval Cues:

- A 30 second RI restores approximately 50% of the depleted ATP/CP.
- A RI of 3-5 minutes or longer allows almost entire restoration of ATP/CP.
- After working to exhaustion, a 4-minute RI is not sufficient to eliminate lactic acid from the working muscles or to replenish the energy stores of glycogen.

Local Muscular and CNS Fatigue

Most research findings point to three causes and sites of fatigue. The motor nerve is the first. The nervous system transmits nerve impulses to muscle fibers via the motor nerves. A nerve impulse has certain degrees of force, speed, and frequency. The higher the force impulse, the stronger the muscle contraction, which gives greater ability to lift heavier loads. Fatigue greatly affects the force of nerve impulses. Therefore, as the level of fatigue increases, the force of contraction decreases. This is why longer RIs of up to 7 minutes are necessary for CNS recovery during the maximum strength phase.

The second site is the neuromuscular junction. This is the nerve attachment on the muscle fiber that relays the nerve impulses to the working muscle. This type of fatigue is largely due to an increased release of chemical transmitters from the nerve endings (Tesch, 1980). Following a set, a 2-3 minute RI usually returns the electrical properties of the nerve to normal levels. However, after work involving powerful contractions, such as maximum strength training, a RI of longer than 5 minutes is needed for sufficient recovery to occur.

Finally, the contractile mechanisms, actin and myosin, also cause fatigue. This fatigue is related to the following factors:

- LA accumulation decreases the peak tension, or the power of the muscle to contract maximally.
- LA accumulation leads to a high acidic concentration in the muscle, which in turn affects the muscle's ability to react to the nerve impulses (Sahlin, 1986; Fox et al., 1989).
- Depletion of the muscle glycogen stores, which occurs during prolonged exercise (i.e., over 30 minutes), causes the fatigue of the contracting muscle (Karlson and Saltin, 1971; Sahlin, 1986; Conlee, 1987).

Other energy sources available to the muscle, including glycogen from the liver, cannot fully cover the energy demands of the working muscle.

The Central Nervous System and Local Muscles

During training, chemical disturbances occur inside the muscle that affect its potential to perform work (Bigland-Ritchie et al., 1983; Hennig and Lomo, 1987). When the effects of the chemical disturbance are signaled back to the CNS, the brain sends weaker nerve impulses to the working muscle to decrease its working capacity in an attempt to protect the body.

During an adequate RI of 4-5 minutes, the muscles can recover almost completely. When the brain senses no danger, it sends more powerful nerve impulses to the muscles, resulting in better muscular performance.

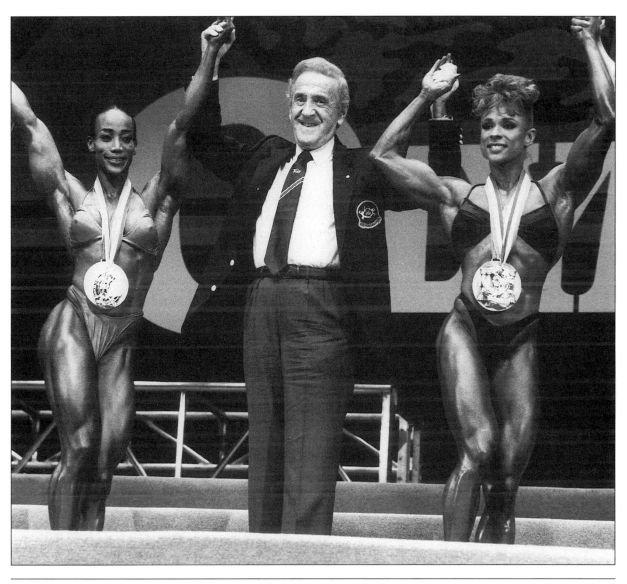

Joe Weider flanked by Lenda Murray and Laura Crevalle at the 9th Olympia.

Rest Interval Between Strength Training Sessions

The athlete's fitness level and recovery ability influence the RI between strength training sessions.Well-conditioned athletes recover more quickly than those with lower fitness levels. We strongly recommend that strength trainers and bodybuilders train their aerobic systems through cardiovascular training in addition to their muscular systems.

Aerobic Training Cue:

> Another benefit of aerobic training is that it helps bodybuilders and strength trainers to stay relatively lean throughout the entire annual plan, not just during contest preparation.

The phase of training and the energy source being tapped during training also play a part in determining a necessary RI between sessions. The energy source being used during training is probably the most important factor to consider when planning the RI between sessions. For example, during the maximum strength phase, when one is taxing primarily the ATP/CP system, daily training is possible, because ATP/CP restoration is complete within 24 hours. If, on the other hand, one is training muscular endurance (for muscle definition), workouts need to be scheduled every second day, because it takes 48 hours for the full restoration of glycogen (Piehl, 1974; Fox et al., 1989). Even with a carbohydrate-rich diet, glycogen levels will not return to normal levels in less than two days.

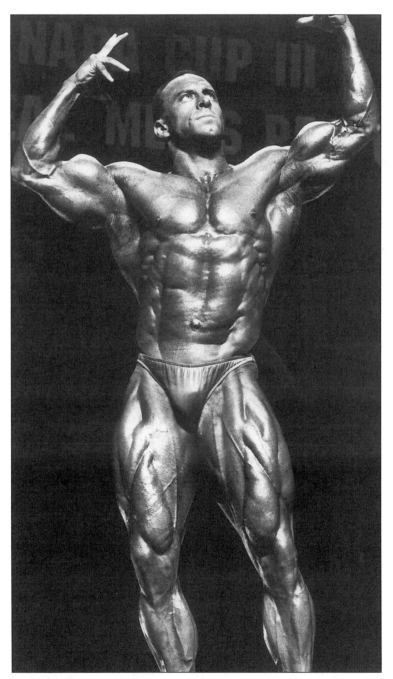

John McGough reaches for the stars.

Activity During Rest

Most athletes do nothing during the RI to facilitate recovery between sets. There are, however, some things that can be done to enhance both the rate and completeness of recovery.

• *Relaxation exercises.* Simple techniques such as shaking the legs, arms, and shoulders and getting a light massage are effective ways to facilitate recovery between sets. Exercises using heavy loads cause an increase in the quantity of muscle protein, mystromin, which causes muscle rigidity (Baroga, 1978). These basic recovery techniques aid in its removal by improving blood circulation within the muscle.

• *Diverting activities.* These activities involve performing light contractions with the nonfatigued muscles (Asmussen & Mazin, 1978) during the RI. Reports have shown that such physical activities can facilitate a faster recovery of the prime movers. The message of local muscular fatigue is sent to the CNS via sensory nerves. The brain then sends inhibitory signals to the fatigued muscle that reduce its work output during the RI. As the muscle becomes more relaxed, this enhances the restoration of energy stores.

Steps for Designing a Training Program

In order to design an effective training program, the athlete should consider these steps, which are described in the following section:

1. Select the type of strength sought.
2. Select the exercises.
3. Test maximum strength.
4. Develop the actual training program.
5. Test to recalculate 1RM.

First, strength training should be phase-specific and designed to meet the needs of the individual (see part 2). Decide on the appropriate percentage of 1RM to be used and the number of reps and sets based on the type of strength sought. Details on training methods and progression are provided in later chapters on planning and training methods.

Next, select the exercises. Identify the prime movers and then select the exercises that can best stimulate these muscles to meet individual needs. These needs might depend upon the background or foundation, individual strengths and weaknesses, or the disproportionate development among muscle groups and body parts. For example, if one has the capacity to develop massive legs quickly and the upper body takes longer to grow, then select exercises to compensate the weaker part to encourage growth and restore symmetry.

The selection of exercises is also phase-specific. For example, during the anatomical adaptation phase, most muscle groups are worked in order to develop a better overall foundation, whereas in the muscle definition phase, training becomes more specific and exercises are selected to target the prime movers.

Third, test maximum strength. As stated earlier, this value is referred to as the 1 repetition maximum, or 1RM, and is the highest load that one can lift in one attempt. Knowing one's 1RM for each exercise is crucial to the concept of Periodization, as each workout is planned using percentages of 1RM.

If for some reason the strength trainer or bodybuilder is unable to test 1RM for each exercise, an attempt should be made to test 1RM for at least the dominant exercise within the training program. Often the load and number of repetitions are chosen randomly, or by following the programs of others, instead of utilizing one's own objective data, which is 1RM for each exercise. Such data is valid for only a short period of time since there is continual improvement in maximum strength, recovery ability, lifting techniques, and other factors from phase to phase.

Among some members of the bodybuilding world, there is an unfounded belief that testing for 1RM is dangerous. They maintain that injury will result if an individual puts forth a maximal effort, but an adequately trained athlete can lift 100% once in a four-week period without danger. Keep in mind, however, that a test for 1RM must be performed following a very thorough and progressive warm-up.

If the athlete is still reluctant to test for 100%, another option is to test for a 3RM or 5RM and then extrapolate to what the 1RM would be. (See appendix 3 for a chart that gives the estimated 1RM from submaximal values.)

The fourth step is to develop the actual training program. By this point, the athlete knows which exercises are to be performed, the 1RM for each exercise, and the type of strength to be developed. With this information, he or she can select the number of exercises, the percentage of 1RM, the number of reps, and the number of sets.

This program cannot, however, be the same for each training phase. The training demand must be progressively increased so one is forced to adapt to increasing work loads, which translates into increases in muscle size, tone, and strength. The training demand might be increased by any of the following means: increase the load, decrease the rest interval, increase the number of repetitions, or increase the number of sets.

Table 2.4 illustrates a hypothetical program to demonstrate how to set up one's own program. Before looking at the chart, it is necessary to understand the notation used to express the load, number of reps, and number of sets.

$$80/10 \cdot 4 = \text{load}/\# \text{ of reps} \cdot \text{sets}$$

The numerator of 80 refers to the load as a percentage of 1RM.
The denominator of 10 represents the number of repetitions per set.
The multiplier of 4 represents the number of sets.

Table 2.4 Hypothetical training program showing format design			
Exercise #	**Exercise**	**Load/# reps · # sets**	**RI (in minutes)**
1	Leg press	80/6·4	3
2	Flat bench press	75/8·4	3
3	Leg curl	60/10·4	2
4	Half squat	80/8·4	3
5	Abdominal curls	15·4	2
6	Dead lifts	60/8·3	2

Reprinted from Bompa 1996.

While many books and articles on this subject actually take the liberty of prescribing the load in lbs/kgs to be used, please notice that we do not. One must surely question the basis upon which someone would actually suggest the poundage that an athlete should use without knowing anything about the athlete. The load must be suggested as a percentage of 1RM. This allows strength trainers and bodybuilders to objectively calculate the load for each exercise according to his or her individual potential within the parameters of a given training phase.

The first column lists the exercises by number, or the order in which they are performed during the training session. The second column lists the exercises. The third column shows the load, number of reps, and number of sets. The last column gives the RI required after each set.

Finally, test to recalculate 1RM. Another test for 1RM is needed prior to the beginning of each new phase, to ensure that progress is acknowledged and new loads are based upon the new gains made in strength. For specific suggestions on testing dates, please examine the microcycle, or the weekly training program in part 2.

3

MICROCYCLES AND WEEKLY TRAINING GOALS

A good strength training or bodybuilding program is one that improves muscle size, tone, density, and definition. A training program is successful only when it has these characteristics:

- It is a part of a longer plan.
- It is based on the scientific knowledge available in the field.
- It uses Periodization as a guideline for planning training throughout the year.

The program must have short-term goals and long-term goals that are *phase specific*. Each training phase has its own objectives, so it is necessary to design the daily and weekly programs to meet these objectives, while coinciding with the overall plan.

The compilation of a plan with both short- and long-term goals must take into account the individual's background, physical potential, and rate of adaptation to the physiological challenges imposed by training. Of all possible plans that can be used, we will make reference in this chapter to only the training session plan and the microcycle.

In part 2, we will introduce you to several types of plans. Since planning theory is very complex, annual planning will be discussed only as it pertains to strength training and bodybuilding.

The Training Session Plan

The training session, or daily program, includes a warm-up, the main workout, and a cool-down.

The Warm-Up

The purpose of the warm-up is to prepare athletes for the program to follow. During the warm-up, the body temperature is raised, which enhances oxygen transport and prevents or reduces ligament sprains and muscle and tendon strains. It also stimulates CNS activity, which coordinates all the systems of the body, speeds up motor reactions through faster transmission of nerve impulses, and improves coordination.

For the purposes of strength and bodybuilding training, the warm-up consists of two parts. *General warm-up* (10-12 minutes) consists of light jogging, cycling, or stair-climbing, followed by stretching exercises. This ritual serves to increase blood flow and body temperature and prepares the muscles and tendons for the workout. During this time, bodybuilders can mentally prepare for the main part of the training session by visualizing the exercises to be performed and motivating themselves for the eventual strain of training.

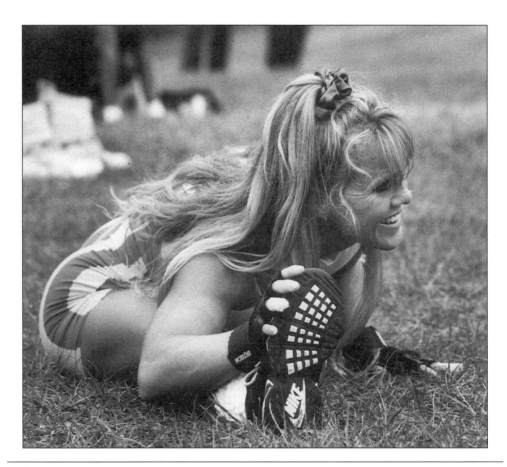

Stretching both before and after a weight-training session prepares the body for action and helps to prevent serious injury.

The second part, the *specific warm-up* (3-5 minutes), is a short transition period that consists of performing a few repetitions of each planned exercise using significantly lighter loads. This prepares the body for the specific work to be done during the main part of the workout.

The Main Workout

This part of the training session is dedicated to performing the actual strength and bodybuilding exercises. For the best results, make up the daily program well in advance of the workout and write it down on paper or, better yet, in a logbook. To know the program in advance is of psychological benefit, because it enables one to better motivate oneself and focus more clearly on the task at hand.

The *duration* of a training session depends on the type of strength being developed, and the specific training phase of the model of Periodization developed by the athlete. For example, the longest workouts are needed for the hypertrophy phase, because there are many sets to perform and the rest interval between sets is relatively long.

The Cool-Down

Just as the warm-up is a transition period to take the body from its normal biological state to a state of high stimulation, the cool-down is also a transition period that produces the opposite effect. The job of the cool-down is to progressively bring the body back to its normal state of functioning.

A cool-down of 10 to 25 minutes consists of performing activities that facilitate *faster recovery and regeneration*. After a tough workout, the muscles are exhausted, tense, and rigid. To overcome this, one must allow for muscle recovery (see chapter 13). Hitting the showers immediately after the last exercise, though tempting, is not the best activity.

The removal of lactic acid from the blood and muscles is also necessary if the effects of fatigue are to be eliminated quickly. The best way to achieve this is by performing 20-25 minutes of light, continuous aerobic activity, such as jogging, cycling, or rowing, which will cause the body to continue perspiring. This will remove about half of the lactic acid from the system and help the athlete to recover more quickly between training sessions. Remember, the faster one recovers, the greater the amount of work that can be performed in the following training session.

The Microcycle

The microcycle refers to the weekly training program and is probably the most important tool in planning. Throughout the annual plan, the nature and dynamics of the microcycles change according to the phase of training, the training objectives, and the physiological and psychological demands of training.

Variations of Load Increments per Microcycle

To plan a program, one must understand how the microcycle fits into a longer training phase, namely the *macrocycle*, or four weeks of training, and how to plan the load of training per microcycle.

Load Increments per Macrocycle

Load increments within the macrocycle must follow a step-type progression. Figure 3.1 illustrates the standard approach. With regard to intensity, microcycles follow the principle of step-type loading.

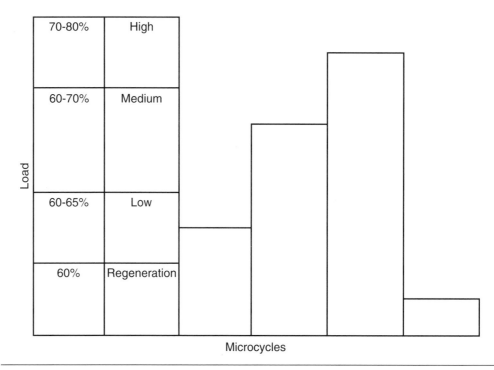

Figure 3.1 The dynamics of increasing the training load over four microcycles (a macrocycle). Reprinted from Bompa 1996.

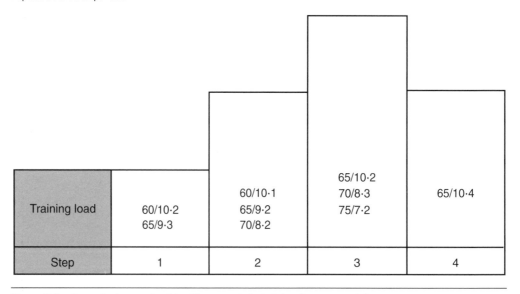

Figure 3.2 A practical example of load increments in training (a macrocycle). Reprinted from Bompa 1996.

As illustrated in figure 3.1, the load is progressively increased over three microcycles (weeks), and then decreased for a regeneration cycle to facilitate recuperation and replenishment of energy before another macrocycle begins.

Based on the model shown in figure 3.1, we give a practical example (figure 3.2) suggesting load increments using the notation explained in chapter 2.

Figure 3.2 illustrates that the work, or the total stress in training, increases in steps, with the highest point being in step 3. To increase the work from step to step, there are two options: increase the load (the highest one being in step 3) and/or increase the number of sets (from five sets in step 1, to seven sets in step 3).

In this example, both options are used at the same time, and this is an appropriate approach for athletes with a solid background in training. Other options can be selected to suit the needs of different classifications. Entry-level athletes, for example, have difficulty tolerating higher loads and an increased number of sets, so it is more important for them to increase the number of exercises. This will serve to develop their entire muscular system and help the ligaments and tendons adapt to strength training.

Step 4 is a regeneration cycle when the load and number of sets are lowered. This lessens the fatigue that has developed during the first three steps and allows the body to replenish its energy stores. This step also allows the athlete to psychologically relax.

Load Increments per Microcycle

The work, or the total stress per microcycle, is increased mainly by increasing the number of days of training per week.

Before discussing options of training per microcycle, we must mention that the total work per week is also planned following the principle of step-type loading. Figures 3.3, 3.4, and 3.5 illustrate the first three microcycles of the macrocycles shown in figures 3.1 and 3.2.

The Role of Low Intensity Days

Due to unscientific theories such as "no pain, no gain" and "overloading," which have dominated the sports of bodybuilding and strength training, the majority of athletes believe in training hard day in and day out regardless of the season. It is not surprising that most of them constantly feel exhausted and frustrated because they do not achieve expected gains. Consequently, many quit because they stop enjoying their sport.

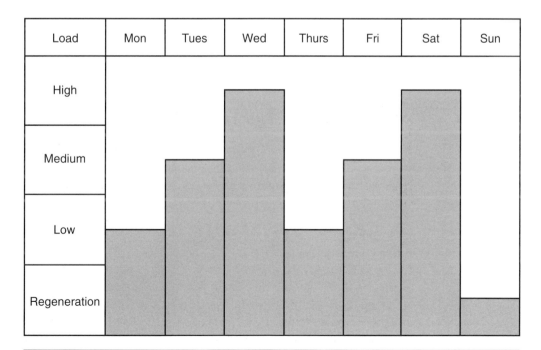

Figure 3.3 A low intensity microcycle (first step as in figures 3.1 and 3.2).
Reprinted from Bompa 1996.

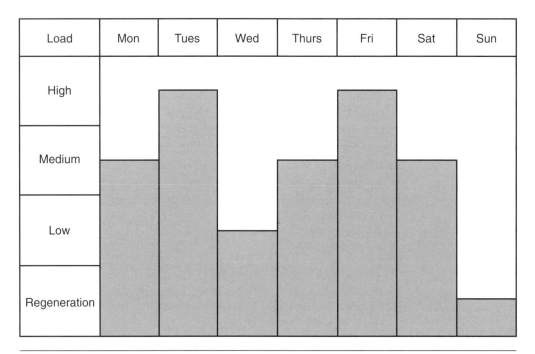

Figure 3.4 A medium intensity microcycle (second step in figures 3.1 and 3.2).
Reprinted from Bompa 1996.

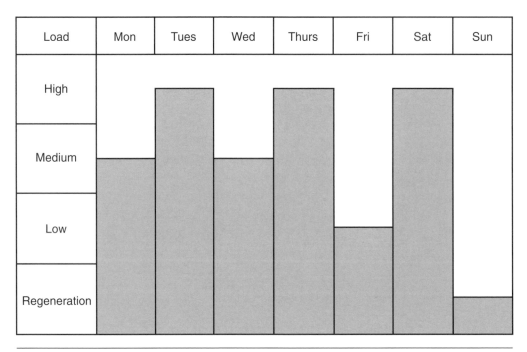

Figure 3.5 A high intensity microcycle (third step in figures 3.1 and 3.2).
Reprinted from Bompa 1996.

To avoid such undesirable outcomes, athletes need to follow the step-type loading pattern and alternate training intensities inside each microcycle. Three such intensity variations are illustrated in figures 3.3 - 3.5. Other variations are possible, depending upon individual circumstances.

In any microcycle variation, there are low-intensity days, and athletes might legitimately question their role. We will explain. The body uses the fuels ATP/CP and glycogen to provide energy. For high intensity workouts that consist of low-rep sets and rest intervals of at least 2-3 minutes, which are typical of maximum strength training, the energy supply is provided by the ATP/CP system. Under these conditions, energy stores can be replenished in about 24 hours, which means that the next day's workout could also be of high intensity.

Every high-intensity workout session, however, creates physiological strain and psychological stress, caused by the intense concentration that is necessary to tackle the challenging loads. Consequently, following such a workout, the athlete must be concerned with two things: whether the energy pools will be replenished before the next workout and whether he or she will be mentally ready for the next session. These reasons make it necessary to plan in advance for low-intensity days following 1-2 days of hard training. Figure 3.6 gives another option for planning a microcycle, where 2 challenging days are planned back-to-back. Please note that this type of microcycle is only for highly-trained strength trainers and bodybuilders who have a high adaptive response and are capable of tolerating intense physiological and psychological strain.

If, however, the session consists of high-rep sets, as proposed for the muscle definition (cuts) phase, or if the workout is especially long (2-3 hours), a large proportion of fuel is supplied by the glycogen system. Following these long and exhausting workouts, the complete restoration of glycogen often takes 48 hours. An appropriate microcycle structure for this type of training is suggested in figure 3.5.

Supercompensation

Supercompensation is the state of physiological and psychological arousal that ideally occurs prior to a day of high intensity training. Supercompensation can only be achieved, however, if work and regeneration are timed perfectly.

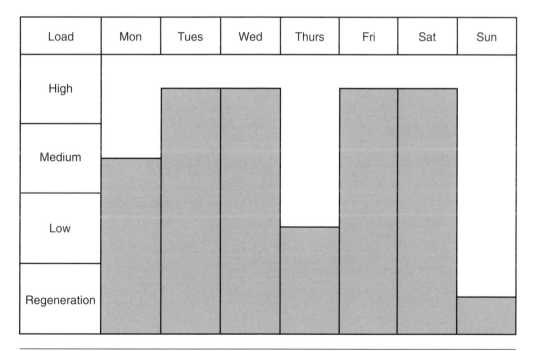

Figure 3.6   A suggested microcycle for the third step, or high-intensity step, of a macrocycle for elite strength trainers and bodybuilders.
Reprinted from Bompa 1996.

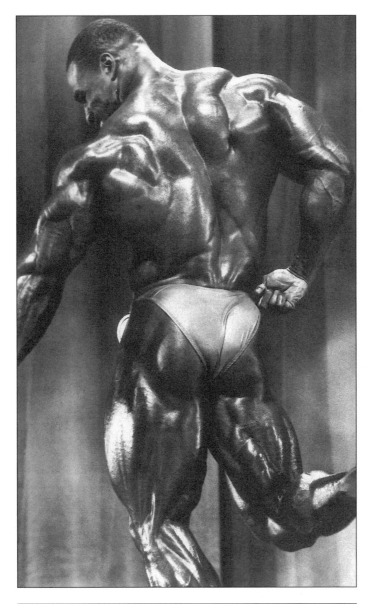

During the maximum strength workouts that are necessary to create a body as massive as Chris Cormier's, the energy system taxed (ATP/CP) can be replenished in approximately 24 hours.

Mistakes in timing are what turn super-charged workouts into daily grind sessions. Figure 3.7 illustrates the super-compensation cycle of a training session.

This is how it works. Under normal conditions of rest and proper diet, an individual is in a balanced state (*homeostasis*). As illustrated by figure 3.7, a certain level of fatigue is reached, both during and at the end of a training session. This is caused by the depletion of fuel stores, lactic acid accumulation in the working muscles, and psychological stress. The abrupt drop of the homeostasis curve illustrates the rapid development of fatigue and a simultaneous reduction of functional capacity, or ability, to train. Following each session, and between two sessions, there is a phase of compensation during which time the biochemical sources of energy are replenished. The return of the curve toward the normal biological state, or homeostasis, is slow and progressive, indicating that the replenishment of lost energy stores requires several hours. If the rest interval between two high-intensity training sessions is planned correctly, the energy sources (especially glycogen) are fully replaced and the body also acquires some fuel reserves. This energy rebound puts the athlete into a state of supercompensation and gives him or her the energy needed to train even harder. This is essential for adaptation to training and, consequently, for improving muscle size, tone,

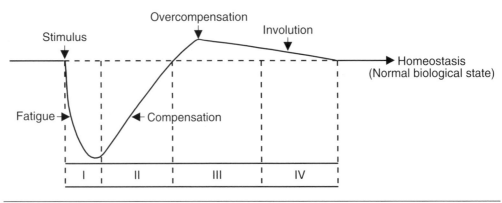

Figure 3.7   The supercompensation cycle of a training session modified from Yakovlev (1967).
Reprinted from Bompa 1983.

and definition. If the time between two workouts is too long, the super-compensation will fade away (*involution*), resulting in little, if any, improvement in work capacity. The optimal recovery period needed for supercompensation varies according to the type and intensity of training. See table 3.1.

The way in which loads are planned directly affects how the body responds to training. For example, if the athlete follows the philosophy of lifting as heavy as possible day in and day out, and the intensity of training per microcycle varies, then the supercompensation curve changes drastically. Under these conditions, the body never has time to replenish its energy stores and comes closer to exhaustion with every workout. Figure 3.8 illustrates what happens to the body and to training potential when continuous exhaustive training is employed over a prolonged period.

As we can see from figure 3.8, it is still possible to reach supercompensation during the first 2-3 days, because fatigue has not yet affected the body's overall potential. As constant overload training continues, more and more fatigue develops, which takes the body farther away from its balanced state (homeostasis). After about 3-4 days, every workout begins in a state of residual fatigue. At this stage, supercompensation is never reached and the athlete's training capacity and growth potential are inhibited. Over the long-term, a very high level of exhaustion is reached and the motivation to train will hit a low. From this point, overtraining and breakdown are only steps away.

In comparison, when one alternates heavy training days with light training days, as suggested in figures 3.3-3.5, and follows the step-loading principle, the

Table 3.1   Time needed for supercompensation to occur following different types of training

Type of training	Energy system	Time needed for supercompensation (in hours)
Aerobic/cardiovascular	Glycogen/fats	6–8
Maximum strength	ATP/CP	24
Hypertrophy/muscle definition	Glycogen	36

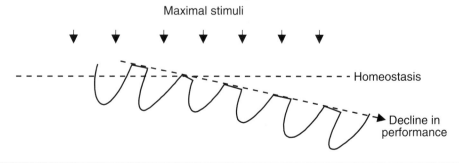

Figure 3.8   The effect of continuous overload training on one's body and one's working capacity. Reprinted from Bompa 1983.

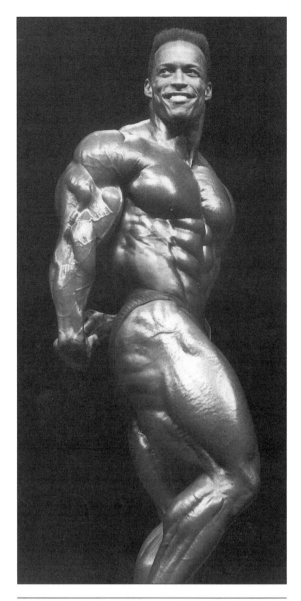

Shawn Ray proves a body that is rested and full of fuel can be pushed to the limits.

supercompensation curve forms a wave-like pattern (figure 3.9) that hovers around and above the body's homeostasis level. This indicates that energy stores are being continuously replenished and the body is not striving to operate in a state of exhaustion or fatigue. When the body is rested and full of fuel, it can be pushed to heights never dreamed of before. By training this way, one can expect supercompensation to occur every 2-4 days.

The improvements in an athlete's working potential and feelings of overall well-being occur mostly on the days when supercompensation is experienced. This is also the time when growth and muscle size increases. Since every bodybuilder and strength trainer wants these positive outcomes, a training program must be carefully planned. A heavy and intense training day should be followed by an easy day, thus encouraging supercompensation.

Training Frequency per Microcycle

The frequency of training sessions depends on the athlete's classification, training phase, and training background. Entry-level athletes must progressively introduce training. At first, they can plan two relatively short strength training sessions per microcycle. Once this training regime is handled easily, the frequency can gradually be increased to 3-4 sessions per microcycle. Higher level athletes who are taking part in shows can plan between 6-10 training sessions per microcycle.

As illustrated in part 2, the number of training sessions also depends on the phase of training: 3-5 for anatomical adaptation, 4-6 or even higher for professional bodybuilders and strength trainers, and 6-10 during the maximum strength and hypertrophy phases.

The athlete's training background and resulting work tolerance are important factors in determining the frequency of training sessions per microcycle.

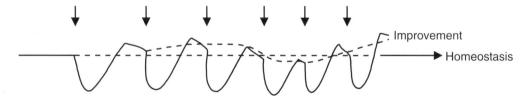

Figure 3.9 The alternation of heavy workouts with low- and medium-intensity workouts produces a wave-like curve of improvement. Reprinted from Bompa 1983.

Obviously, well-trained athletes with 2-3 years experience can train with ease at least 4 times per microcycle, which translates into visible improvements in size and muscle tone. These athletes can tolerate more work than novices.

The Split Routines

Although split routines are a virtual necessity for seriously committed bodybuilders and strength trainers, they are not necessarily appropriate for recreational athletes whose goals are to look fit, strong, and toned. These bodybuilders will probably get the best results from training three times a week with a total body routine. Less training frequency than this would decrease training efficiency and reduce the necessary adaptive responses.

Most serious strength trainers and bodybuilders train very frequently, from 4-6 times a week. But it is difficult to challenge the same muscles in consecutive training sessions. Therefore, split routines are very important to these athletes because they allow them to train the various muscle groups every second day or so to achieve better recovery between workouts. Box 3.1 is a classic example of a six-day split routine.

Many athletes believe that a program such as the classic split routine shown in box 3.1, which trains each muscle group twice per week, is sufficient to stimulate an optimal adaptive response to training. Even worse, others believe that training a muscle group to exhaustion once a week is sufficient stimulus to make the desired gains in muscle size, tone, and definition. We question both these modes of thinking very seriously because, in our opinion, neither is enough. For continual improvements, workouts must constantly challenge your present state of adaptation. In order to provoke a new adaptive response, you should progressively increase your training load using the step-type loading method. As a result, depending on the load used, your training will stimulate either an increase in size or an increase in muscle tone and strength.

In order to accomplish this response, competitive bodybuilders and strength trainers should work some muscle groups three times a week during certain training phases. (Please note that this is feasible only if you decrease the number of sets and exercises per muscle group to the lowest level possible to ensure that your energy is spent most effectively.) In box 3.2, suggestions are offered for number of sets for each muscle or muscle group per workout.

Box 3.1	Classic Six-Day Split
Day	**Body Part**
1	Legs, calves, and shoulders
2	Chest and biceps
3	Back and triceps
4	Legs, calves, and shoulders
5	Chest and biceps
6	Back and triceps
7	Rest

Box 3.2	Suggested Sets per Workout	
Muscle		**Number of sets/workout**
Chest		8
Back		10
Legs:	Quadriceps	6
	Hamstrings	4-6
	Calves	6-8
Arms:	Biceps	6
	Triceps	6
Shoulders		10-12
Abdominal		6

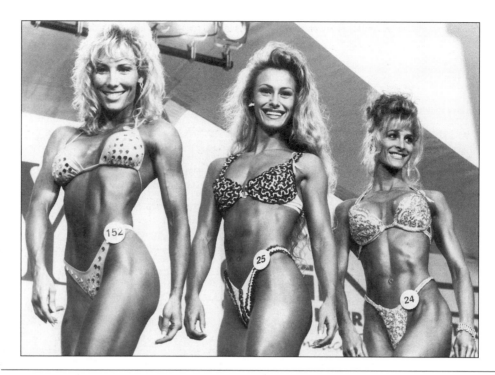

A strong and fit look can be achieved with total body routines as opposed to the split routines favored by many "hard core" bodybuilders.

Box 3.3 High-Adaptive Response Six-Day Split	
Day	**Body Part**
1	Chest, back, and arms
2	Legs, calves, shoulders, and abdominals
3	Chest, back, and arms
4	Legs, calves, shoulders, and abdominals
5	Chest, back, and arms
6	Legs, calves, shoulders, and abdominals
7	Rest

Box 3.4 High-Adaptive Response Six-Day Double Split	
Day	**Body Part**
1 a.m.	Legs and calves
p.m.	Chest and biceps
2 a.m.	Shoulders and triceps
p.m.	Back and abdominals
3 a.m.	Legs and calves
p.m.	Chest and biceps
4 a.m.	Shoulders and triceps
p.m.	Back and abdominals
5 a.m.	Legs and calves
p.m.	Chest and biceps
6 a.m.	Shoulders and triceps
p.m.	Back and abdominals
7 a.m.	Rest

The High-Adaptive Response Six-Day Split outlined in box 3.3 trains each body part three times per week and allows each muscle group 48 hours of recovery before it is trained again. The same approach can be used on a double-split routine. Box 3.4 shows one of many possible combinations.

Although most bodybuilders and strength trainers believe that the split routine allows sufficient recovery to occur between training sessions, this theory does not meet the needs of the energy systems. While the implementation of a split routine facilitates the elimination of local muscular fatigue (the fatigue acquired by a group of muscles worked to exhaustion), it does little to facilitate the overall replenishment of the body's energy stores. If, as is often the case, exhaustive workouts are performed every day, glycogen stores become depleted regardless of whether or not a split routine is used. Remember, exhaustive workouts use glycogen as the main fuel source and take it from the working muscles as well as the liver. The body needs 48 hours to fully restore glycogen levels and cannot operate optimally if exhaustive training is planned every 24 hours.

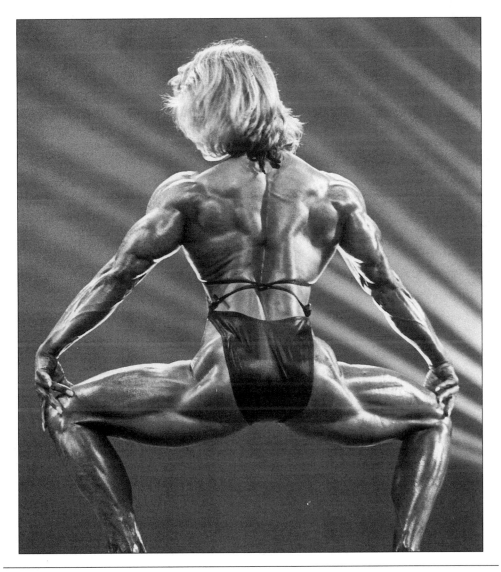

The famous Laura Crevalle.

PERIODIZED WORKOUTS

In training nothing happens
by accident, but rather by design.

Do you want to be successful?

Plan for it!

PART 2

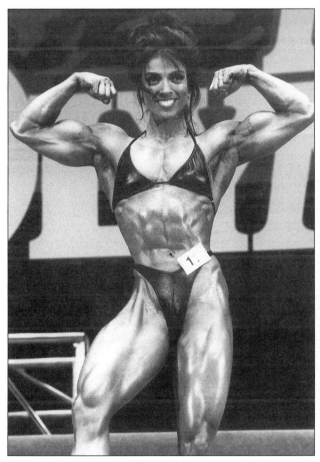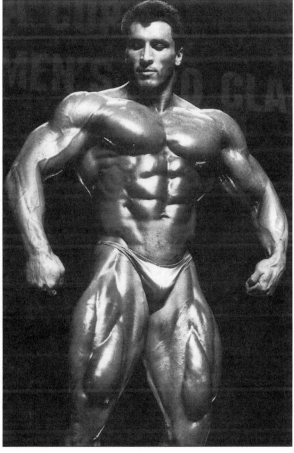

The ideal for every strength trainer and bodybuilder is to acquire the desired amount of muscle mass—without sacrificing one's physical appearance. Bruneau and Sarcev, both perfectly muscled and perfectly symmetrical.

Very few strength trainers and bodybuilders, it seems, follow a well-adjusted and carefully thought-out plan. Through Periodization, we intend to promote a new type of athlete—one who is in control of his or her body and whose training leads to complete body development. The new athlete will have impressive muscular development and will cultivate muscle density, tone, definition, symmetry, and strength superior to that of "traditional" strength trainers and bodybuilders who use antiquated training philosophies. Regardless of whether you are training just to look gorgeous or to compete professionally, the ideal for each and every athlete is to acquire the desired amount of muscle mass without sacrificing physical appearance.

Periodization is a training concept that allows you to accomplish your goals through the strategic implementation of specific phases: *anatomical adaptation, hypertrophy, mixed, maximum strength, muscle definition, and transition.*

Figure 4.1 illustrates the basic model of Periodization. Many variations of this plan are possible, however, to meet the different needs of each bodybuilder and strength trainer.

Nutrition Cue:

> To significantly enhance the effects of each phase of training, you must match your nutritional needs with your training requirements. The nutrition strategies we promote in this book are part of "Periodization of Nutrition." They are explained at the end of each training phase, except for the anatomical adaptation phase.

The basic model of Periodization of Bodybuilding and Strength Training presented in figure 4.1 illustrates the proper sequence of training phases and may be adapted to address the specific needs of individual athletes. This particular plan uses September as the starting point, although any month of the year can be used when developing your own individual plan. The small blocks beneath each month represent the weeks, or microcycles. One must plan how many weeks are appropriate for each particular phase. The bottom row of the chart divides the year into training phases. The athlete should organize these phases in a way that assures him or her of meeting goals at the appropriate time. For example, a competitive athlete might design an annual plan to peak for major shows. On the other hand, recreational bodybuilders and strength trainers who are concerned with aesthetics might wish to plan for vacations and other activities.

Dates	Sept	Oct	Nov	Dec	Jan	Feb	Mar	Apr	May	June	July	Aug
Weeks												
Phase	AA	H1	T	H2	T	M	T	MxS	T	MD1	T	MD2	T

Figure 4.1 The basic model of the annual plan for "Periodization of Bodybuilding and Strength Training." AA = Anatomical Adaptation; H = Hypertrophy; M = Mixed Training; MxS = Maximum Strength; MD = Muscle Definition; T = Transition.

CHAPTER

4

PHASE ONE: ANATOMICAL ADAPTATION (AA)

Most strength training and bodybuilding athletes commence new rigorous training programs without being mentally and physically prepared. This book proposes a better method, where time is taken for a progressive adaptation in the form of anatomical adaptation.

This phase represents the foundation of training for the new annual plan. Following a period of rest or low-activity training, it is vital to begin the new module of training with a short phase of involvement, or activation of the main body parts. As the term anatomical adaptation (AA) implies, the body needs time to adapt to a new stimulus. This non-stressful progressive training stage is designed to encourage this adaptation. One must remember that vigorous strength training always develops the strength of the ligaments and tendons, which can lead to serious injury. The AA stage allows for careful, progressive strengthening of the tendons, ligaments, and muscle tissues, helping the athlete to move injury-free into the next, more strenuous phase of training.

Scope of AA Training

- Activate all of the muscles, ligaments, and tendons of the body, so they will better cope with the heavy loads of subsequent training phases.
- Bring all of the body parts into balance. That is, to begin to develop previously neglected muscles or body parts and restore symmetry.
- Prevent injuries through the progressive adaptation to heavy loads.
- Progressively increase the athlete's cardiorespiratory endurance.

Duration and Frequency of AA Training

For entry-level bodybuilders and strength trainers, 6 to 12 weeks are necessary to train the tendons and ligaments. Although the program is not a stressful one, some beginners might experience an increase in muscle size. A lengthy AA phase will give the novice time to improve his or her lifting skills before introducing heavy loads. Six weeks are sufficient for recreational bodybuilders and strength trainers with 2-3 years of training. Advanced bodybuilders and strength trainers can make do with three to six weeks of training. Any longer than six weeks will not produce a training effect. At this point the body has nothing to adapt to, so it is a waste of time.

The frequency depends on one's training background and overall commitment to training. Two to three sessions per week are expected for entry-level and recreational bodybuilders, while 4-5 sessions per week are appropriate for advanced and elite bodybuilders.

Exercises that use one's own body weight are perfect for AA training.

Training Method for AA Phase

As previously mentioned, the purpose of the AA phase is to progressively adapt the body to work—to develop the muscles as well as their attachments to the bones. The best training method for the AA phase is *circuit training (CT),* mainly because it alternates muscle groups and involves most or all of the body parts and muscles.

Circuit Training

The first variant of CT was proposed by Morgan and Adamson (1959) from Leeds University, and was used as a method to develop general fitness. Initially, CT utilized several stations all arranged in a circle, hence the name, circuit training. The exercises were organized in such a way that the muscle groups used were constantly alternating from station to station.

There are a huge variety of exercises to use when developing a CT program, including those that utilize one's own body weight, such as dips and pull-ups; and those requiring dumbbells, barbells, and strength training machines, such as leg extensions, bench presses, and others.

Exercise to Alternate Muscle Groups

A circuit may be repeated several times depending on the number of exercises involved, number of repetitions per station, the load used, and the individual's work tolerance and fitness level. Select CT exercises to *alternate muscle groups*, thus facilitating a better and faster recovery between stations. The rest interval (RI) should be 60-90 seconds between stations, and 1-3 minutes between circuits. A normal gym offers many different apparatuses, workstations, and strength training machines that make it possible to create circuits that will involve most or all of the muscle groups. This will continually challenge the athlete's skills and maintain his or her interest.

Program Design for the AA Phase

From the first week of training, athletes must plan their workouts based on objective data. This means testing your 1RM for at least the main exercises or prime movers, so you can objectively calculate your training loads as a percentage of maximum. (See chapter 2.)

During the first 1-2 weeks, it is normal to experience some discomfort in the way of muscle soreness and fatigue. This is especially true for individuals who have not been very active in the past. Once the muscles become accustomed to working again, this quickly disappears. As the program continues, you will begin to feel good and the program will seem easy! The best thing you can do for yourself is to continue to train as per the original plan.

Adaptation Cue:

> Resist the temptation to increase the load! There will be plenty of time to do that in the next phase. Remember that even though your muscles feel as if they have adapted, your tendons and ligaments need more time.

The total physical demand per circuit must be progressively and individually increased. Figure 4.2 demonstrates how load patterning differs between entry-level and advanced athletes. Entry-level athletes need a more gradual adaptation and, therefore, the load remains the same for 2 weeks (2 microcycles) before increasing the demand. Advanced athletes can change their load every microcycle. Use these guidelines when creating your own plan.

To better monitor improvements in training, and be constantly able to calculate the load, we suggest testing for 1RM at the beginning of weeks 1 and 4, and at the beginning of week 1 of the next training phase.

As illustrated in figure 4.2, toward the end of the AA phase the load reaches a percentage of maximum that allows the athlete to immediately make the transition to the H phase. Please use table 4.1 as a guideline for creating your own AA plan.

Table 4.2 illustrates a suggested 6-week AA training program for a recreational bodybuilder or strength trainer. To perform the circuit, follow the exercises from the top down, performing just one set before moving to the next station. This facilitates a better recovery for each muscle group since they are being constantly alternated. If, however, too many bodybuilders are using the same equipment, or you have to wait too long between sets, then perform all the sets at one station before moving to the next.

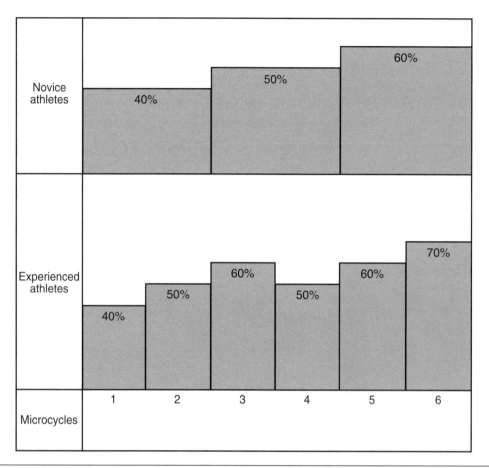

Figure 4.2 A suggested pattern of load increments for CT for entry-level and advanced bodybuilders and strength trainers.
Reprinted from Bompa 1996.

If a high number of exercises are being done per session, you can follow a split routine, so the same muscle groups are trained every second day. Conversely, if the numbers are lower, you can perform all of the exercises in one day, and repeat as many times as you train per week.

Anatomical Adaptation Cues:

- Other exercises may be selected.
- Test for 1RM: early week 1, and at the end of week 4 and week 7 (first week of the next phase).
- Progression over the 6 weeks occurs in the form of increased load, and increased number of sets and reps. Please observe and apply the progression from table 4.2.
- Load increments for "leg curls" start at a lower load and have a slower progression, because the hamstring muscles are easier to injure, therefore, "go slowly on hams"!!
- Do 20-25 minutes of aerobic work as part of your warm-up.
- Remember 40/15·3 means load/# of reps·sets.

Table 4.1   Guidelines for creating an individual anatomical adaptation plan

Bodybuilder's classification	Entry level	Recreational	Advanced
Duration of AA phase (weeks)	6–12	6	3–6
# of stations	9–12	9	9
# of sets/training sessions	2	3	3–4
RI between sets (minutes)	2–3	2	2
Frequency/week	2–3	3–4	3–5
Aerobic training sessions/week	1	1–2	2

Reprinted from Bompa 1996.

Table 4.2   An example of a six-week AA phase for recreational bodybuilders and strength trainers

No.	Exercise	Week 1	Week 2	Week 3	Week 4	Week 5	Week 6
1	Leg extensions	40/15·3	50/12·3	60/8·3	50/15·4	60/12·4	70/10·4
2	Flat bench press	40/15·3	50/12·3	60/8·3	50/15·4	60/12·4	70/10·4
3	Seated pulley rows	40/15·3	50/12·3	60/8·3	50/15·4	60/12·4	70/10·4
4	Back extensions	40/15·3	50/12·3	60/8·3	50/15·4	60/12·4	70/10·4
5	Standing leg curls	40/12·3	40/15·3	50/12·3	40/12·4	50/12·4	50/12·4
6	Donkey calf raises	40/15·3	50/12·3	60/8·3	50/15·4	60/12·4	70/10·4
7	Nautilus crunches	3·12	3·15	3·15	4·12	4·15	4·15

5
PHASE TWO: HYPERTROPHY (H)

In the standard model (figure 4.1), we propose two six-week hypertrophy phases (H1 and H2). This is to provide sufficient time for you to meticulously address your own needs regarding the improvement of muscle size and refinement. A one-week transition phase is recommended between these two H phases. During this time, the volume and intensity of training are sizably reduced. This week of lower intensity training helps to remove the fatigue accumulated during the first H phase, and gives the body a chance to fully replenish its energy stores before commencing the next H phase.

Similar short transition phases are planned between all of the suggested training phases of the basic model of Periodization (figure 4.1).

Scope of H Training

- Increase muscle size to the desired level by constantly taxing the ATP/CP stores.
- Refine all the muscle groups of the body.
- Improve the proportion among all the muscles of the body, and especially between arms and legs, back and chest, leg flexors and extensors.

Duration of H Training

The duration of H training depends upon several factors. These include the athlete's classification, training background, specific body goals—such as

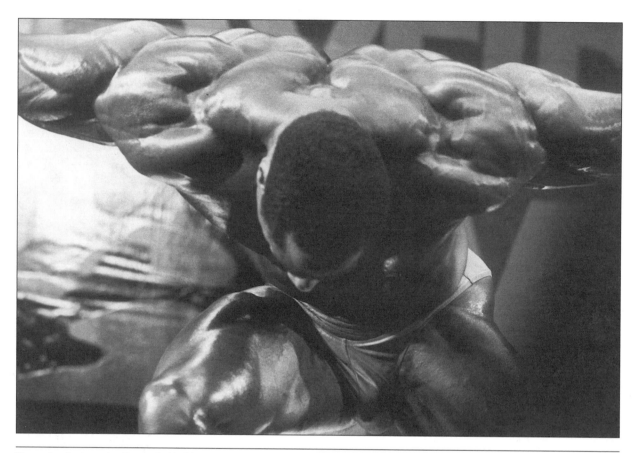

The recipe for muscles that look this big: 1) Start with hypertrophy training; 2) Add just enough protein; 3) Get cookin!

increased size versus density, or muscle definition, and the type of Periodization being followed. To learn how to customize your plan, please refer to chapter 10, Yearly Training Programs.

To achieve substantial gains in muscle size, one should plan at least one six-week or, better yet, two six-week H phases. During this time, the athlete must apply the training methods that best suit him or her. Variations of training methods, which we will discuss shortly, should be carefully selected in order to achieve the planned training goals.

The RI between sets is perhaps the most important element of training if hypertrophy is to be stimulated. The RI must be calculated in such a way that it brings the body to exhaustion following each set, as well as at the end of a workout. It is necessary to plan such exhaustion days mostly during the second, and especially during the third steps, as per the step-type loading method. (See figures 3.1 and 3.2).

Training Methods for H Phase

An enlargement of muscle size (hypertrophy) is best achieved by applying the methodology of bodybuilding. Two methods can be employed by strength trainers and bodybuilders. The first method we describe is the hypertrophy method. The second is the isokinetic method.

Hypertrophy (Bodybuilding) Method

The main objective of bodybuilding is to provoke significant chemical changes in the muscles necessary for the development of mass. Unfortunately, for some bodybuilders, increased muscle size is often the result of an increase of fluid/plasma within the muscles rather than enlarged contractile elements within the muscle fibers (the myosin filaments). In other words, the enlargement of the muscles might be due to a shift in the body fluids to the worked muscle, as opposed to an actual increase in muscle fiber size. This is why the strength of some bodybuilders is not always proportional to their size—a problem that can be corrected by applying the Periodization concept of training.

Submaximal loads are employed in hypertrophy training as opposed to maximal loads (100% 1RM) and, therefore, maximum tension is not being provoked within the muscles. The training objective when using submaximal loads is to contract the muscles to exhaustion in an effort to recruit all of the muscle fibers. As you "rep-out" to exhaustion, muscle fiber recruitment increases, because as some fibers begin to fatigue, others start to function, and so on, until exhaustion is reached.

In order to achieve optimum training benefits, it is crucial to perform the greatest number of repetitions possible during each set. A bodybuilder should, therefore, always reach the state of local muscular exhaustion that prevents him or her from performing one more repetition, even when applying maximum

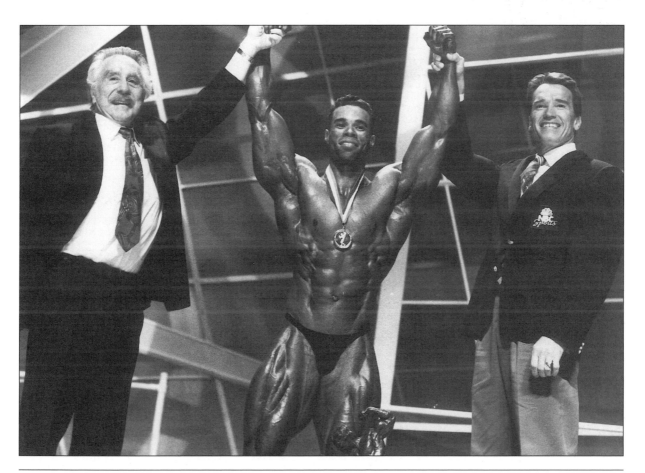

Three heavy-hitters in the world of bodybuilding: Joe Weider, Kevin Levrone, Arnold Schwarzenegger.

force. If the individual sets are not performed to exhaustion, muscle hypertrophy will not reach the expected level because the first repetitions do not produce the stimulus necessary to increase muscle mass. The key element in hypertrophy training is the cumulative effect of exhaustion over the total number of sets, and not just exhaustion per set. This cumulative exhaustion stimulates the chemical reactions and protein metabolism responsible for optimal muscle hypertrophy.

Bodybuilding/hypertrophy training mostly utilizes the fuels specific to the anaerobic system (ATP/CP). Therefore, training should be designed to exhaust or deplete these energy stores, thereby threatening the energy available for the working muscle. This can be achieved by taking shorter RIs between sets (30-45 seconds). The rationale behind this thinking is that when the body is given only a limited amount of rest, the muscles have less time to restore the energy reserves, namely the ATP/CP. As an exhaustive set depletes ATP/CP stores, and the short RI does not allow for its complete restoration, the body is forced to adapt by increasing its energy transport capacity, which in turn stimulates muscle growth. This occurs as a result of increasing the CP content in muscle cells and activating protein metabolism, which stimulates hypertrophy.

Variations of Training Methods for Hypertrophy

Repetitions to exhaustion represent the main element of success in bodybuilding and strength training, therefore, several variations of the original method

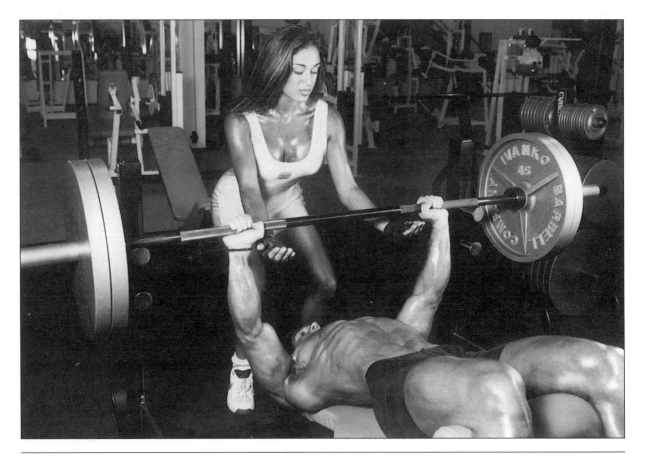

Spotter provides resistance for the eccentric segments of contraction.

are presented. Each of the following variations has the same objective, which is to achieve 2-3 more repetitions after one reaches exhaustion, through sweat and tears. The result is increased muscle growth and increased hypertrophy.

Assisted Repetitions: Once the athlete has performed a set to temporary exhaustion of the neuromuscular system, a partner gives sufficient support to enable 2-3 more repetitions to be performed.

Resisted Repetitions: Once the athlete performs a set to temporary exhaustion, a partner helps to execute 2-3 more repetitions concentrically and provides

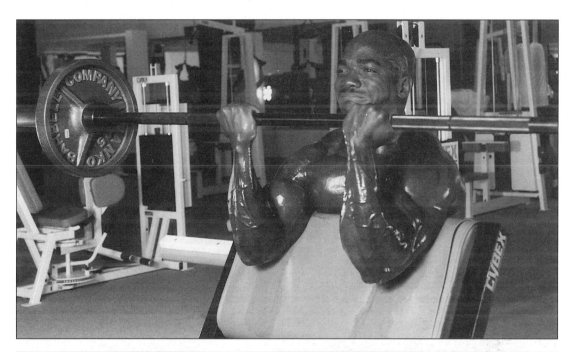

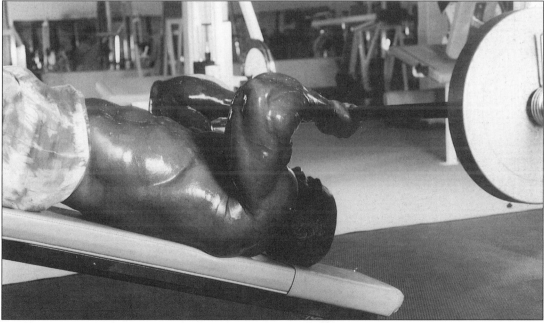

Wesley Mohammed performing a superset with biceps preacher curls followed immediately by decline triceps extensions.

resistance for the eccentric segments of contraction, hence the name, *resisted repetitions*. During these last 2-3 reps, the eccentric part of the contraction is twice as long as the concentric part of the contraction, which overloads the muscles involved beyond the standard level.

We caution athletes performing resisted repetitions that the longer active muscle fibers are held in tension, the higher the nervous tension and energy expenditure becomes. If a normal contraction is 2-4 seconds in duration, a repetition performed against resistance can be 6-8 seconds long, consuming 20-40% more energy (Hartman and Tünnemann, 1988). The longer the muscles remain in tension, the more strongly activated the muscle's metabolism becomes, which stimulates muscle growth to new highs.

Superset: The superset is a training method in which a set is performed for the agonistic muscles of a given joint and followed, without a rest period, by a set for the antagonistic muscles. For example, an elbow flexion or biceps preacher curl, followed immediately by an elbow extension or decline triceps extension.

Variation of the Superset: Perform a set to exhaustion followed, after 20-30 seconds, by another set for the same muscle group. For example, triceps extensions and then dips. Of course, due to exhaustion, one might not be able to perform the same number of repetitions in the second set as were performed in the first set.

Cheated Repetitions: An athlete will normally resort to this technique when there is no spotter available. When unable to perform another repetition with proper form through the entire range of motion, the action is completed by jerking another segment of the body toward the performing limb. For example, perform elbow flexions to exhaustion, then jerk the trunk toward the forearm to trick or "cheat" the body into performing additional reps. This sustains the crucial tension in the exhausted muscle. This method is limited to certain limbs and exercises and should only be attempted by athletes with a sound training base.

Helpful Tips for Employing the Hypertrophy Method

Bodybuilding books, and especially some magazines, often refer to many other methods, some of them promising miracles! Care must be taken to recognize the fine line separating reality from fantasy.

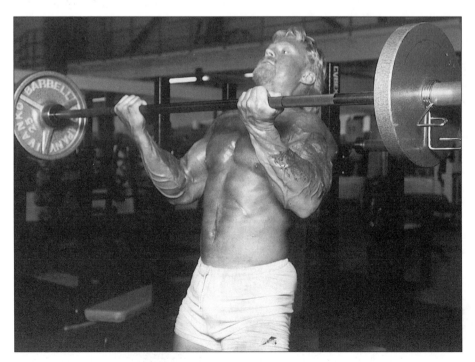

Trevor Butler performing cheated repetitions.

Even if the split routine method is employed, hypertrophy workouts are very exhausting to those who might perform upwards of 75-160 repetitions per training session. Such high muscle loading requires a long recovery period following a session. The type of training specific to this phase exhausts most, if not all, of the ATP/CP and glycogen stores during a demanding training session. We must remember that although ATP/CP is restored very quickly, the exhausted liver glycogen takes approximately 46-48 hours to replenish. It is logical, therefore, that heavy hypertrophy workouts to complete exhaustion be performed no more than 3 times per microcycle—preferably in the second, and especially in the third step of the 4-step loading pattern. (See figures 3.5 and 3.6.)

Constant exhaustive training depletes the body's energy stores and puts wear and tear on the contractile protein (myosin), accelerating its rate of *anabolism* (the myosins' protein building rate). The undesirable outcome of such overloading can be that the muscles involved no longer increase in size. Maybe we should change the old adage to "too much pain, no gain!" If you now use the overload technique, we urge you to do your body a favor and try the step-type approach to loading, and watch your body evolve. In addition, be sure to alternate intensities within each microcycle. Your body will respond to proper sequences of loading and regeneration.

The Isokinetic Method

The term isokinetic means "equal motion," or "same velocity of motion throughout the range of motion." Isokinetic training is performed on specially designed equipment that provides the muscles with the same resistance for both the concentric and eccentric parts of the contraction. This provides maximum activation of the muscles involved. Training velocity is very important in this type of training. Training at slower speeds seems to increase contractile strength, but *only* at slow speeds, and the major gains tend to be in muscle hypertrophy. On the other hand, training at higher speeds may increase the contractile strength at all speeds of contraction, either at or below the training speed, with major benefits being reaped for maximum strength (MxS). The more advanced computerized equipment allows the athlete to select and set the desired training velocity. These machines are often used as strength measuring devices.

Isokinetic equipment provides several key benefits:

- It offers a safe way to train and is, therefore, suitable for entry-level athletes during their early years.
- It is well suited for the AA phase when overall strength development and muscle attachment adaptation are the main purposes of training.
- It is a good training device for the rehabilitation of injured athletes.
- It can be used for gains in muscle hypertrophy if the load and number of repetitions are performed as suggested by this training method.
- With a higher velocity, it can result in gains in MxS.

Program Design for the H Phase

As with any new training phase, H training should start with a test for 1RM. The test must be performed in the second part of the first week, because this is the lowest intensity week in the step-type loading pattern. If it is performed in the early part of the week, the athlete is slightly fatigued from the previous high-intensity week. The brief delay ensures that fatigue does not affect the accuracy of the measurement.

One of the main objectives of H training is to consistently train all of the muscle groups in order to achieve the ultimate symmetrical shape. There are, however, two muscle groups to which additional reference should be made.

Hamstrings

The hams are often neglected and, in many instances, might not be developed proportionately to the quads. When planning your own program, please keep this in mind. Furthermore, power loading is too often used for the hams in the same way it is for other muscles, despite the fact that most muscle strains and injuries occur in the hamstrings. In sprinting, the hams are called "nervous" muscles since they have more nerve end plates per square inch than the quads and many other muscles. The programs we suggest often propose a 10-20% lower load for the hams than for the quads. Work slowly and carefully on the hams!

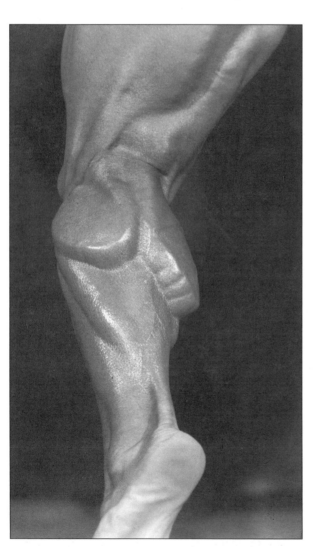

The impressive calf of Roger Stewart.

Calves

These muscles, along with the quads, support the human form in the standing or walking positions. Due to incessant low-level stimulation, they have biologically adapted by developing a higher proportion of slow-twitch (76%) fibers than fast-twitch (24%) fibers (Fox et al., 1989). As a result, it is difficult to stimulate the same growth in the calves as most of the other muscle groups. The special physiological composition of the calves prevents them from responding well to traditional bodybuilding and strength training programs, in which the same loading and RI are used for the calves as for other muscles.

The calves have a higher capillarization than other muscles because of their genetic adaptation to human needs, and are able to resupply their energy needs (ATP/CP stores) more quickly. In order to offset the energy balance of the calves, training must be slightly different. The RI should be no longer than 30-45 seconds, in order to inhibit immediate ATP and CP restoration. This forces the body to increase its energy transport capacity, which increases the CP content of the cells and activates protein metabolism. As a result, the hypertrophy of the

Table 5.1 Training guidelines for the H phase

Bodybuilder's classification	Entry level	Recreational	Advanced	Professional
Duration of H* phase (weeks)	6	3–6	3–6	12
# of reps/set	6–12	9–12	9–12	9–12
# of sets/exercise	2–3	4–5	4–5	3–7
RI between sets (seconds)	60–120	45–60	45–60	30–45
Workouts/week	2–3	3–5	4–5	5–6
Aerobic training sessions/week	1	1	1–2	2–3

calves is better stimulated, allowing the athlete to build the calves in proportion to the rest of the body. Table 5.1 suggests training guidelines for the hypertrophy phase.

Program Examples

Suggested programs for the H phase are presented in tables 5.2-5.5 for four different classifications of bodybuilders and strength trainers. Let's look at table 5.2 as an example.

- The top row of the chart is for the "date." In our example, we simply numbered the six weeks of the program, but when making your individual program use this space to indicate the date of the week (e.g., September 1-7).

- The second row is the "step" row, which contains information about the load intensity, as per the step-type loading method. The first step is "low," indicating a low intensity and volume of training. Programs for the second step are of "medium" intensity. Finally, programs for the third step are of "high" intensity. The same pattern is repeated for weeks 4, 5, and 6.

- The third row shows the "day" of training. For example, in table 5.2, days 1 and 4 will consist of the top program, while days 2 and 5 will consist of the bottom program. Days 3, 6, and 7 are for rest.

As you can see, this is an example of a 2-day split routine, in which there are two groups of exercises, each being performed twice a week. This simple split routine is superior to the traditional routines because the muscles receive more stimulation when trained twice a week than only once a week. The obvious outcome is a more dramatic increase in muscle size.

- All of the exercises numbered from 1 to 6 are listed. If you follow one exercise for all six weeks, you can see the difference in the amount of work between the "low-," "medium-," and "high-" intensity training days, as well as the progression of expected strength gains. Changes in loading are done mostly by altering the load and number of sets.

Table 5.2 A suggested training program for the H phase of an entry-level bodybuilder or strength trainer*

Exercise no.	Step / Day	1 Low		2 Medium		3 High		4 Low		5 Medium		6 High	
	Day	1	4	1	4	1	4	1	4	1	4	1	4
1	Leg press	40/10·2	40/12·2	40/15·2	40/15·2	50/12·2	50/10·3	40/12·2	40/12·3	50/12·3	50/12·3	60/10·2	60/10·3
2	Seated leg curls	40/8·2	40/10·2	40/10·2	40/8·3	50/10·2	50/8·3	40/10·3	40/10·2	50/10·3	50/10·3	50/10·3	50/10·3
3	Front dumbbell press	40/8·2	40/10·2	40/12·2	40/15·2	50/10·3	50/10·3	40/12·3	40/10·3	50/12·3	50/12·3	60/10·3	60/10·3
4	Incline side laterals	40/8·2	40/8·2	40/10·2	40/8·3	50/10·2	50/8·3	40/10·2	40/10·2	50/10·3	50/10·3	50/10·3	50/10·3
5	Back extensions	2·10	2·12	2·15	2·15	3·10	3·10	2·15	3·10	3·12	3·15	3·15	3·15
6	Diagonal curl-ups	2·12	2·12	2·15	2·15	3·10	3·10	2·12	3·10	3·12	3·15	3·15	3·15
7	?												
8	?												
	Day	2	5	2	5	2	5	2	5	2	5	2	5
1	Shrugs	40/10·2	40/10·2	40/12·2	40/15·2	50/10·2	50/10·3	40/12·2	40/10·3	50/12·3	50/12·3	60/10·3	60/10·3
2	Incline bench press	40/10·2	40/10·2	40/12·2	40/15·2	50/10·2	50/10·3	40/12·2	40/10·3	50/12·3	50/10·3	60/10·3	60/10·3
3	Seated pulley rows	40/10·2	40/10·2	40/12·2	40/15·2	50/10·2	50/10·3	40/12·2	40/10·3	50/12·3	50/12·3	60/10·3	60/10·3
4	Triceps push-downs	40/10·2	40/10·2	40/12·2	40/15·2	50/10·2	50/10·3	40/12·2	40/10·3	50/12·3	50/12·3	60/10·3	60/10·3
5	Standing calf raises	40/10·2	40/12·2	40/15·2	40/15·2	50/12·2	50/10·3	40/10·2	40/10·3	50/12·3	50/12·3	60/10·3	60/10·3
6	Seated calf raises	40/12·2	40/12·2	40/15·2	40/15·2	50/12·2	50/12·3	40/12·2	40/12·3	50/12·3	50/12·3	60/10·2	60/10·3
7	?												
8	?												

*RI between sets should be 1–2 minutes. ? = You may add any exercise(s) you would like.

Table 5.3 A suggested training program for the H phase for a recreational bodybuilder or strength trainer*

Column structure — the twelve data columns are two repeated week‑progressions:

Week #	1	1	2	2	3	3	1	1	2	2	3	3
Step	Low	Low	Medium	Medium	High	High	Low	Low	Medium	Medium	High	High
Day	1	4	1	4	1	4	1	4	1	4	1	4

Day 2

Exercise no.	Exercise	1/Low·1	1/Low·4	2/Med·1	2/Med·4	3/High·1	3/High·4	1/Low·1	1/Low·4	2/Med·1	2/Med·4	3/High·1	3/High·4
1	Hack squats	50/12·3	50/12·3	60/12·3	60/12·3	60/15·3	60/12·4	50/12·3	50/12·3	60/12·4	60/12·4	70/10·4	70/10·4
2	Standing leg curls	50/10·3	50/10·3	50/12·3	50/12·3	50/10·4	50/10·4	50/10·3	50/10·3	60/10·3	60/10·3	60/8·4	60/8·4
3	Lunges	50/12·3	50/12·3	60/12·3	60/12·3	60/15·3	60/12·4	50/12·3	50/12·3	60/12·4	60/12·4	70/10·4	70/10·4
4	Back extensions	3·12	3·12	3·15	3·15	4·12	4·15	3·15	3·15	4·15	4·15	4·15	4·15
5	Diagonal curl-ups	3·12	3·12	3·15	3·15	4·12	4·15	3·15	3·15	4·15	4·15	4·15	4·15
6	Biceps preacher curls	50/12·3	50/12·3	60/12·3	60/12·3	60/15·3	60/12·4	50/12·3	50/12·3	60/12·4	60/12·4	70/10·4	70/10·4
7	Triceps push-downs	50/12·3	50/12·3	60/12·3	60/12·3	60/15·3	60/12·4	50/12·3	50/12·3	60/10·3	60/10·3	70/10·4	70/10·4
8	?												

Day 5

Exercise no.	Exercise	1/Low·1	1/Low·4	2/Med·1	2/Med·4	3/High·1	3/High·4	1/Low·1	1/Low·4	2/Med·1	2/Med·4	3/High·1	3/High·4
1	Flat bench press	50/12·3	50/12·3	60/12·3	60/12·3	60/15·3	60/12·4	50/12·3	50/12·3	60/10·3	60/10·3	70/10·4	70/10·4
2	Incline dumbbell bench press	50/12·3	50/12·3	60/12·3	60/12·3	60/15·3	60/12·4	50/12·3	50/12·3	60/12·4	60/10·3	60/8·4	70/10·4
3	Front dumbbell press	50/12·3	50/12·3	60/12·3	60/12·3	60/15·3	60/12·4	50/12·3	50/12·3	60/12·4	60/12·4	70/10·4	70/10·4
4	Standing dumbbell side laterals	50/10·3	50/10·3	50/12·3	50/12·3	50/10·4	50/10·4	50/10·3	50/10·3	60/10·3	60/10·3	60/8·4	60/8·4
5	Shrugs	50/12·3	50/12·3	60/12·3	60/12·3	60/15·3	60/12·4	50/12·3	50/12·3	60/12·4	60/12·4	70/10·4	70/10·4
6	Seated pulley rows	50/12·3	50/12·3	60/12·3	60/12·3	60/15·3	60/12·4	50/12·3	50/12·3	60/10·3	60/12·4	60/10·3	60/8·4
7	Seated calf raises	50/12·3	50/12·3	60/12·3	60/12·3	60/15·3	60/12·4	50/12·3	50/12·3	60/12·4	60/12·4	70/10·4	70/10·4
8	Standing calf raises	50/12·3	50/12·3	60/12·3	60/12·3	60/15·3	60/12·4	50/12·3	50/12·3	60/12·4	60/12·4	70/10·4	70/10·4
9	?												

*RI between sets should be 45–60 seconds.

Table 5.4　Hypertrophy training program for an advanced bodybuilder or strength trainer with 5 workouts per week*

	Week #	1 Low			2 Medium			3 High			4 Low			5 Medium			6 High		
Exercise no.	Day	1	3	5	1	3	5	1	3	5	1	3	5	1	3	5	1	3	5
1	Safety squats	60/12-4	Off	60/15-4	60/15-4	70/10-4	70/10-4	75/10-4	Off	75/10-4	60/12-4	70/10-4	70/10-4	75/10-4	Off	80/8-4	80/8-5	85/5-5	85/5-5
2	Standing leg curls	60/8-3	Off	60/8-3	60/8-4	60/8-4	60/8-4	65/7-4	Off	65/7-4	60/10-3	60/10-3	60/10-4	65/7-4	Off	65/10-4	70/8-4	70/8-4	70/8-4
3	Lunges	60/12-4	Off	60/15-4	60/15-4	70/10-4	70/10-4	75/10-4	Off	75/10-4	60/12-4	70/10-4	70/10-4	75/10-4	Off	80/8-4	80/8-5	85/5-5	85/5-5
4	B. bent-over row	60/12-4	Off	60/15-4	60/15-4	60/15-4	70/10-4	75/10-4	Off	75/10-4	60/12-4	60/12-4	70/10-4	75/10-4	Off	80/8-4	80/8-5	85/5-5	85/5-5
5	Back extensions	3-15	Off	4-15	4-12	4-12	4-15	4-15	Off	4-15	3-15	3-15	4-12	4-15	Off	4-15	5-15	5-15	5-15
6	Diagonal curl-ups	3-15	Off	4-15	4-12	4-12	4-12	4-15	Off	4-15	3-15	3-15	4-12	4-15	Off	4-15	5-15	5-15	5-15
7	Decline triceps extensions	60/12-4	Off	60/15-4	60/15-4	60/15-4	70/10-4	75/10-4	Off	75/10-4	60/12-4	60/12-4	70/10-4	75/10-4	Off	80/8-4	80/8-5	85/5-5	85/5-5
8	?																		

	Week #	1 Low			2 Medium			3 High			4 Low			5 Medium			6 High		
Exercise no.	Day	2	4	6	2	4	6	2	4	6	2	4	6	2	4	6	2	4	6
1	Flat bench press	60/12-4	60/12-4	60/15-4	60/15-4	Off	70/10-4	75/10-4	75/10-4	75/10-4	60/12-4	Off	70/10-4	75/10-4	75/10-4	80/8-4	80/8-5	Off	85/5-5
2	Incline flys	60/12-4	60/12-4	60/15-4	60/15-4	Off	70/10-4	75/10-4	75/10-4	75/10-4	60/12-4	Off	70/10-4	75/10-4	75/10-4	80/8-5	80/8-5	Off	85/5-5
3	Front dumbbell press	60/12-4	60/12-4	60/15-4	60/15-4	Off	70/10-4	75/10-4	75/10-4	75/10-4	60/12-4	Off	70/10-4	75/10-4	75/10-4	80/8-5	80/8-5	Off	85/5-5
4	Incline side laterals	60/10-3	60/10-3	60/10-3	65/8-4	Off	65/8-4	70/8-4	70/8-4	70/8-4	60/10-4	Off	60/10-4	75/6-4	75/6-4	75/6-4	75/6-4	Off	75/6-4
5	Shrugs	60/12-4	60/12-4	60/15-4	60/15-4	Off	70/10-4	75/10-4	75/10-4	75/10-4	60/12-4	Off	70/10-4	75/10-4	75/10-4	80/8-4	80/8-5	Off	85/5-5
6	Biceps preacher curls	60/12-4	60/12-4	60/15-4	60/15-4	Off	70/10-4	75/10-4	75/10-4	75/10-4	60/12-4	Off	70/10-4	75/10-4	75/10-4	80/8-4	80/8-5	Off	85/5-5
7	Donkey calf raises	60/12-4	60/12-4	70/10-4	60/15-4	Off	70/10-4	75/10-4	75/10-4	75/10-4	60/12-4	Off	70/10-4	75/10-4	75/10-4	80/8-4	80/8-5	Off	85/5-5
8	?																		

*You may decrease the number of workouts to 4, but maintain the same loading. If the number of workouts is reduced, an aerobic training session should be added. RI between sets should be 45 seconds.

Table 5.5   Suggested three-week H training program for a professional bodybuilder*

Exercise no.	Week #	1			2			3		
	Step	Low			Medium			High		
	Day	1	3	5	1	3	5	1	3	5
1	Safety squats	70/12·4	70/15·4	75/10·5	75/10·5	70/15·5	75/8·3	80/7·6	80/6·6	85/4·7
2	Standing leg curls	70/8·4	70/15·4	75/10·5	75/10·5	70/15·5	80/7·5	80/7·6	80/6·6	85/4·6
3	Lunges	70/12·3	70/15·3	75/10·3	75/10·3	70/15·3	75/8·1	80/7·3	80/6·3	85/4·3
4	Back extensions	4·15	4·15	4·18	4·18	4·12	4·12	4·15	4·15	4·15
5	Biceps preacher curls	70/12·4	70/15·4	75/10·5	75/10·5	70/15·5	75/8·3	80/7·6	80/7·6	85/4·6
6	Decline triceps extensions	70/12·4	70/15·4	75/10·5	75/10·5	70/15·5	75/8·3	80/7·6	80/7·6	85/4·6
7	?									
	Day	2	4	6	2	4	6	2	4	6
1	Flat bench press	70/12·4	70/15·4	75/10·5	75/10·5	70/15·3	75/8·1	80/7·6	80/7·6	85/4·6
2	Incline flys	70/12·3	70/15·3	75/10·3	75/10·3	70/15·3	75/8·1	80/7·3	80/7·3	85/4·3
3	One-arm dumbbell rows	70/12·4	70/15·4	75/10·4	75/10·4	70/15·4	75/8·2	80/7·4	80/7·4	85/4·4
4	Incline side laterals	70/12·4	70/15·4	75/10·4	75/10·4	70/15·5	75/7·4	80/6·4	80/6·4	80/4·4
5	Front dumbbell press	70/12·3	70/15·3	75/10·3	75/10·3	70/15·4	75/8·1	80/7·3	80/7·3	85/4·3
6	Shrugs	70/12·3	70/15·3	75/10·3	75/10·3	70/15·3	75/8·1	80/7·3	80/7·3	85/4·3
7	Two abdominal exercises	4·15	4·15	6·18	6·18	6·12	6·12	6·15	6·15	6·15
8	Donkey calf raises	70/12·4	70/15·4	75/10·5	75/10·5	70/15·5	75/8·3	80/7·6	80/6·6	85/4·6
9	?									

*RI between sets should be 30–45 seconds.

Hypertrophy Cues:

- Test for 1RM: (1) during week 1; (2) during the second part of week 4; (3) during the first week of the next program.

- A few spaces are left open at the end of the lists so the athlete can add a preferred or needed exercise.

- The number of exercises can be slightly increased or decreased according to one's needs.

- Regardless of any of the above changes that might be made, always apply the suggested loading pattern.

- Decrease the load if it is too high, but maintain the same number of reps.

- The number of sets could be increased or decreased in response to the particular potential and needs of an individual.

- Do not forget to do 20-25 minutes of aerobic work!

- During the hypertrophy phase, all of the sets per exercise are performed before moving on to the next exercise. (This is different from the AA phase.)

Nutrition Strategy for the H Phase

Since the goal of the hypertrophy training is to increase muscle size, food must provide the body with what it needs to support tissue growth and maintenance under intensive training. Protein intake must be high in relation to body weight and carbohydrate intake must be high in relation to protein intake. Such a diet will provide sufficient energy for the workouts and spare body protein from being used as an energy source.

During this phase, 20% of the diet is allotted to fat. Fat helps to lubricate the joints during this strenuous training phase, and is important to the workings of fat soluble vitamins. Traditional bodybuilders and strength trainers may consume far greater amounts of fat. However, excess fat that becomes useless body weight only has to be shed later.

To create the appropriate diet for your own training, refer to tables 5.6, 5.7, and 5.8, which represent low, medium, and high days, respectively. To use these charts, find your present weight in the left hand column and use the protein, carbohydrate, and fat gram values specified for that weight.

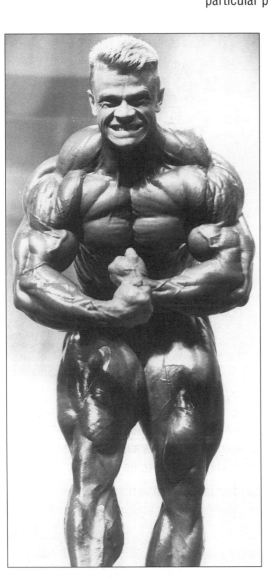

Roland Cziurlok knows how to eat for muscle size.

Table 5.6   Hypertrophy diet: Low-calorie day

Body weight (lbs.)	Protein (g)	Carbs (g)	Fat (g)	Total calories
90	72	162	26	1,170
100	80	180	28	1,290
110	88	198	31	1,425
120	96	216	34	1,555
130	104	234	37	1,685
140	112	252	40	1,815
150	120	270	43	1,950
160	128	288	46	2,080
170	136	306	48	2,220
180	144	324	51	2,330
190	152	342	54	2,460
200	160	360	57	2,595
210	168	370	60	2,725
220	176	396	63	2,855
230	184	414	65	2,975
240	192	432	68	3,110
250	200	450	71	3,240
260	208	468	74	3,370
270	216	486	77	3,500
280	224	504	80	3,630
290	232	522	82	3,755
300	240	540	85	3,885

H Phase Nutrition Cues:

- This is a hypertrophy diet, so weight gain can be expected. The low fat content will, however, cause most of the gain to be in muscle.

- Everyone's body is different and variables such as the amount of cardio performed per week, actual workout intensity, and genetic physiology, will affect how each individual responds.

- A constant diet must be maintained in terms of keeping the same recommended percentages of proteins, carbohydrates, and fats. Do this by moving either up or down the weight scale on the chart.

Table 5.7 Hypertrophy diet: Medium-calorie day

Body weight (lbs.)	Protein (g)	Carbs (g)	Fat (g)	Total calories
90	90	198	32	1,440
100	100	220	36	1,605
110	110	242	39	1,760
120	120	264	43	1,925
130	130	286	46	2,080
140	140	308	50	2,240
150	150	330	53	2,400
160	160	352	57	2,560
170	170	374	60	2,715
180	180	396	64	2,880
190	190	418	68	3,045
200	200	440	71	3,200
210	210	462	75	3,365
220	220	484	78	3,520
230	230	506	82	3,680
240	240	528	85	3,835
250	250	550	89	4,000
260	260	572	92	4,255
270	270	594	96	4,320
280	280	616	100	4,485
290	290	638	103	4,640
300	300	660	106	4,795

If you begin to lose weight, are continuously hungry, or are not making muscle gain, increase food intake. Do this by eating the protein and carbohydrate values recommended for the next heavier weight group. Only if you are fighting for every ounce of body weight should you use the fat values for the next heavier weight group. Continue to monitor progress and adjust the diet until you are achieving the desired results.

If you begin to gain weight in terms of excess body fat, which can occur if you lead a sedentary life outside the gym or do no cardiovascular work, then lower food intake. Do this by eating the food values for the next lower weight group. Continue to monitor progress and adjust the diet until you find the level that works for you.

Table 5.8   Hypertrophy diet: High-calorie day

Body weight (lbs.)	Protein (g)	Carbs (g)	Fat (g)	Total calories
90	108	234	38	1,710
100	120	260	43	1,905
110	132	286	47	2,095
120	144	312	51	2,285
130	156	338	55	2,470
140	168	364	59	2,660
150	180	390	64	2,855
160	192	416	68	3,045
170	204	442	72	3,230
180	216	468	76	3,420
190	228	494	81	3,615
200	240	520	85	3,805
210	252	546	89	3,995
220	264	572	93	4,180
230	276	598	98	4,380
240	288	624	102	4,565
250	300	650	106	5,755
260	312	676	110	4,940
270	324	702	115	5,140
280	336	728	119	5,325
290	348	754	123	5,515
300	360	780	128	5,710

CHAPTER

6

PHASE THREE: MIXED TRAINING (M)

Before entering the maximum strength (MxS) phase, it is necessary to gradually introduce some specific training elements for the development of MxS. As the name implies, mixed training incorporates some workouts specific to H training and applies MxS methods for other sessions, therefore, programs must be planned.

Scope of M Training

- Continue to improve muscle hypertrophy.
- Introduce MxS methods in order to increase "chronic hypertrophy," or long-term muscle tone and density.

Use desired proportions between the two types of training depending on the needs of the athlete.

> For example: 40% H and 60% MxS
> 50% H and 50% MxS
> 60% H and 40% MxS

Duration of M Training— The Progressive Transition

Regardless of the proportions used, M training ensures a more progressive transition into the maximum strength phase, where extremely heavy loads might challenge the athlete's ability to cope with the stress and strains of high intensity workouts.

Program Design for the M Phase

Table 6.1 presents the proportions of an H and MxS mixed training program for four classifications of bodybuilders. The program can be repeated as many times as necessary, depending upon the length of the M phase. As shown in the chart, MxS training is consistently recommended for the first workout of the week, and/or following a rest day. The reason is a scientific one. Since MxS training employs loads that come close to maximum potential, the CNS and the athlete's ability to reach maximum concentration before and during training become important elements in planning these sessions.

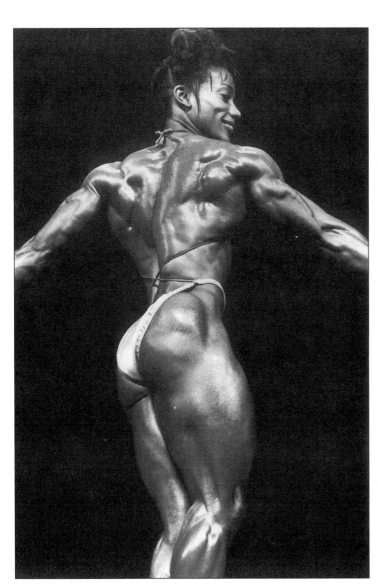

The elegant Lenda Murray.

The Fatigue Factor

It is well known that fatigue affects one's ability to lift heavy loads, such as those used in MxS (Grimby, 1992; Sale, 1986; Hakkinen, 1991; Schmidt-bleicher, 1992). If, for example, an athlete performs a MxS workout following an H workout, he or she will have decreased lifting efficiency for the heavy loads. On the other hand, if H training starts with slight residual fatigue, this tends to have a stimulating effect on the development of muscle. A slightly fatigued muscle seems to exhaust the ATP/CP stores more quickly and appears to stimulate muscle growth. In the case of mixed training, therefore, always plan MxS workouts before H workouts.

In Tables 6.2-6.9, we offer M training programs for entry-level, recreational, advanced, and professional athletes. To follow the same sequence of H and MxS training days shown in table 6.1, a plan for each level of athlete must be split into two parts—one for the H portion and one for the MxS portion. For example, table 6.2 shows the H portion of the M program for entry-level athletes, with 3 days planned for the development of H—days 1, 2, and 6. Table 6.3 shows the MxS portion of the M program for entry-level athletes, with only 1 day planned for MxS training. Day 6 consists of a selection of exercises from both programs. Please perform only those exercises you have chosen and NOT both complete programs.

Table 6.1   Suggested proportion between MxS and H training for the M phase

No.	Classification	Mon	Tues	Wed	Thur	Fri	Sat	Sun
1	Entry level	H	H	Off	MxS	Off	H	Off
2	Recreational	MxS	H	Off	MxS	Off	H	Off
3	Advanced	MxS	H	MxS	H	Off	H	Off
4	Professional	MxS	H	H	Off	MxS	H	Off

Mixed Training Cues:

- The exercises that we have recommended may be substituted with similar exercises according to one's needs and preferences.
- The recommended programs for the M phase are all 3 weeks in duration, however, if a longer M phase is needed, the entire program can be repeated.

Achieve Optimum Recovery

Unlike the exercise pattern for H training, where all the planned sets for one exercise are performed before moving on to the next exercise, MxS training requires that the athlete always reach optimum recovery between sets. The MxS exercise pattern, therefore, is to perform one set for the first exercise, and then move on to perform one set for the next exercise, and so on. Always work the exercises from the top down! In order to enhance the recovery process further, the exercises are planned in such a way that the muscle groups are constantly being alternated.

It is extremely important to religiously observe the proposed RI! Do not make the mistake of performing your sets too soon. Regardless of whether you feel ready before the RI is up, your body needs the time to recover from this type of training. Your last set should be as good as your first set.

Mixed Training Cues:

- Test for 1RM as suggested for the other training phases.
- You may select exercises other than those suggested, but apply the same loading pattern.
- The suggested loading is not carved in stone. If a given load is too high for you, reduce it slightly until you can perform the recommended number of reps.
- The number of sets can be increased or decreased according to your own potential.
- Do your aerobic training.
- Follow the nutrition strategy suggested for the H phase.

Table 6.2 Mixed phase, H training portion for an entry-level bodybuilder or strength trainer*

Exercise no.	Week # Step Day	1 Low 1	3	6	2 Medium 1	3	6	3 High 1	3	6
1	Leg extension	40/15·3	Off		50/12·3	Off		60/12·3	Off	
2	Leg press	40/12·3	Off	40/12·3	50/12·3	Off	50/12·3	60/10·3	Off	60/10·3
3	Lunges	40/12·3	Off	40/12·3	50/12·3	Off	50/12·3	60/10·3	Off	60/10·3
4	Standing leg curls	40/10·3	Off	40/10·3	50/10·3	Off	50/10·3	50/10·3	Off	50/10·3
5	T-B rows	40/12·3	Off		50/12·3	Off		60/10·3	Off	
6	Back extensions	3·10	Off		3·12	Off		3·15	Off	
7	Seated calf raises	40/12·3	Off		50/12·3	Off		60/10·3	Off	
8	Flat flys	40/12·3	Off	40/12·3	50/12·3	Off	50/12·3	60/10·3	Off	60/10·3
9	?									

Exercise no.	Day	2	5	6	2	5	6	2	5	6
1	Front dumbbell press	40/12·3	Off		50/12·3	Off		60/10·3	Off	
2	Incline side laterals	40/12·3	Off	40/12·3	50/12·3	Off	50/12·3	60/10·3	Off	60/10·3
3	Upright rows	40/12·3	Off		50/12·3	Off		60/10·3	Off	
4	Shrugs	40/12·3	Off	40/12·3	50/12·3	Off	50/12·3	60/10·3	Off	60/10·3
5	Decline triceps extensions	40/12·3	Off	40/12·3	50/12·3	Off	50/12·3	60/10·3	Off	60/10·3
6	Diagonal curl-ups	3·10	Off	3·10	3·12	Off	3·12	3·15	Off	3·15
7	?									

*RI between sets should be 1–2 minutes.

Table 6.3   Mixed phase, MxS training portion for entry-level bodybuilders or strength trainers

Exercise no.	Week #	1	2		3
	Step	Low	Medium		High
	Day	4	4		5
1	Leg press	70/7·3	70/8·1	80/6·2	80/6·3
2	Flat bench press	70/7·3	70/8·1	80/6·2	80/6·3
3	Supine leg curls	50/10·3	60/10·3		70/7·3
4	T-B rows	50/10·3	60/10·3		70/8·3
5	Seated calf raises	70/7·3	70/8·1	80/6·2	80/6·3
6	?				

Table 6.4   Mixed phase, H training portion for recreational bodybuilders and strength trainers

Exercise no.	Week #	1	2	3
	Step	Low	Medium	High
	Day	2	2	2
1	Front dumbbell press	50/12·3	60/12·3	70/8·4
2	Incline side laterals	50/12·3	60/12·3	70/8·4
3	Biceps: preacher curls	50/12·3	60/12·3	70/8·4
4	Shrugs	50/12·3	60/12·3	70/8·4
5	Seated calf raises	50/12·3	60/12·3	70/8·4
6	?			
	Day	6	6	6
1	Hack squats	50/12·3	60/12·3	70/8·4
2	Supine leg curls	50/12·3	60/12·3	70/8·4
3	Seated pulley rows	50/12·3	60/12·3	70/8·4
4	Incline flys	50/10·3	60/10·3	60/8·4
5	Triceps push-downs	50/12·3	60/12·3	70/8·4
6	Crunches	3·10	3·12	4·15

Table 6.5 Mixed phase, MxS training portion for recreational bodybuilders and strength trainers*

Exercise no.	Week #	1			2			3	
	Step	Low			Medium			High	
	Day	1	4		1	4		1	4
1	Leg press	70/8·3	70/8·2	80/6·1	70/8·1	80/7·2	80/7·3	80/8·4	80/8·4
2	Flat bench press	70/8·3	70/8·2	80/6·1	70/8·1	80/7·2	80/7·3	80/8·4	80/8·4
3	Supine leg curls	60/10·3	60/10·3		70/8·3		70/8·3	70/8·4	70/8·4
4	Lat. pull-downs	70/8·3	70/8·2	80/6·1	70/8·1	80/7·2	80/7·3	80/8·4	80/8·4
5	?								

*RI between sets should be 3 minutes.

Table 6.6 Mixed phase, MxS training for advanced bodybuilders and strength trainers*

Exercise no.	Week #	1			2			3	
	Step	Low			Medium			High	
	Day	1	3		1	3		1	3
1	Safety squats	70/8·4	80/7·1	80/7·5	80/6·2	90/3·3	85/4·2	90/3·3	90/3·5	90/2·5
2	Standing leg curls	60/8·5		60/8·5	70/7·5		70/7·5		80/6·5	80/6·5
3	Flat bench press	70/8·4	80/7·1	80/7·5	80/6·2	90/3·3	85/4·2	90/3·3	90/3·5	90/2·5
4	B. bent over rows	70/8·4	80/7·1	80/7·5	80/6·2	90/3·3	85/4·2	90/3·3	90/3·5	90/2·5
5	Front dumbbell press	70/8·4	80/7·1	80/7·5	80/6·2	90/3·3	85/4·2	90/3·3	90/3·5	90/2·5
6	Donkey calf raises	60/8·5		60/8·5	70/7·5		70/7·5		80/6·5	80/6·5
7	?								

*RI between sets should be 3–4 minutes.

Table 6.7   An example of H training program for the M phase for advanced bodybuilders and strength trainers*

Exercise no.	Week #	1		2		3			
	Step	Low		Medium		High			
	Day		6		6			6	
1	Lunges		70/8·4		80/9·5			85/5·5	
2	Diagonal curl-ups		4·12		5·15			5·15	
3	Biceps: preacher curls		70/8·4		80/7·5			85/5·5	
4	?								
5	?								
	Day	2/4	6	2/4	6	2/4		6	
1	Decline triceps extensions	70/8·4	70/8·4	80/7·5	80/7·5	80/7·2	85/5·3	80/7·2	85/5·3
2	Pull-downs behind neck	70/8·4	70/8·4	80/7·5	80/7·5	80/7·2	85/5·3	80/7·2	85/5·3
3	Standing dumbbell bent laterals	60/10·4	70/8·4	70/7·5	80/7·5	75/6·5			
4	Shrugs	70/8·4		80/7·5		80/7·2	85/5·3		
5	Back extensions	4·12		4·15		5·15			
6	?								

RI between sets should be 30–45 seconds.

Table 6.8 Suggested H training program for the M phase for professional bodybuilders and strength trainers*

Exercise no.	Week #	1		2		3	
	Step	Low		Medium		High	
	Day	2	6	2	6	2	6
1	Front dumbbell press	60/12·3	60/12·3	70/10·3	75/8·3	80/7·2	80/7·2
2	Incline side laterals	60/12·4	60/12·4	70/10·4	75/8·4	80/7·3	80/7·3
3	Shrugs	60/12·6	60/12·6	70/10·6	75/8·6	80/7·6	80/7·6
4	Decline triceps extensions	60/12·4	60/12·4	70/10·6	75/8·6	80/7·6	80/7·6
5	Biceps preacher curls	60/12·3	60/12·3	70/10·3	70/10·3	80/7·3	80/7·3
	Day	**3**		**3**		**3**	
1	Safety squats	60/12·6		70/10·7		80/7·8	
2	Standing leg curls	60/12·6		70/10·7		70/7·8	
3	Flat bench press	60/12·6		70/10·7		80/7·8	
4	Barbell bent-over rows	60/12·6		70/10·7		80/7·8	
5	Back extensions	60/12·3		70/10·3		80/7·3	
6	Nautilus crunches	60/12·3		70/10·3		80/7·3	
7	Donkey calf raises	60/12·6		70/10·7		80/7·8	

RI between sets should be 30–45 seconds.

Table 6.9 Mixed phase, MxS training portion for professional bodybuilders and strength trainers

Exercise no.	Week #	1		2		3	
	Step	Low		Medium		High	
	Day	1	5	1	5	1	5
1	Safety squats	80/7·6	80/7·6	85/4·3	90/3·3	90/3·6	90/3·2	95/2·4	80/3·2	95/2·4
2	Standing leg curls	70/6·5	70/6·5	80/6·5		80/6·5	80/6·5		80/6·5	
3	Barbell bent-over rows	80/7·6	80/7·6	85/4·3	90/3·3	90/3·6	90/3·2	95/2·4	80/3·2	95/2·4
4	Flat bench press	80/7·6	80/7·6	85/4·3	90/3·3	90/3·6	90/3·2	95/2·4	80/3·2	95/2·4

CHAPTER 7

PHASE FOUR: MAXIMUM STRENGTH (MxS)

The MxS phase is one of the original elements introduced by the Periodization concept, and its application in a training program results in better symmetry, stronger muscles, and a more aesthetically pleasing body.

Scope of MxS Training

- Increase the protein content of the muscle in order to induce chronic hypertrophy, thus increasing muscle tone and density.
- Increase the thickness of the cross-bridges and myosin filaments since this is the only way to improve chronic hypertrophy.
- Condition the muscles to recruit as many fast-twitch muscle fibers as possible, through the application of heavy loads since this develops maximum strength and improves muscle tone and density.

The duration of this phase is recommended to be six weeks, although other variations are possible.

The Physiology Behind MxS Training

An athlete's ability to develop MxS depends, to a high degree, on the following factors:

- The diameter, or cross-sectional area, of the muscle involved. More specifically, this means the diameter of the myosin filaments, including their cross-bridges.

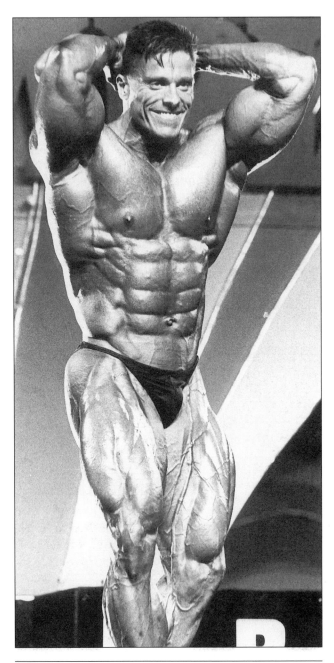

The muscular symmetry of Achim Albrecht.

Although muscle size depends largely upon the duration of the H phase, the diameter of the myosin filaments depends specifically on the volume and duration of the MxS phase. This is because MxS training is responsible for increasing the protein content of the muscles.

• The capacity to recruit FT muscle fibers.

This ability depends largely on training content. Maximum loads, with high application of force against resistance, is the only type of training that results in the complete involvement of the powerful FT motor units.

• The ability to successfully synchronize all of the muscles involved in the action.

This develops over time as a function of learning, which is based on performing many repetitions of the same exercise, with heavy loads. Most North American bodybuilders use only bodybuilding (i.e., H) methods for increasing muscle size. What is very neglected, therefore, is the type of training that stimulates the recruitment of FT muscle fibers to build high-density, tight muscle tone, and impressive muscle separation with more visible muscle striations. While North American bodybuilders do increase their muscle size, it is usually not chronic, because the growth is largely due to fluid displacement within the muscles rather than a thickening of the muscle fibers. The MxS phase in the Periodized Workouts program can correct this deficiency. Maximum strength improves as a result of creating high tension in the muscle that can only be achieved by utilizing loads that result in higher FT muscle fiber recruitment (loads over 80-85% of 1RM).

Training Methods and Duration for MxS

Exercises used for the development of MxS must not be carried out under the conditions of exhaustion as in the H phase. During MxS training, the muscles should be allowed to recover maximally between sets. Due to the maximum activation of the CNS, and the high levels of concentration and motivation required, MxS training improves the links with the CNS that lead to improved muscle coordination and synchronization. Strength, therefore, is dependent upon the size of the muscle and the total number of cross-bridges as well as the capacity of the CNS to "drive" that muscle.

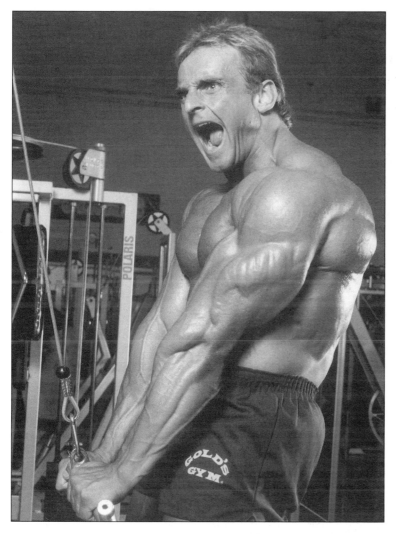

Training with intensity: the late Andreas Munzer.

High activation of the CNS (i.e., muscle synchronization) also results in an inhibition of the antagonistic muscles. When maximum force is applied, therefore, the antagonistic muscles are coordinated in such a way that they do not contract to oppose the movement, and this allows the athlete to lift even heavier weights.

Most changes in strength are said to occur at the level of muscle tissue. Little is said, however, about the involvement of the nervous system during MxS training. In fact, very little research has been conducted on the subject. The research that has been done suggests that the CNS acts as a stimulus for gains in strength. The CNS normally acts as an inhibitor of motor units during contraction. Under extreme circumstances, such as a life-and-death situation, this inhibition is removed and all the motor units are activated (Fox et al., 1989), giving the person what seems to be superhuman strength. One of the main objectives of MxS training is to teach the body to eliminate CNS inhibition, which will result in a huge improvement of strength potential.

The Maximum Load Method (MLM)

MxS improvement occurs almost solely through the *maximum load method (MLM)*. This method should only be performed after a minimum of 2-3 years of general bodybuilding or strength training programs, because of the strain of training and the utilization of maximum loads. The gains will be largely due to motor learning whereby athletes learn to use and coordinate the muscles involved in training more efficiently.

Benefits of MLM

1. MLM increases motor unit activation, resulting in high recruitment and firing frequency of FT muscle fibers.
2. Increases the secretion of growth hormones and increases catecholamine levels (a chemical compound that acts like a hormone), increasing the strong physiological response to this type of training (Tesch et al., 1986).

3. The coordination and synchronization of muscle groups during perfor-
    mance improves. The better the coordination and synchronization of
    the muscles involved in contraction, and the more they learn to recruit
    FT muscles, the better the performance.

4. The diameter of the contractile elements of the muscle increases.

5. The body's testosterone level naturally increases.

The gains obtained through MLM will be predominantly gains in MxS, with
muscle hypertrophy being a secondary benefit. Large gains in muscle size
through MLM are possible, but this generally occurs only in athletes who are
just beginning to experience MLM. For athletes with a more solid background,
gains in muscle size will not be as noticeable as the gains made in MxS. The MxS
phase will serve to set the stage for future growth explosions as a result of better
synchronization and increased recruitment of FT fibers. Highly-trained athletes, with a background in MLM of 3-4 years, are so well adapted to such
training that they are able to recruit approximately 85% of the FT fibers. The
remaining 15% represent a "latent reserve" that is not easily tapped through
training (Hartman and Tünnemann, 1989).

Once an athlete has reached such an advanced level, he or she might find it
very difficult to further increase MxS. In order to avoid stagnating and further
improve muscle density and separation, alternative methods must be used to
provide greater stimulation to the muscles. One method is to increase the
eccentric component of contractions, because the increased tension helps the
body to continue developing MxS despite an already high level of adaptation.

The most important elements to be considered in MLM training are the load
utilized in training, the RI, and the speed of performing the contraction. A brief
explanation of these factors will help clarify this statement.

The Load

As already mentioned, MxS is developed only when maximum tension is
created in the muscle. While the lower loads stimulate the ST muscle fibers,
loads exceeding 85% max are necessary if most muscle fibers, and especially
FT fibers, are to be recruited in contraction. Maximum loads with low repetitions result in significant nervous system adaptation, better synchronization of
the muscles involved, and an increased capacity to recruit the FT muscle fibers.

If, as suggested by Goldberg et al. (1975), the stimulus for protein synthesis
is the tension that is developed within the myofilaments, then this further
illustrates why training for MxS should be performed only with maximum loads.
It is because the load for the MLM is maximum that the number of repetitions
per set is low: 1-4(6).

The Rest Interval

The RI between sets depends partially on the athlete's fitness level and should
be carefully calculated to ensure adequate recovery of the neuromuscular
system. For MLM, a 3-5 minute RI is necessary because maximum loads involve
the CNS system, which recovers more slowly than the skeletal system. If the RI
is too short, nervous system participation in the form of maximum concentration, motivation, and the power of the nerve impulses sent to the contracting
muscle could be less than optimal. In addition, complete restoration of the

required fuel for contraction (ATP/CP) can also be jeopardized if the RI is too brief.

The Speed

The speed of execution plays an important role in MLM. Even when using the typical maximum loads, the athlete's force against resistance must be exerted as quickly as possible. Although the magnitude of the load restricts the speed of contraction, the athlete must concentrate on activating the muscles as briskly as possible.

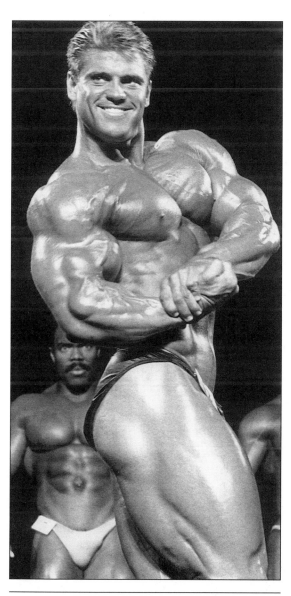

A splendid physique and dazzling personality have given Eddie Robinson longevity in the sport.

The Eccentric Method

Strength exercises, using either free weights or most isokinetic apparatuses, involve both concentric and eccentric types of contraction. During the concentric phase, force is produced while the muscle shortens, whereas during the eccentric segment, force is produced while the muscle lengthens, or returns to the resting position.

Everyone knows that the eccentric phase is easier than the concentric phase. For example, when performing the bench press, the lowering of the barbell to the chest (eccentric part of the lift) is easier than pressing the bar upward. Due to the fact that eccentric work is easier, it allows athletes to work with heavier loads than if they were only performing concentric work, and heavier training loads translate into greater strength gains. Strength training specialists and researchers have arrived at the same conclusion, which is that eccentric training creates a higher tension in the muscles than the isometric or isotonic contractions. Since higher muscle tension is normally equated with greater strength development (Goldberg et al., 1975), eccentric training should be considered a superior training method. Training specialists from the former East Germany claim that the eccentric strength training method results in a 10-35% higher strength gain than that of the other methods (Hartman and Tünnemann, 1989).

The load in eccentric training is much higher than the athlete's 1RM, so the speed of performance is quite slow. Such a slow rate of contraction produces a larger stimulus for protein synthesis and, therefore, normally results in muscle hypertrophy and greater strength development.

During the first few days of using the eccentric method, the athlete might experience muscle soreness, because higher tensions provoke some minor muscle damage. As the athlete adapts, muscle soreness disappears in about 7-10 days. In any case, this short-term discomfort can be avoided if the load is increased progressively, using the step-type approach.

Program Design for the MxS Phase

Since the eccentric method employs the heaviest loads in strength training (110-160%), only athletes with a solid strength training background (i.e., 2-4 years of strength or bodybuilding experience) should be exposed to it.

The eccentric method can be used alone or in combination with the MLM for only a short period of time. Eccentric training should not be abused. When overused it might have its limitations, and can lead to a plateau that might be difficult to break. In addition, because eccentric training requires such intense mental concentration, every time maximum or super maximum loads are used, there is a great deal of psychological wear.

For maximum training benefits, an athlete should use the MLM for as long as practically possible. When a plateau is reached and little or no improvement is being achieved, then the athlete should begin using the eccentric method. This training approach will break through the ceiling of adaptation created by the plateau and enable new heights of strength improvement to be achieved.

During eccentric training, which is usually performed with free weights, the assistance of two spotters is always necessary because the weights are always greater than the athlete can lift concentrically by him- or herself. The spotters'

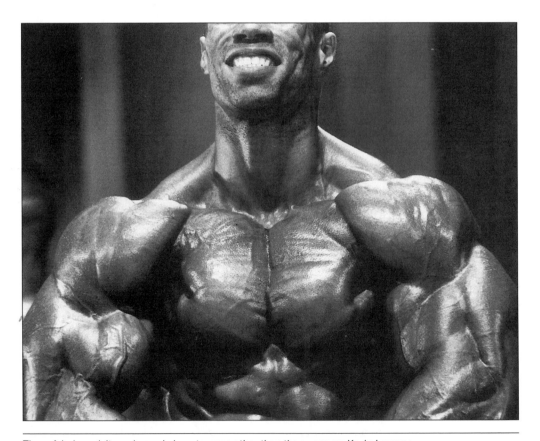

These fabulous delts and pecs belong to none other than the awesome Kevin Levrone.

job is to help the performer lift the weight during the concentric portion and watch the lifter carefully during the eccentric portion to ensure that the huge load can be handled.

If muscular soreness is experienced, use active recovery techniques to eliminate the discomfort and hasten regeneration. For further information, please refer to chapter 13, Muscle Recovery Between Workouts.

Training parameters for the eccentric method are presented in table 7.1. The load is expressed as a percentage of 1RM for the concentric contraction and is recommended to be between 110-160%. The most effective load for athletes of high caliber is around 130-140%. Lesser experienced athletes need to use lower loads. These loads are to be used after at least two phases of MxS training where the eccentric contraction is employed as well. They are not to be used in the first few months of training.

The number of sets per exercise and training session recommended in table 7.1 is a guideline for experienced athletes. Entry-level and recreational athletes need fewer sets depending upon their training potential.

The RI is an important element in the capacity to perform highly-demanding work. If, following a set, the athlete does not recover sufficiently to perform the next set at the same level, the RI must be slightly increased.

As eccentric contraction utilizes extremely heavy loads, the athlete must be highly motivated and have maximum concentration before performing each set. Only under such mental and psychological conditions will the athlete be capable of performing eccentric contraction effectively.

The eccentric method is rarely performed in isolation from the other MxS methods. Even during the MxS phase, the eccentric method is used together with MLM. Only one eccentric training session per week, therefore, is recommended. The frequency may eventually be increased for high caliber athletes during the third step of the step-type approach to load patterning.

Maximum Strength Cues:

- Test for 1RM during the second part of the first week and during the first week of the next phase.

Table 7.1   Training guidelines for the MxS phase

Bodybuilder's classification	Entry level	Recreational	Advanced	Professional
# of reps/set	1–4	3–8	3–8	2–8
# of sets/session	10–15	15–20	20–32	25–40
RI between sets (minutes)	4–5	3–5	3–5	3–5
Frequency/week:				
MLM	None	2–3	2–3	2–3
Eccentric	None	None	1	1–2
Rhythm/speed of contraction	Slow	Slow	Active	Active

- Since MxS training is very taxing for the neuromuscular system, the number of exercises should be reduced to the lowest level realistically possible. As much as possible, such exercises should be multijoint exercises, involving several muscle groups. However, this does not exclude the use of "single-joint" exercises.

  - Because of the physiological and psychological stress of MxS training, the RI between sets must be 3-5 minutes long. Throughout the RI, one should relax the muscles, keep them warm with dry clothing, and do mild stretching exercises.

  - If the suggested load is too high, then lower it, and maintain the recommended number of repetitions.

  - Adjust the program and exercises to meet your own needs and training potential.

  - Remember to do 20-25 minutes of aerobic training for most training sessions.

  - Advanced/Professional bodybuilders and strength trainers may use more complex exercises such as deadlifts or powerlifts, which involve up to six joints.

Tables 7.2-7.4 illustrate MxS programs for recreational, advanced, and professional bodybuilders and strength trainers. The load differs quite visibly among the three groups, as it must match ability and training potential.

Table 7.2 A suggested training program for the MxS phase for recreational bodybuilders or strength trainers*

Exercise no.	Week # Step Day	1 Low			2 Medium			3 High		
		1	3	5	1	3	5	1	3	5
1	Leg press	70/8·3	75/8·4	75/8·4	80/6·4	80/6·4	80/6·3 90/3·1	90/3·4	90/3·4	90/3·4
2	Supine leg curls	60/10·3	60/10·3	70/7·4	70/7·4	70/7·4	70/7·4	70/7·4	70/7·4	70/7·4
3	Lat pull-downs	70/8·3	75/8·4	75/8·4	80/6·4	80/6·4	80/6·3 90/3·1	90/3·4	90/3·4	90/3·4
4	Front dumbbell press	70/8·3	75/8·4	75/8·4	80/6·4	80/6·4	80/6·3 90/3·1	90/3·4	90/3·4	90/3·4
5	Donkey calf raises	70/8·3	75/8·4	75/8·4	80/6·4	80/6·4	80/6·3 90/3·1	90/3·4	90/3·4	90/3·4
6	?									

*Combining programs is possible, such as 4 MxS, 3 MxS, plus 1 H training.

Table 7.3 An illustration of a MxS training program for advanced bodybuilders or strength trainers*

Exercise no.	Day	Week 1 — Low				Week 2 — Medium				Week 3 — High				
		1	3	5	7	1	3	5	7	1	3	5	7	
1	Safety squats	75/8×4	75/8×4	75/8×4	75/8×4	80/6×5	85/5×5	90/3×5	90/3×5	90/3×5	95/2×5	95/2×3	100/1×2	120/3×5
2	Standing leg curls	60/10×4	60/10×4	65/10×4	65/10×4	70/7×5	85/5×5	90/3×5	90/3×5	80/6×5	80/6×5	80/6×5	80/6×5	
3	Incline bench press	75/8×4	75/8×4	75/8×4	75/8×4	80/6×5	85/5×5	90/3×5	90/3×5	90/3×5	95/2×5	95/2×3	100/1×2	120/3×5
4	B. bent-over row	75/8×4	75/8×4	75/8×4	75/8×4	80/6×5	85/5×5	90/3×5	90/3×5	90/3×5	95/2×5	95/2×3	100/1×2	120/3×5
5	Donkey calf raises	75/8×4	75/8×4	75/8×4	75/8×4	80/6×5	85/5×5	90/3×5	90/3×5	90/3×5	95/2×5	95/2×3	100/1×2	120/3×5
6	Nautilus crunches	60/10×4	60/10×4	65/10×4	65/10×4	70/7×5	85/5×5	90/3×5	90/3×5	80/6×5	80/6×5	80/6×5	80/6×5	
7	?													

*Note that in the last workout of the third week there is a session entirely dedicated to the Eccentric Method.

Table 7.4   A suggested MxS program for a professional bodybuilder, with a mixture of MLM and eccentric method*

Exercise no.	Week #	1						
	Step	Low						
	Day	1	2	3	4		5	6
1	Safety squats	70/8·6	70/8·6	Off	75/8·3	80/6·3	80/6·5	Off
2	Standing leg curls	70/8·5	70/8·5	Off	75/8·6		75/8·6	Off
3	T-B rows	70/8·6	70/8·6	Off	75/8·3	80/6·3	80/6·5	Off
4	Flat bench press	70/8·6	70/8·6	Off	75/8·3	80/6·3	80/6·5	Off
5	Donkey calf raises	70/8·6	70/8·5	Off	75/8·3	80/6·3	80/6·5	Off
6	Nautilus crunches	70/8·5	70/8·5	Off	75/8·6		75/8·6	Off
7	?							

*For exercises 2, 3, and 6, where the load is lower, use only MLM, since they are inappropriate for eccentric training.

Nutrition Strategy for the MxS Phase

The goal of MxS training is to increase muscle density and tone to induce chronic hypertrophy. This is accomplished by increasing the protein content of the muscle through MxS training and proper nutrition. (See chapter 12.)

During the MxS phase, overall daily caloric intake is decreased. This decrease comes from lowering the amount of carbohydrates and fats, in response to the reduced need for glycogen and fats. Protein intake, on the other hand, must remain high and is raised slightly from the H phase, in order to support the increasing protein content within the muscles.

Remember to cycle calories on low, medium, and high days (see tables 7.5, 7.6, and 7.7).

MxS Phase Nutrition Cues:

- When consuming large amounts of protein, it is extremely important to drink plenty of water. This helps to flush the kidneys and rid the body of uric acid, which is a by-product of protein metabolism.
- No two people will respond to the diet plan in the same way.

If you are losing weight or are constantly hungry, you may use the protein and carbohydrate values for the next heavier weight group. Only if you are fighting for every ounce of body weight should you use the fat values for the next heavier weight group. Continue to monitor your progress and experiment until you find a diet that produces the desired results.

If you find that you are gaining fat, first check to ensure that your diet is strictly within the carbohydrate and fat limits. The fat values prescribed for this

| | 2 | | | | | | 3 | | | | | | |
| | Medium | | | | | | High | | | | | | |
1	2	3	4	5	6	1	2		3	4	5	6
80/8·6	85/4·6	120/4·6	Off	90/3·7	120/3·7	90/3·6	95/2·3	100/1·4	130/3·7	Off	95/2·7	130/3·7
75/8·6	75/8·6	80/6·5	Off	80/6·6	80/6·6	80/6·6	80/6·6		85/4·5	Off	85/4·5	85/4·5
80/8·6	85/4·6	85/4·6	Off	90/3·7	90/3·7	90/3·6	95/2·3	100/1·3	100/1·3	Off	95/2·7	95/2·7
80/8·6	85/4·6	120/4·6	Off	90/3·7	120/3·7	90/3·6	95/2·3	100/1·3	130/3·7	Off	95/2·7	130/3·7
80/8·6	85/4·6	120/4·6	Off	90/3·7	120/3·7	90/3·6	95/2·3	100/1·3	130/3·7	Off	95/2·7	130/3·7
75/8·6	75/8·6	80/6·5	Off	80/6·6	80/6·6	80/6·6	80/6·6		85/4·5	Off	85/4·5	85/4·5

phase are very low—designed to keep you lean. If the diet is accurate and you are still gaining weight from fat, drop down a weight group and use those values. Continue to monitor your progress and make adjustments until you are achieving the desired results.

Table 7.5 Maximum strength diet: Low-calorie day

Body weight (lbs)	Protein (g)	Carbs (g)	Fat (g)	Total calories
90	81	153	18	1,100
100	90	170	20	1,220
110	99	187	22	1,340
120	108	204	24	1,465
130	117	221	26	1,585
140	126	238	28	1,710
150	135	255	30	1,830
160	144	272	32	1,950
170	153	289	34	2,075
180	162	306	36	2,195
190	171	323	38	2,320
200	180	340	40	2,440
210	189	357	42	2,560
220	198	374	44	2,685
230	207	391	46	2,805
240	216	408	48	2,930
250	225	425	50	3,050
260	234	442	52	3,170
270	243	459	54	3,295
280	252	476	56	3,415
290	261	493	58	3,540
300	270	510	60	3,660

Table 7.6   Maximum strength diet: Medium-calorie day

Body weight (lbs.)	Protein (g)	Carbs (g)	Fat (g)	Total calories
90	99	180	22	1,315
100	110	200	24	1,455
110	121	220	26	1,600
120	132	240	29	1,750
130	143	260	31	1,890
140	154	280	34	2,040
150	165	300	36	2,185
160	176	320	39	2,335
170	187	340	41	2,477
180	198	360	44	2,630
190	209	380	46	2,770
200	220	400	48	2,910
210	231	420	51	3,065
220	242	440	53	3,205
230	253	460	56	3,385
240	264	480	58	3,500
250	275	500	61	3,650
260	286	520	63	3,790
270	297	540	66	3,940
280	308	560	68	4,085
290	319	580	70	4,225
300	330	600	73	4,375

Table 7.7   Maximum strength diet: High-calorie day

Body weight (lbs.)	Protein (g)	Carbs (g)	Fat (g)	Total calories
90	117	207	26	1,530
100	130	230	28	1,690
110	143	253	29	1,795
120	156	276	34	2,035
130	169	299	37	2,205
140	182	322	40	2,376
150	195	345	43	2,545
160	208	368	46	2,720
170	221	391	49	2,890
180	234	414	52	3,060
190	247	437	54	3,220
200	260	460	57	3,395
210	273	483	60	3,565
220	286	506	63	3,735
230	299	529	66	3,905
240	312	552	69	4,075
250	325	575	72	4,250
260	338	598	75	4,420
270	351	621	78	4,590
280	364	644	80	4,750
290	377	667	83	4,925
300	390	690	86	5,095

8

PHASE FIVE: MUSCLE DEFINITION (MD)

During this training phase, the athlete strives to develop the most refined, polished, and visible muscles possible—known as "getting ripped." Through specific training methods featuring high repetitions, fatty acids act as a fuel source and help to burn the subcutaneous fat that is responsible for hiding those precious "cuts."

Scope of MD Training

- Burn off subcutaneous fat and increase the visibility of muscle striations.

- Increase the protein content of muscles through the performance of long, high-rep sets, which will result in better definition, and in some instances will also create increments in muscle strength (as was the case with some of the subjects used to test the efficiency of our model).

- Clearly increase capillary density within the muscle through increased adaptation to aerobic work, which may result in a slight increase in muscle size.

The duration of the MD phase depends upon the needs of the individual. The phase can be either 3 weeks, 6 weeks or, as in our model (figure 4.1) a 2 x 6 weeks phase. The latter ensures better achievement of MD. A bodybuilder preparing for a contest would probably wish to extend the MD phase to 2 x 6 weeks.

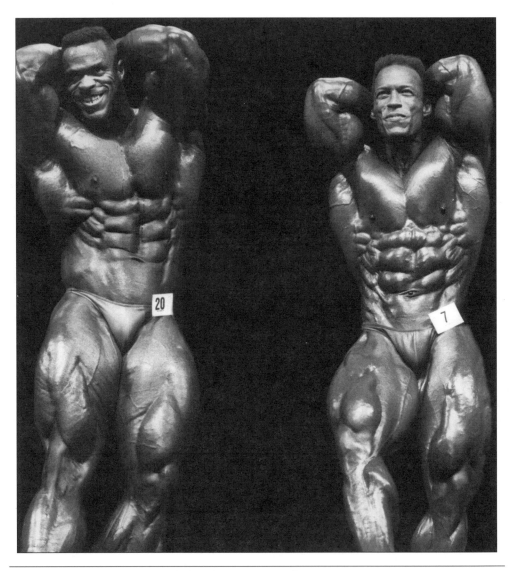

Dillet and Ray display the results of dedicated contest preparation.

Training Methods and Duration for MD

The vast majority of today's bodybuilders and strength trainers are convinced that the highest number of repetitions they ever need to perform is 12-15. These traditionalists believe that in order to increase muscle size, a larger number of repetitions are not necessary and this is certainly true.

The difference is that we are breaking away from the traditional approach to bodybuilding and strength training, and believe that the overall body package is more important than plain mass. We want to promote better looking bodies with higher muscle density, perfect symmetry, and increased muscle separation and striations. The type of training we promote will revolutionize the training philosophy of many bodybuilders and strength trainers. Those who decide to use the Periodization technique will never want to go back to the traditional methods. The MD phase plays a very important role in sculpting the ideal body.

Burn Off That Fat

In order to maximize muscle separation, striation, and definition, one must burn off as much fat as possible. To accomplish this, the duration of nonstop muscular contraction must be increased. Traditionally, bodybuilders attempted to do this through aerobic work such as running or using rowing machines, stationary bikes, or stair-climbers. This type of work, however, does not and should not satisfy most bodybuilders who want to become extremely lean. This type of work does not entirely achieve the goal of burning off most of the body's subcutaneous fat.

The training methods we promote will result in the elimination of fat from the overall body and, more importantly, the local muscle groups involved in activity. To achieve this, the number of repetitions per muscle group and per workout must be drastically, but progressively, increased. It is equally important to perform the program in a nonstop fashion—to perform hundreds of repetitions per muscle group per workout. Since it is impossible to do work of such long duration nonstop for only one muscle group, the exercises must be continually alternated during the workout. Please refer to the suggested training programs.

Decrease Load With More Reps

In order to perform extremely high repetitions per muscle group, the load must be decreased to 30-50% of 1RM. At the beginning of a high-rep, low-load set, only a limited number of muscle fibers are active. The other fibers are at rest, and they become activated as the contracting fibers become fatigued. This progressively increasing recruitment of muscle fibers allows one to perform work for a prolonged period of time. Prolonged work exhausts the ATP/CP and glycogen energy supplies, which means that the only fuel available to sustain this activity is fatty acids. The use of this fuel source burns fat from the body, especially the subcutaneous fat. The burning off of this type of fat increases muscle striations and muscle definition.

Program Design for the MD Phase

As previously mentioned, in order to use fatty acids as fuel, the athlete must perform a high number of repetitions per set nonstop. The best way to achieve the goal of using fatty acids for fuel is by having short RIs, because this prevents ATP/CP and glycogen from being restored. This condition forces the body to tap its fatty acid reserves. The MD program must be carefully designed. It is necessary to select exercises and work stations so it takes no more than 2-3 seconds to move from one station to another.

Pair Exercises

Exercises are often paired together, so it is advisable to select an even number of exercises for each session, as illustrated in our sample programs. (See tables 8.1 and 8.2.)

Tables 8.1 and 8.2 present MD programs for recreational and advanced or professional athletes. The suggested exercises are for reference only and the

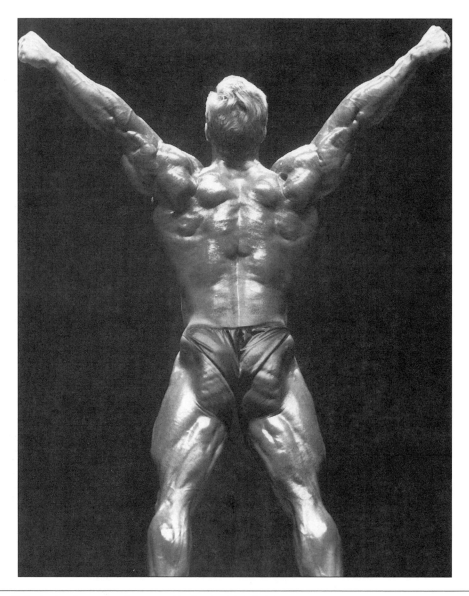

Dave Fisher's signature pose showcases his deeply striated glutes.

user has the choice of employing other exercises if needed. In the first three weeks, the purpose of training is to increase the number of reps to 50 or more for each exercise. When this is accomplished, the exercises are grouped into two, then four, and so on, until eventually, all eight exercises can be performed together without stopping. For maximum MD benefits, the ideal program is the one containing two 6-week MD phases, as those suggested in figures 4.1 and 10.9. The longer the time spent on MD, the greater the amount of fat burned and, consequently, the better the muscles will show their striations.

Exercise Examples

We will illustrate how to apply the MD training method using the eight exercises suggested in tables 8.1 and 8.2.

Table 8.1   An MD training program for recreational bodybuilders and strength trainers*

No.	Exercise/week #	1	2	3	4	5	6
1	Leg press	Increase number of reps to 30 for each exercise. RI between exercises: 1 min	Perform 40 reps per exercise. RI between exercises: 1 min	Perform 50 reps per exercise. RI between exercises: 1 min	Perform 2 exercises together nonstop, or 100 reps (i.e., 50 leg press and 50 upright rowing). Do the same for the other 3 pairs. RI between exercises: 1 min	Perform 4 exercises together nonstop, or 200 reps. Same for the other 4. RI between set of 4 exercises: 1 min	Perform all 8 exercises together nonstop, or 400 reps. RI between set of 8 exercises: 1 min
2	Front barbell press						
3	Crunches						
4	Biceps preacher curls						
5	Flat bench press						
6	Leg extensions						
7	Supine leg curls						
8	Lat. pull-downs						

*Duration, 6 weeks; load, 30%; number of sets, 2–3.

Table 8.2   An MD training program for advanced or professional bodybuilders and strength trainers*

Week #	1–4	5–6	7	8–9	10–12
Training program	First 4 weeks as per figure 8.1.	Perform 4 exercises together nonstop, or 200 reps. Then do the other 4.	A light week of training for regeneration.	Perform 4 exercises together nonstop, or 200 reps. Then do the other 4.	Perform 8 exercises together nonstop, or 400 reps.

*Duration: 6 + 6 weeks = total of 12 weeks. Load: 40–50% depending on individual's ability and work tolerance. Number of sets: 3–5. RI between sets: 1 minute (if too short, increase slightly and reduce to 1 minute at a later date). RI between exercises: none.

In the first week, the load is dropped to 30-50% 1RM, with lower loads for recreational athletes and higher loads for advanced and professional athletes. Using table 8.1 as an example, the actual program is performed as follows:

1. Perform 30 reps with the appropriate load on the leg press machine. Without any rest, perform 30 reps of the front barbell press.

2. Place a bar with the appropriate load on the preacher curl bench and then perform 30 crunches, followed immediately by 30 preacher curls.

3.   Next, lie down on a bench and perform 30 bench presses, followed by 30 leg extensions, 30 supine leg curls, and finally 30 lat pulldowns.

For the MD program, a set is the performance of all eight exercises. The suggested number of sets is not a standard or a limitation. Depending on one's working potential and motivation, the number of sets can be slightly increased. One may perform a higher number of sets if the number of exercises and work stations are lower, or fewer sets if 8-12 exercises are being used.

Muscle Definition Cues:

- MD training requires that muscle groups be constantly alternated.

- The same exercise may be performed twice per set, especially one targeting a desired muscle group.

- The number of reps might not be exactly the same for each exercise. The decision depends on individual strengths and weaknesses for given muscle groups, or individual choice in the targeting of a specific muscle(s).

- Maintain a moderate speed throughout the set. A fast lifting rhythm may produce a high level of lactic acid, which can hamper ability to finish the entire set.

- In order to avoid wasting time between exercises, set up all the equipment needed before training, if possible.

- Since the physiological demand of MD training may be quite severe, we do not suggest such a program for entry-level athletes.

- The total number of MD workouts per week could be from 2-4, depending on the classification: lower for recreational and higher for advanced or professional. The additional 1-2 workouts could be divided between aerobic, H, or MxS training.

- The number of reps per exercise should not be restricted to 50, as shown in our example. A very well-trained athlete might go as high as 60-75.

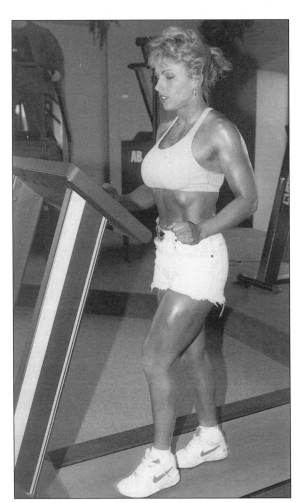

Cardiovascular exercise is a very important component in bodybuilding and strength training.

Nutrition Strategy for the MD Phase

The purpose of the MD phase is to strip the body of its subcutaneous fat in order to achieve that hard, lean, striated look. To attain this low level of body fat, the diet must be altered to put the body into a *negative caloric balance*. This means that the body must burn off more calories than it takes in, so it is forced to rely on energy reserves. To help the body reach a negative caloric balance, one must increase cardiovascular exercise to one or two sessions per day.

General MD Diet

The general muscle definition diet is for those who are cutting down for aesthetics, photos, or even fitness shows. These people want to look lean, with visible muscle striations, without looking "shredded."

Negative Caloric Balance

To achieve the necessary negative caloric balance, calorie intake for this phase is lowered largely through decreasing the percentages of fat and carbohydrates in the diet. MD training is extremely strenuous, and the energy needed to sustain long exhaustive sets as well as increased cardio work, is drawn from the body's glycogen and fat stores. When carbohydrate intake is restricted, this energy source is quickly depleted, which forces the body to draw more heavily on its fat stores to produce energy. When the body reaches a negative caloric balance, more and more fat is used to produce energy, which results in more and more muscle definition.

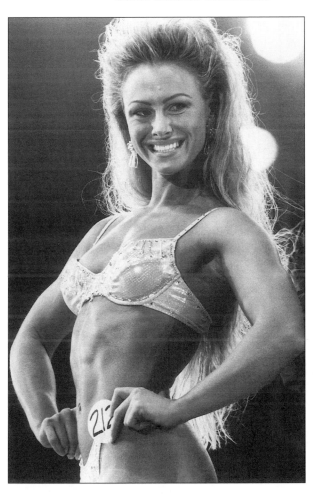

Slim and lean.

It is a surprising fact that the percentage of the diet allotted to protein actually increases during this phase. Research shows that when calories are restricted to decrease body fat, protein requirements increase (Munro, 1951; Walberg, 1988). Increased protein is needed to prevent the body from breaking down muscle tissue for energy and to repair tissue damage and maintain muscle size.

MD Phase Nutrition Cues:

- Muscle hypertrophy is unlikely to occur during this phase. At this stage, the goal is to maintain existing muscle size. See tables 8.3, 8.4, and 8.5 for general muscle definition nutrition plans.

- It takes a lot of discipline to eat this way and "get ripped." Many of us are addicted to high-fat and high-carbohydrate diets that we must abandon to reach this goal.

- The amount of carbs might look small on paper, but when you are eating "clean," that is, low- or no-fat, it is still a substantial amount of food.

- The general muscle definition diet calls for very little fat. It is easy to reach the allowed amount from the trace amounts found in meats, cooking spray, and other products. So, add NO extra fats during this phase.

Table 8.3   General MD diet: Low-calorie day

Body weight (lbs.)	Protein (g)	Carbs (g)	Fat (g)	Total calories
90	80	108	5	795
100	90	120	5	885
110	99	132	6	980
120	108	144	6	1,060
130	117	156	7	1,145
140	126	168	7	1,240
150	135	180	7	1,325
160	144	192	8	1,350
170	153	204	8	1,500
180	162	216	9	1,595
190	171	228	9	1,675
200	180	240	10	1,770
210	189	252	10	1,855
220	198	264	11	1,945
230	207	276	11	2,030
240	216	288	12	2,125
250	225	300	12	2,210
260	234	312	13	2,300
270	243	324	13	2,385
280	252	336	14	2,480
290	261	348	14	2,560
300	270	360	15	2,655

Table 8.4   General MD diet: Medium-calorie day

Body weight (lbs.)	Protein (g)	Carbs (g)	Fat (g)	Total calories
90	90	126	5	910
100	100	140	5	1,005
110	110	154	6	1,110
120	120	168	6	1,205
130	130	182	7	1,310
140	140	196	7	1,405
150	150	210	8	1,510
160	160	224	8	1,610
170	170	238	9	1,715
180	180	252	10	1,820
190	190	266	10	1,915
200	200	280	11	2,020
210	210	294	11	2,115
220	220	308	12	2,220
230	230	322	12	2,315
240	240	336	13	2,420
250	250	350	13	2,515
260	260	364	14	2,620
270	270	378	15	2,725
280	280	392	15	2,825
290	290	406	16	2,930
300	300	420	16	3,025

Table 8.5   General MD diet: High-calorie day

Body weight (lbs.)	Protein (g)	Carbs (g)	Fat (g)	Total calories
90	99	144	5	1,015
100	110	160	6	1,135
110	121	176	6	1,240
120	132	192	7	1,360
130	143	208	7	1,465
140	154	224	8	1,585
150	165	240	9	1,700
160	176	256	9	1,810
170	187	272	10	1,925
180	198	288	11	2,045
190	209	304	11	2,150
200	220	320	12	2,305
210	231	336	12	2,375
220	242	352	13	2,495
230	253	368	14	2,610
240	264	384	14	2,720
250	275	400	15	2,835
260	286	416	15	2,945
270	297	432	16	3,060
280	308	448	17	3,175
290	319	464	17	3,285
300	330	480	18	3,400

PHASE SIX: TRANSITION (T)

An annual plan, as suggested in our examples, should finish with a transition phase. Following many months of intensive training, an athlete must give his or her body a respite to allow recovery and regeneration to occur prior to beginning a new year of training.

In addition to a year-end transition phase, we recommend employing brief transition periods between each different training phase.

Scope of T Training

- Decrease the volume and intensity of training to facilitate removal of the fatigue acquired during the previous phase or annual plan.
- Replenish exhausted energy stores.
- Relax the body and the mind.

Duration of T Training

If the year-end T phase exceeds 4-6 weeks, the hard sought training benefits will fade away and the athlete will experience a detraining effect. Also, the athlete who adheres to the 4-6 week time frame, but does no strength training during the T phase, might experience a decrease in muscle size together with a considerable loss in power (Wilmore and Costill, 1988).

During transition, physical activity is reduced by 60-70%. It is advisable, however, to lightly train those muscles that are or might become asymmetrically developed during a period of low-intensity training.

The body needs a period of one week to recover completely before beginning a new phase of training. This week rids the body of fatigue, replenishes energy stores, and helps the athlete to prepare mentally for the next phase.

Program Design for T Phase: Detraining

The improvement or maintenance of muscle size and strength is possible only if the body is constantly exposed to an adequate training stimulus. When training decreases or stops, as it does during a long transition phase, there is a disturbance in the biological state of the muscle cell and of bodily organs. Consequently, there is a marked decrease in the athlete's physiological well-being and work output (Kuipers and Keizer, 1988; Fry et al., 1991).

This state of diminished training can leave the athlete vulnerable to the *detraining syndrome* (Israel, 1972) or *exercise-dependency syndrome* (Kuipers and Keizer, 1988), the extent of which depends upon the length of time away from training.

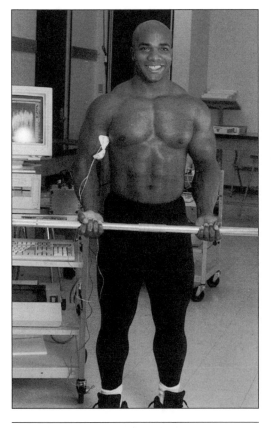

Wesley Mohammed in the laboratory during the transition phase (off season).

Effects of Detraining

A decrease in the cross-sectional area of the muscle fibers becomes visible after only a couple weeks of inactivity. These changes are the result of an increased rate of protein degradation (catabolism) breaking down the muscle gains that were made during training (Edgerton, 1976; Appell, 1990) and increased levels of some chemicals (Na^+ and Cl^-) in the muscle also play a role in the breakdown of muscle fibers (Appell, 1990).

Strength loss occurs during periods of inactivity at a rate of roughly 3-4% per day for the first week (Appell, 1990). For some individuals this can represent a substantial loss. Decreases in strength are largely due to the degeneration of the motor units. Slow-twitch fibers are usually the first to lose their force-producing capabilities, while fast-twitch fibers generally take longer to be affected by inactivity. During the state of detraining, the body cannot recruit the same number of motor units that it once could, resulting in a net decrease in the amount of force that can be generated within the muscle (Edgerton, 1976; Hainaut, 1989; Houmard, 1991).

The body's natural testosterone levels fall as a result of detraining. The presence of testosterone in the body is crucial for gains in size and strength, and as these levels fall, protein synthesis or building within the muscles diminishes (Houmard, 1991).

Headaches, insomnia, feelings of exhaustion, loss of appetite, increased tension, mood disturbances, and depression are among the usual symptoms associated with total abstinence from training. An athlete might develop any number of these symptoms, all of which appear to be associated with the lowered levels of testosterone and beta-endorphin (a neuroendocrine compound that is the main forerunner to euphoric post-exercise feelings) (Houmard, 1991).

10 YEARLY TRAINING PROGRAMS

It is important to understand that Periodization is not a rigid concept. Figure 4.1 is a basic structure that will not apply to every bodybuilder and strength trainer. We recognize that each athlete has different personal and professional commitments, so we offer various training plans. Please keep in mind that the suggested variations do not exhaust all of the possible options. Each athlete can construct an individualized Periodization plan according to his or her unique set of needs and obligations. The options presented below are intended to help implement the concept of Periodization according to individual needs.

Double-Periodization: Design and Duration

This is an option for individuals who cannot commit themselves to a year-round training program, as recommended on page 54 in figure 4.1. It is also an option for individuals with better training backgrounds or for those seeking more variety in training.

In the Double-Periodization model, illustrated in figure 10.1, the months of the year are numbered rather than named to allow the athlete to commence training at any time during the year. The phases in this model follow the same sequence as those in the basic model (figure 4.1), except that the annual plan is divided into two halves and the sequence is repeated. Also, for each training phase in figure 10.1, there is a number on the upper right-hand side that refers to the actual number of weeks for each phase.

Double-Periodization for Athletes With Family Obligations

Figure 10.2 presents another variation of the basic model that revolves around the busiest times of the year for a family person. During Christmas and summer vacation periods, training is often disorganized and interrupted because of

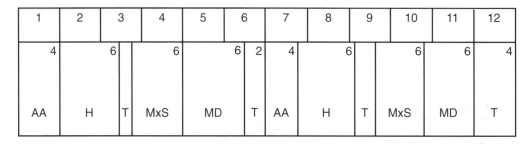

1	2	3	4	5	6	7	8	9	10	11	12
4	6	6	6	2	4	6	6	6	4		
AA	H	T	MxS	MD	T	AA	H	T	MxS	MD	T

Figure 10.1   A Double-Periodization model.

Sept	Oct	Nov	Dec	Jan	Feb	Mar	Apr	May	June	July	Aug
4	6	6	2	4	6	6	6	6	4		
AA	H	MxS	T	AA	H1	T	H2	MxS	T	MD	T

Figure 10.2   A Double-Periodization model revolving around the holidays of the year.

family commitments. In order to avoid the frustration that accompanies periods of fragmented training, it is better to actually structure an annual plan around the main holidays of the year.

As indicated by figure 10.2, mini-transition phases are planned during holiday times. The second part of the plan prescribes two hypertrophy (H) phases, in which the purpose of training is to increase muscle size.

Certainly, other variations of the basic structure are possible, for instance:

- H2 could be replaced by a mixed program of H and MxS in proportions decided by the athlete.

- H2 could be replaced by MxS, if the development of this strength quality is your goal.

- H2 could be divided into 3 weeks of MxS, followed by 3 weeks of H.

Periodization Program for Entry-Level Bodybuilders and Strength Trainers

We strongly recommend that entry-level bodybuilders and strength trainers create their own programs, or follow a model such as the one we present in figure 10.3. This figure presents months by name rather than number. Please resist the temptation to copy the programs of experienced bodybuilders. Entry-level athletes have fragile bodies that are not ready for the challenge of programs designed for experienced individuals. These beginning athletes must be extra careful to progressively increase the training load. This is done by performing a lower number of training sessions and hours per week, planning longer AA phases, and confronting the body with less overall stress in training.

In this entry-level program, AA is 8 weeks long, giving the muscle tissue, ligaments, and tendons adequate time to prepare for the phases to come. In

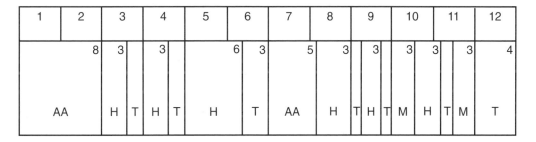

1	2	3	4	5	6	7	8	9	10	11	12
	8	3	3		6	3	5	3	3	3	3	3	4
AA		H	T	H	T	H	T	AA	H	T	H	T	M	H	T	M	T

Figure 10.3 A recommended periodization program for entry-level bodybuilders or strength trainers.

order to make the adaptation to hypertrophy a careful and gradual process, the first two H phases are only 3 weeks in duration, separated by a 1-week regeneration T phase.

After four months, we can assume that the anatomy of an entry-level athlete has progressively adapted to training and, at this time, it is possible to plan longer H phases. The first half of the program ends with a 3-week T phase, giving the body a long regeneration phase before a new and slightly more difficult program begins.

Periodization Program for Recreational Bodybuilders and Strength Trainers

Those who have completed 1-2 years of bodybuilding or strength training could follow an annual plan such as the one presented in figure 10.4. During the Christmas and summer holidays, T phases are planned to allow recreational bodybuilders the time to enjoy other activities.

Sept	Oct	Nov	Dec	Jan	Feb	Mar	Apr	May	June	July	Aug
	8	3	3	2	5		6	3	3	3	3	3	5
AA		H	T	H	T	AA	T	H		M	T	H	M	T	H	T	MxS	T

Figure 10.4 A recommended periodization program for recreational bodybuilders or strength trainers.

Non-Bulk Program for Female Athletes

As suggested by figure 10.5, some athletes might wish to have more variety in training. This high-variety program has many alternations of training phases. It was created for those bodybuilders and strength trainers who want to sculpt a toned, muscular, and symmetrical body without packing on massive, bulky muscles.

A Triple-Periodization Plan: Design and Duration

This plan is suggested for recreational bodybuilders or strength trainers, or for busy professionals who cannot easily commit themselves to a year-long plan,

Sept	Oct	Nov	Dec	Jan	Feb	Mar	Apr	May	June	July	Aug
3	3 3	3	3 3	3	4	3 3	3	3 3	3	4	4
AA	H MxS	T	M MD	T	AA	H M	T	MD MxS	T MD M	T MD	T

Figure 10.5 A recommended periodization program for female bodybuilders or strength trainers, or those who do not want to train for bulk.

Sept	Oct	Nov	Dec	Jan	Feb	Mar	Apr	May	June	July	Aug
7	3	3 2	3	6	3	3 2	3 3	3 3	5		
AA	H T	M T	AA	H	T M	MD T	AA H	T MxS MD	T		

Figure 10.6 Triple-Periodization: A recommended program for recreational or busy professional bodybuilders or strength trainers.

such as the basic model (figure 4.1), or even to a Double-Periodization plan (figure 10.1). Shorter modules, such as the ones presented in figures 10.5 and 10.6, help these athletes to achieve the basic goals of a well-developed body and good fitness, while taking into account their social needs during the main holidays of the year.

Hypertrophy (Mass) Program

An athlete who sees the building of muscle size as the primary training objective could use this program, as outlined in figure 10.7. It follows a Double-Periodization plan, whereby most of the training program is dedicated to the development of muscle hypertrophy. Longer H phases, alternated with M training toward the end of each segment, will stimulate the highest possible development of muscle size. Our periodized approach to

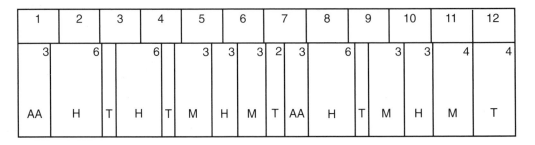

1	2	3	4	5	6	7	8	9	10	11	12
3	6	6	3	3	3 2	3	6	3	3	4	4
AA	H	T H	T	M	H M	T AA	H	T	M	H	M T

Figure 10.7 A hypertrophy (mass) training program.

mass training differs from "traditional" programs in that the M phases, which mix hypertrophy with maximum strength training, have the important merit of developing short-term and, more significantly, chronic hypertrophy.

Periodization Plan Stressing Maximum Strength

There are many strength athletes who would like to develop large muscles and, more importantly, muscle tone, high muscle density, and certainly stronger muscles. Increased chronic hypertrophy results from following a training program such as the one presented in figure 10.8.

As illustrated by figure 10.8, the program follows a Double-Periodization plan. The fact that MxS dominates this program means that more fast-twitch muscle fibers are recruited during training. This will result in chronic hypertrophy and muscles that are well defined and visibly striated.

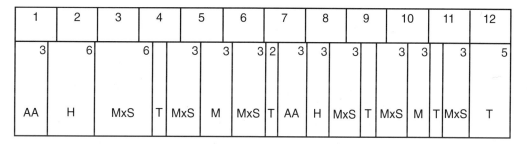

1	2	3	4	5	6	7	8	9	10	11	12
3	6	6	3	3	3 2	3	3	3	3 3	3	5
AA	H	MxS	T MxS	M	MxS T	AA	H	MxS T	MxS M	T MxS	T

Figure 10.8 A periodization plan stressing maximum strength.

Periodization Plan Stressing Muscle Definition

For those athletes who have already reached their desired level of muscle hypertrophy, the scope of their training might be to improve muscle definition in order to achieve total body development. The subjects who have already tested our program have reported incredible body changes, especially the female subjects. The majority found that they drastically trimmed their waists, while at the same time significantly increasing muscle definition in the upper body, buttocks, and legs. Some have even reported increases in strength. In one of our female groups, 68% lost substantial weight and changed their overall body shape so much that they had to change their wardrobe as well. They achieved this weight loss by natural means and not as a result of some diet gimmick—just natural, honest, and dedicated training. This is the healthy way.

The plan illustrated in figure 10.9 is a Double-Periodization program with the focus on burning more subcutaneous fat, allowing for better striated and visible muscles.

1	2	3	4	5	6	7	8	9	10	11	12
3	6	3	4	6	2	3	6	3	4	3	4
AA	H	MxS T	MD T	MD	T	AA	H	MxS T	MD	MD	T

Figure 10.9 A Periodization plan stressing muscle definition.

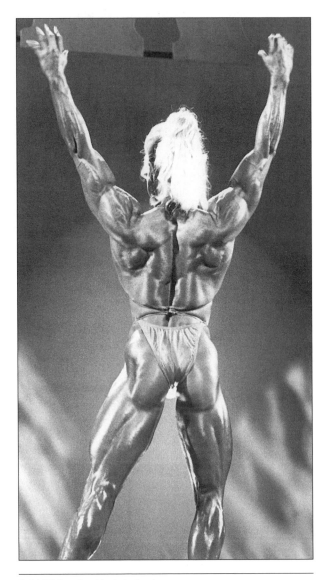

Astrid Falconi's chiseled physique.

## PART 3

SCULPTING THE ULTIMATE PHYSIQUE

CHAPTER 11

MAXIMUM STIMULATION LIFTS

Unlike strength training, very little research has been done in the area of bodybuilding. Much of the "knowledge" put forth by self-proclaimed experts in the industry is primarily the product of trial and error, scientifically void experiments, and the passing on of belief systems from one generation to the next. This history of tradition, which is unsupported by scientific information, has created, validated, and perpetuated a number of myths in the world of bodybuilding and even in strength training. In the interest of safety, and for the development of our sport, we went to the lab to put some of these myths to the test.

Electromyographical (EMG) Research

Electromyography has become an essential research tool, allowing physiologists and medical experts to determine the role of muscles during specific movements (Melo and Cafarelli, 1994/1995). Electromyography is a scientific method of measuring the level of excitation (electrical signal) of a muscle group. Muscle contraction is initiated by electrical charges that travel across the membrane of muscle fibers and this movement of ion flow can be measured on the skin by a *surface electromyogram (SEMG)* (Kobayashi, 1983; Moritani et al., 1986.) An SEMG is representative of the entire electrical activity of the motor units and the frequency of their firing rates for each muscle being examined (DeLuca et al., 1982; Moritani et al., 1987).

The purpose of this series of studies was to find, through EMG recordings, which exercises cause the greatest amount of stimulation within each muscle

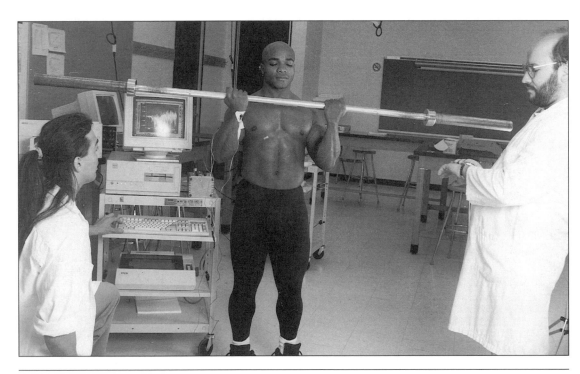

Co-author Lorenzo Cornacchia (left) with exercise physiologist Louis Melo (right) determining the electromyographical activity of a "biceps curl."

group and, consequently, to determine which exercises will produce the greatest gains in mass and strength. Figure 11.1 shows the EMG activity during a standing barbell biceps curl.

Methods

For each study, we used both male and female bodybuilders and strength trainers who were free of neuromuscular disease, had at least two years of bodybuilding experience, and were free of performance-enhancing drugs for at least two years.

Testing was performed on two separate days. On the first day, 1RM was determined for all exercises. Each subject underwent a warm-up of 10 reps at 50% 1RM, 5 reps at 80% 1RM, and 2 reps at 90% 1RM, interspaced with a 5-minute rest interval between sets. 1RM was then performed 3 times, interspaced with a 5-minute rest interval between each repetition. On the second day, the subjects performed 80% 1RM 5 times, interspaced with 3-minute rest intervals.

Electromyographical activity was measured during all exercises. All EMG data was rectified and integrated (IEMG) for one second. For each muscle, the exercise that yielded the highest IEMG determined at 1RM was designated as IEMG max for the specified muscle. IEMG at 80% 1RM was determined by taking the average of the five 80% 1RM trials.

Data was analyzed using two one-way repeated measures analysis of variance to determine which exercise yields the greatest percent IEMG max for each muscle. Differences among exercises were determined with the Newman post hoc test.

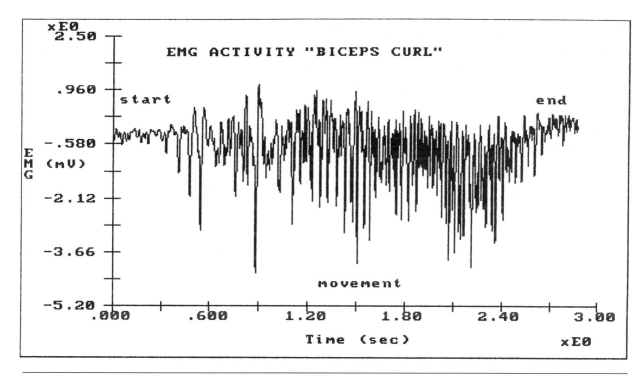

Figure 11.1   EMG activity during a standing barbell biceps curl.

Results of EMG Research

The results of our EMG studies show which exercises produce the greatest amount of stimulation within each target muscle group. Table 11.1 displays the results of the EMG studies. Refer to figures 11.2 and 11.3 for anterior and posterior views of the human muscular system.

Most Effective Exercises for Increasing Muscle Strength and Size

The effectiveness of a program is strongly related to the exercises performed. Exercises that produce the greatest amount of electrical activity during muscular contraction will produce the greatest amount of muscular efficiency. The exercises beginning on page 126 must be clearly recognized for their potential to increase muscular strength and size.

Table 11.1   IEMG max motor-unit activation

Exercise	% IEMG max	Exercise	% IEMG max
Pectoralis major		**Triceps brachii (outer head)** *(continued)*	
Decline dumbbell bench press	93	Triceps dip between benches	87
Decline bench press (Olympic bar)	89	One-arm cable triceps extensions (reverse grip)	85
Push-ups between benches	88	Overhead rope triceps extensions	84
Flat dumbbell bench press	87	Seated one-arm dumbbell triceps extensions (neutral grip)	82
Flat bench press (Olympic bar)	85	Close-grip bench press (Olympic bar)	72
Flat dumbbell flys	84	**Latissimus dorsi**	
Pectoralis minor		Bent-over barbell rows	93
Incline dumbbell bench press	91	One-arm dumbbell rows (alternate)	91
Incline bench press (Olympic bar)	85	T-bar rows	89
Incline dumbbell flys	83	Lat pulldowns to the front	86
Incline bench press (Smith machine)	81	Seated pulley rows	83
Medial deltoids		**Rectus femoris (quadriceps)**	
Incline dumbbell side laterals	66	Safety squats (90° angle, shoulder-width stance)	88
Standing dumbbell side laterals	63	Seated leg extensions (toes straight)	86
Seated dumbbell side laterals	62	Hack squats (90° angle, shoulder-width stance)	78
Cable side laterals	47	Leg press (110° angle)	76
Posterior deltoids		Smith machine squats (90° angle, shoulder-width stance)	60
Standing dumbbell bent laterals	85	**Biceps femoris (hamstring)**	
Seated dumbbell bent laterals	83	Standing leg curls	82
Standing cable bent laterals	77	Lying leg curls	71
Anterior deltoids		Seated leg curls	58
Seated front dumbbell press	79	Modified hamstring deadlifts	56
Standing front dumbbell raises	73	**Semitendinosus (hamstring)**	
Seated front barbell press	61	Seated leg curls	88
Biceps brachii (long head)		Standing leg curls	79
Biceps preacher curls (Olympic bar)	90	Lying leg curls	70
Incline seated dumbbell curls (alternate)	88	Modified hamstring deadlifts	63
Standing biceps curls (Olympic bar/narrow grip)	86	**Gastrocnemius (calf muscle)**	
Standing dumbbell curls (alternate)	84	Donkey calf raises	80
Concentration dumbbell curls	80	Standing one-leg calf raises	79
Standing biceps curls (Olympic bar/wide grip)	63	Standing two-leg calf raises	68
Standing E-Z biceps curls (wide grip)	61	Seated calf raises	61
Triceps brachii (outer head)			
Decline triceps extensions (Olympic bar)	92		
Triceps pressdowns (angled bar)	90		

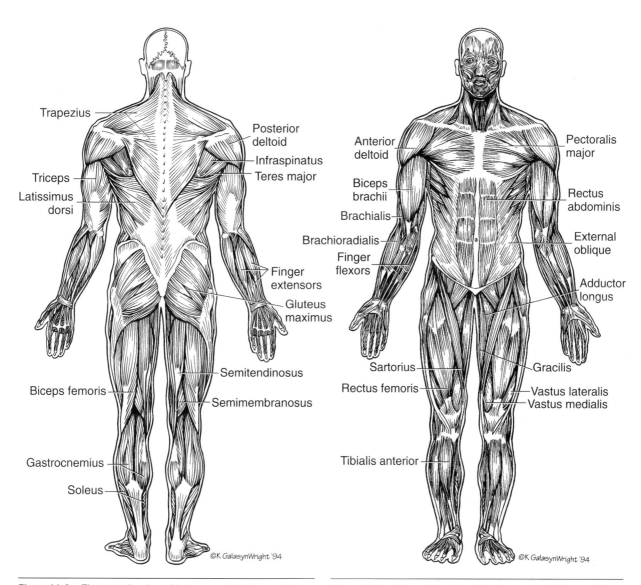

Figure 11.2   The posterior view of the human skeletal musculature.
© K. Gasalyn-Wright, Champaign, IL 1994.

Figure 11.3   The anterior view of the human skeletal musculature.
© K. Gasalyn-Wright, Champaign, IL 1994.

CHEST EXERCISES

Decline Dumbbell Bench Press

Primary Muscles Worked
- Pectoralis Major (Lower Chest)
- Anterior Deltoids

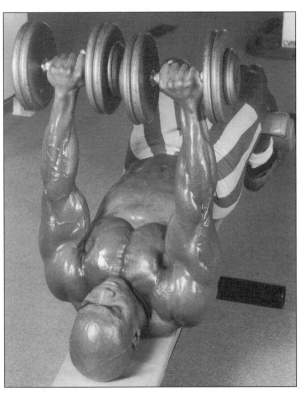

◄Starting Position

1. Grasp two dumbbells using an overhand grip while sitting at the high end of a decline bench.
2. Secure ankles and feet underneath the pads.
3. Rest the dumbbells in an upright position on the knees.
4. Lie on a decline bench, simultaneously bringing the dumbbells so they are held at the sides of the torso at the chest level.
5. Raise the dumbbells to a position of straight arm's length (elbows not locked), with palms facing forward.
6. At this point, the dumbbells are positioned directly over the chest in contact with each other.

Exercise Technique►

1. Slowly bend the arms and lower the dumbbells until they are at either side of the chest.
2. Dumbbells are lowered to a position where a comfortable but maximum stretch is achieved.
3. Raise the dumbbells from the sides of the chest to the starting position.
4. Perform the desired number of repetitions while keeping the movement fluent, slow, and controlled.

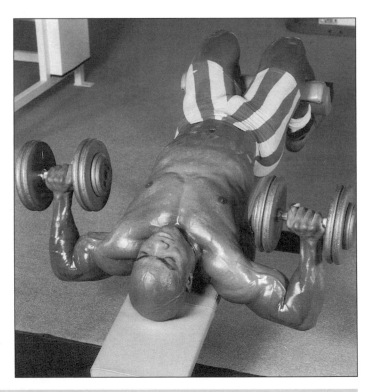

CHEST EXERCISES

Decline Bench Press (Olympic Bar)

Primary Muscles Worked
- Pectoralis Major (Lower Chest)
- Anterior Deltoids

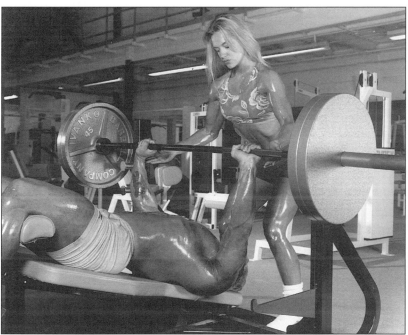

◄Starting Position

1. Lie down on a decline bench with back pressed firmly against the padding and feet and ankles secured underneath the pads.

2. Grasp the Olympic bar using an overhand grip with hands 3-5 inches wider than shoulder-width apart, and lift the bar from the standards.

3. Arms should be fully extended (not locked) as the bar is held over the chest area.

Exercise Technique ►

1. Slowly lower the bar to touch the nipple line of the chest.

2. Once the bar lightly touches the chest, push it upward and slightly back so the bar ends up over the shoulders.

3. Remember never to lock the elbows during this movement. This will allow continuous tension to remain on the working muscles.

4. Perform the desired number of repetitions while keeping the movement fluent, slow, and controlled.

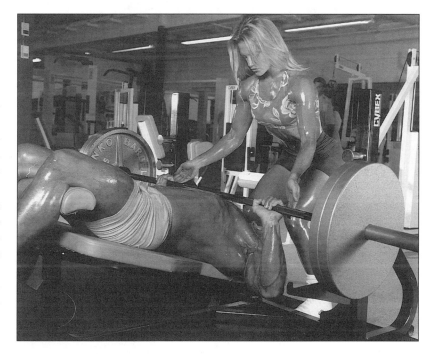

CHEST EXERCISES

Push-Ups Between Benches

Primary Muscles Worked
• Pectoralis Major (Mid Chest)
• Anterior Deltoids

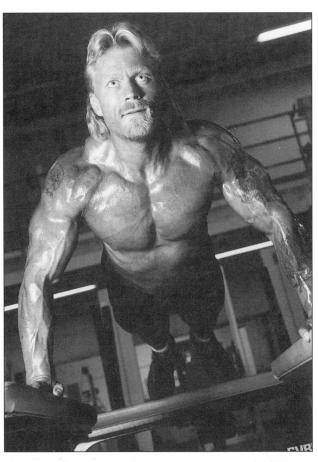

◄Starting Position

1. Arrange three benches; two parallel to each other, and slightly wider than chest-width apart, and one perpendicular to, and behind the other two benches.

2. Place both feet on the rear bench, and one hand on each of the parallel benches.

3. At this point, you are in a supported position ready to perform push-ups.

Exercise Technique►

1. Lower the body as far down between the benches as possible until a comfortable stretch (mid-chest area) is achieved.

2. Then, push the body upward to the starting position.

3. Perform the desired number of repetitions while keeping the movement fluent, slow, and controlled.

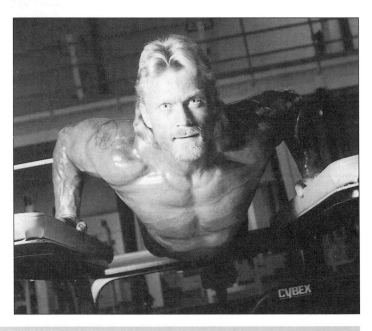

CHEST EXERCISES

Flat Dumbbell Bench Press

Primary Muscles Worked
- Pectoralis Major (Mid Chest)
- Anterior Deltoids

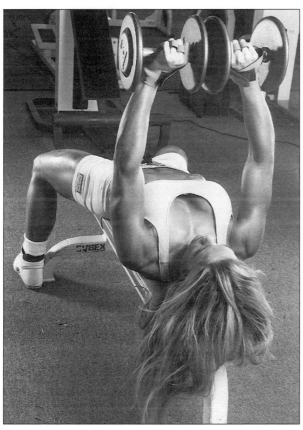

◄Starting Position

1. Grasp two dumbbells using an overhand grip while sitting at the edge of the flat bench.
2. Rest the dumbbells in an upright position on the knees.
3. Lie on the flat bench, simultaneously bringing the dumbbells to a position where they are held at the sides of the torso at chest level.
4. Raise the dumbbells to a position of straight arm's length (elbows not locked).
5. At this point, the dumbbells are held directly over the chest area, in contact with each other, with palms facing forward.

Exercise Technique►

1. Slowly bend the arms and lower the dumbbells until they are at either side of the chest.
2. Dumbbells are lowered to a position where a comfortable but maximum stretch is achieved.
3. Raise the dumbbells from the sides of the chest to the starting position.
4. Perform the desired number of repetitions while keeping the movement fluent, slow, and controlled.

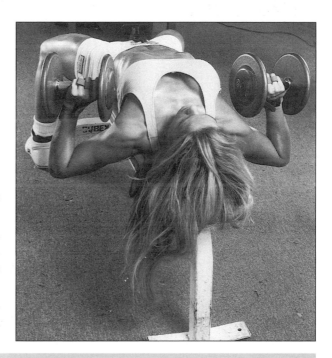

CHEST EXERCISES

Flat Bench Press (Olympic Bar)

Primary Muscles Worked
- Pectoralis Major (Mid Chest)
- Anterior Deltoids

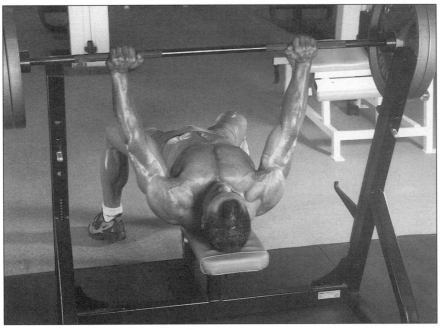

◄Starting Position

1. Lie on the flat bench with back pressed firmly against the padding and feet placed flat on the floor.

2. Grasp the bar using an overhand grip, with hands 3-5 inches wider than shoulder-width apart, and lift the bar from the standards.

3. Arms should be fully extended (not locked) as the bar is held over the chest area.

Exercise Technique►

1. Slowly lower the barbell to touch the nipple line of the chest.

2. Once the bar lightly touches the chest, push it upward and slightly back so the bar ends up over the shoulders. If you push the bar straight up, this shifts the tension off of your pecs and onto the triceps.

3. Repeat the movement until the desired number of repetitions is completed keeping the movement fluent, slow, and controlled.

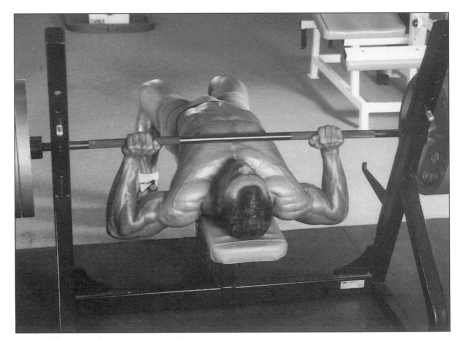

CHEST EXERCISES

Flat Dumbbell Flys

Primary Muscles Worked
- Pectoralis Major (Mid Chest)
- Anterior Deltoids

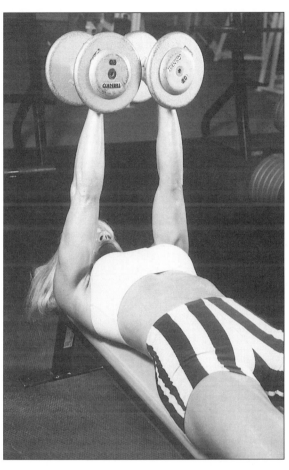

◄Starting Position

1. Grasp the dumbbells using an overhand grip while sitting at the end of the flat bench.
2. Rest the dumbbells in an upright position on the knees.
3. Lie on the flat bench, simultaneously bringing the dumbbells to a position where they are held at the sides of the torso at chest level.
4. Raise the dumbbells to a position of straight arm's length.
5. At this point, the dumbbells are held directly over the chest, in contact with each other, while the palms are facing inward.
6. Elbows must remain flexed throughout the entire movement.

Exercise Technique►

1. Slowly lower the dumbbells in an arc-like motion toward the floor until the chest is comfortably stretched (visualize opening a book).
2. Once this stretch is reached (dumbbells at either side of the chest), return the dumbbells to the starting position, using the same arc-like motion.
3. Perform the desired number of repetitions while keeping the movement fluent, slow, and controlled.

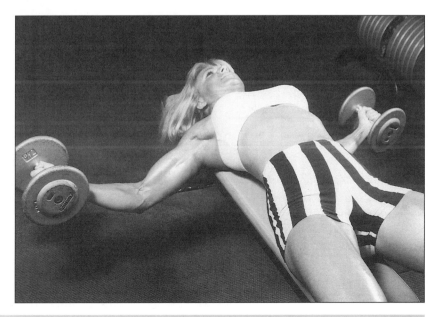

CHEST EXERCISES

Incline Dumbbell Bench Press

Primary Muscles Worked
- Pectoralis Minor (Upper Chest)
- Anterior Deltoids

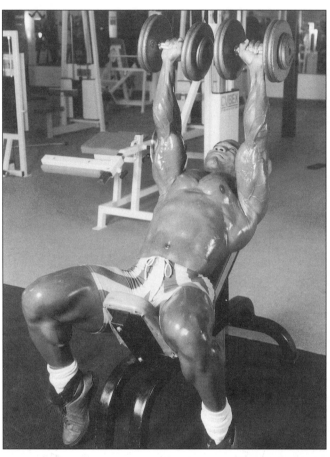

◄Starting Position

1. Grasp the dumbbells using an overhand grip while sitting at the edge of the incline bench.
2. Rest the dumbbells in an upright position on the knees.
3. Lie on the incline bench, simultaneously bringing the dumbbells to a position where they are held at the sides of the torso at chest level.
4. Raise the dumbbells to a position of straight arm's length (elbows not locked).
5. At this point, the dumbbells are held directly over the upper chest, in contact with each other, while the palms are facing forward.

Exercise Technique ►

1. Slowly bend the arms and lower the dumbbells until they are at either side of the chest.
2. Dumbbells are lowered to a position where a comfortable stretch is achieved.
3. Raise the dumbbells from the sides of the chest to the starting position.
4. Perform the desired number of repetitions while keeping the movement fluent, slow, and controlled.

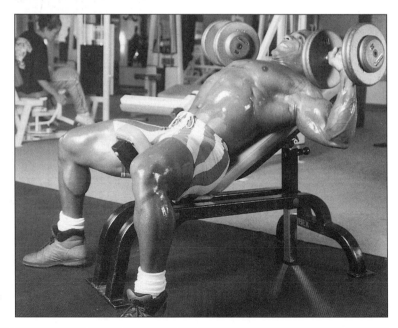

CHEST EXERCISES

Incline Bench Press (Olympic Bar)

Primary Muscles Worked
- Pectoralis Minor (Upper Chest)
- Anterior Deltoids

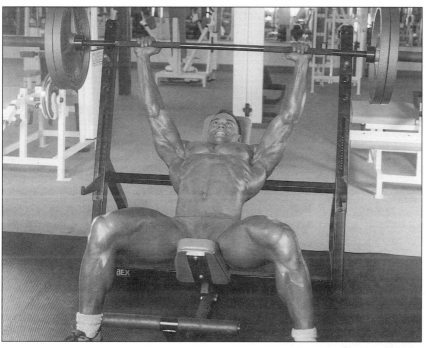

◄Starting Position

1. Lie down on an incline bench with back pressed firmly against the padding and feet placed flat on the floor.
2. Grasp the Olympic bar using an overhand grip, with hands slightly wider than shoulder-width apart, and lift the bar from the standards.
3. Arms should be fully extended (not locked) as the bar is held over the chest area.

Exercise Technique ►

1. Slowly lower the Olympic bar to touch the upper pectoral area.
2. Once the bar lightly touches the nipple line of the chest, push it upward to the starting position.
3. Remember the higher you place the bar on your chest, the greater the stress on the anterior deltoids (secondary movers) rather than the pectoralis minor (primary movers).
4. Remember never lock the elbows. This will allow the tension to remain on the upper chest area.

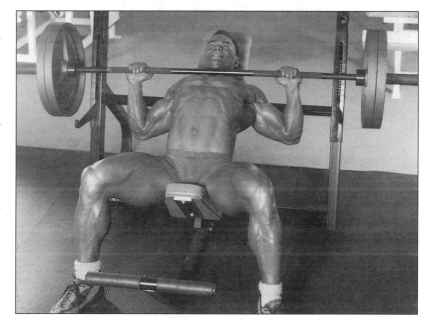

5. Repeat the movement until the desired number of repetitions is completed keeping the movement fluent, slow, and controlled.

CHEST EXERCISES

Incline Dumbbell Flys

Primary Muscles Worked
- Pectoralis Minor (Upper Chest)
- Anterior Deltoids

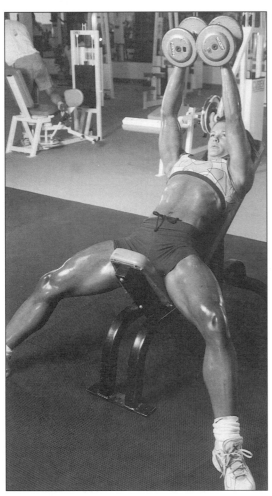

◀Starting Position

1. Grasp the dumbbells using an overhand grip while sitting on an incline bench.
2. Rest the dumbbells in an upright position on the knees.
3. Lie on the incline bench, simultaneously bringing the dumbbells to a position where they are held at the sides of the torso at chest level.
4. Raise the dumbbells to a position of straight arm's length.
5. At this point, the dumbbells are held directly over the upper chest, in contact with each other, while the palms are facing inward.
6. Elbows must remain flexed throughout the entire movement.

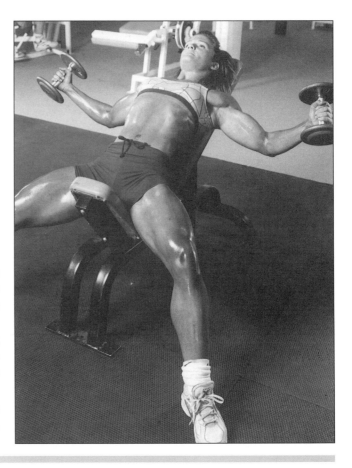

Exercise Technique▶

1. Slowly lower the dumbbells in an arc-like motion toward the floor until the chest is comfortably stretched (visualize opening a book).
2. Once this stretch is reached (dumbbells at either side of the chest), return the dumbbells to the starting position, using the same arc-like motion.
3. Perform the desired number of repetitions while keeping the movement fluent, slow, and controlled.

CHEST EXERCISES

Incline Bench Press (Smith Machine)

Primary Muscles Worked
- Pectoralis Minor (Upper Chest)
- Anterior Deltoids

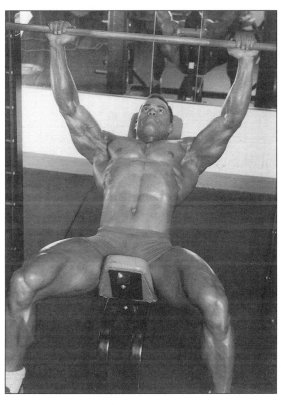

◄Starting Position

1. Lie down on an incline bench (inside Smith machine work station) with back pressed firmly against the padding and feet placed flat on the floor.
2. Grasp the Olympic bar using an overhand grip, with hands 3-5 inches wider than shoulder-width apart, and unlock the bar from the safety standards.
3. Arms should be fully extended (not locked) as the bar is held over the upper chest area.

Exercise Technique►

1. Slowly lower the Olympic bar (Smith machine) to lightly touch the upper pectoral area.
2. Once the bar lightly touches the nipple line of the chest, push it upward to the starting position.
3. Remember that placing the bar at the highest point on your upper pecs may overstretch the joint capsules, muscles, or tendons in the shoulder girdle.
4. Remember never lock the elbows. This will allow the tension to remain on the upper chest area.
5. Repeat the movement until the desired number of repetitions is completed keeping the movement fluent, slow, and controlled.

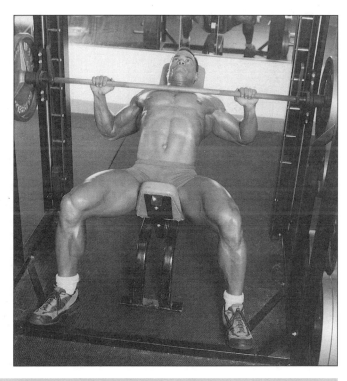

CHEST EXERCISES

Cable Crossovers

Primary Muscles Worked
- Pectoralis Major (Lower and Mid Chest)
- Anterior Deltoids

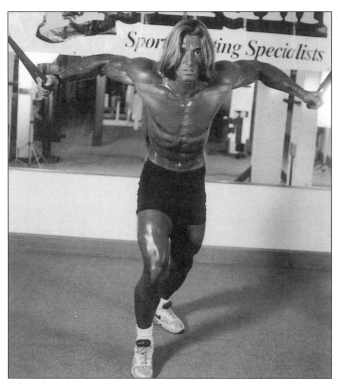

◄Starting Position

1. Grasp each cable using an overhand grip with palms facing inward.
2. Stand in the middle of the cable machine with feet slightly wider than shoulder-width apart, or with one foot slightly in front of the other (stance is up to the individual, whatever you are comfortable with).
3. Keep back erect and elbows slightly bent throughout the entire motion.
4. To begin exercise, extend the cables to the point where the chest is completely stretched (arms wide open).

Exercise Technique►

1. Move the cables in a downward arcing motion until hands make contact (6-8 inches from front aspect of pelvis).
2. Hold this position for approximately 1-2 seconds to fully contract the pectoral muscles.
3. Slowly resist as the cables are returned to their starting position.
4. Repeat the movement until the desired number of repetitions is completed keeping the movement fluent, slow, and controlled.

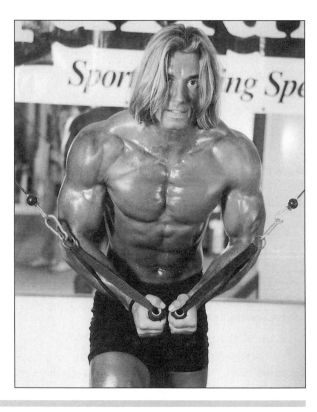

CHEST EXERCISES

Parallel Bar Dip

Primary Muscles Worked
- Pectoralis Major and Minor
- Anterior Deltoids

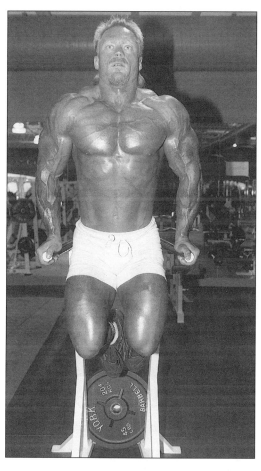

◄Starting Position

1. Support the body at straight arm's length with the chin down.
2. Keep knees flexed, feet behind, and torso erect at starting position.

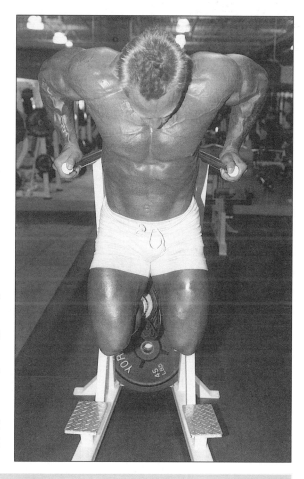

Exercise Technique▶

1. Bend the arms allowing the elbows to travel slightly out to the sides while the torso inclines forward.
2. Lower the body to a point where a comfortable stretch is achieved.
3. When this occurs, slowly push the torso upward to the starting position.
4. Remember never lock the elbows.
5. Repeat the movement until the desired number of repetitions is completed keeping the movement fluent, slow, and controlled.

TRAPEZIUS, DELTOID

Standing Dumbbell Side Laterals

Primary Muscles Worked
• Medial Deltoids

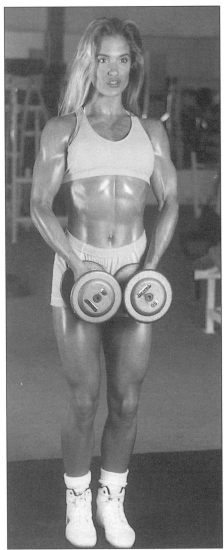

◄ Starting Position

1. Stand with back straight, knees slightly bent, and feet slightly less than shoulder-width apart.
2. Keep back erect and elbows slightly flexed throughout the entire movement.
3. Grasp the dumbbells using an overhand grip, with palms facing each other.
4. Press dumbbells together approximately 4-6 inches in front of the hips.

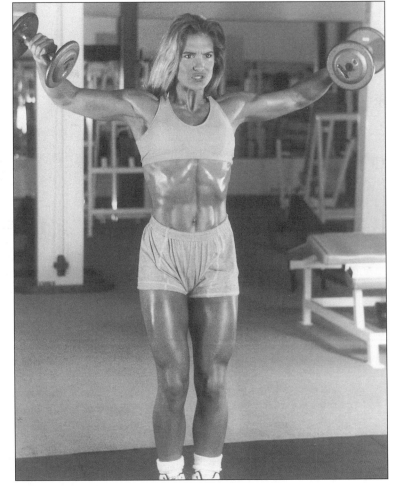

Exercise Technique ►

1. Keeping elbows slightly bent, raise the dumbbells laterally, in an arc toward the ceiling until arms are parallel to the floor, and hold briefly.
2. Slowly lower the dumbbells to the starting position and repeat the movement until the desired number of repetitions is completed.

TRAPEZIUS, DELTOID

Standing Dumbbell Bent Laterals

Primary Muscles Worked
- Posterior Deltoids • Medial Deltoids
- Upper Trapezius

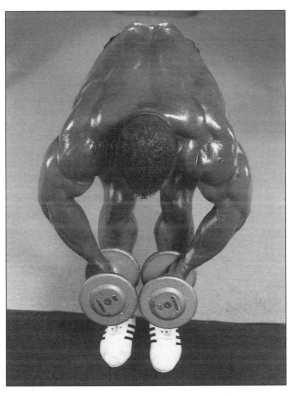

◄Starting Position

1. Stand with back straight, knees bent, and feet shoulder-width apart.
2. Grasp the dumbbells using an overhand grip, with palms facing each other.
3. Bend at the hips until back is parallel to the floor and arms are hanging down in an extended position (arms perpendicular to the floor).

Exercise Technique►

1. Keeping elbows slightly bent, raise the dumbbells laterally in an arc-like motion until arms are parallel to the floor.
2. Slowly lower the dumbbells to the starting position, and repeat the movement until the desired number of repetitions is completed.

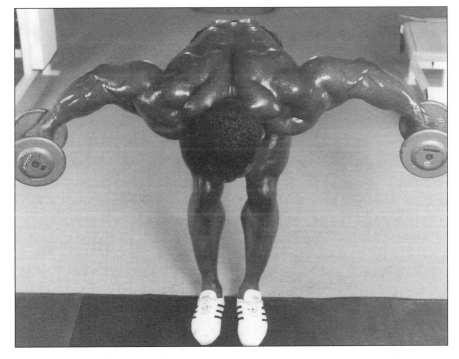

TRAPEZIUS, DELTOID | Seated Front Dumbbell Press

Primary Muscles Worked
• Anterior Deltoids

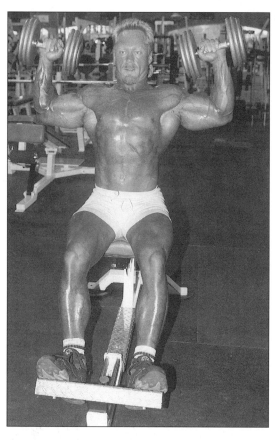

◄Starting Position

1. Grasp two dumbbells using an overhand grip, and sit down on an upright bench.
2. Lift the dumbbells to shoulder level.
3. Rotate palms so they are facing forward.

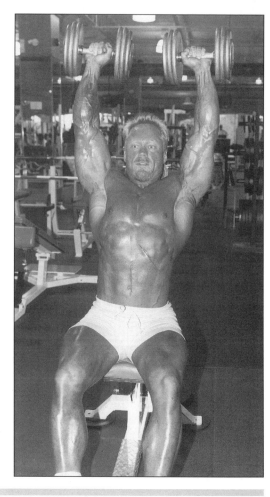

Exercise Technique►

1. Slowly push the dumbbells directly upward until they touch each other at straight arm's length, and slowly return the dumbbells to the starting position.
2. Remember never to lock the elbows at the top of the movement.
3. Repeat the movement until the desired number of repetitions is completed.

TRAPEZIUS, DELTOID | Standing Front Dumbbell Raises

Primary Muscles Worked
• Anterior Deltoids

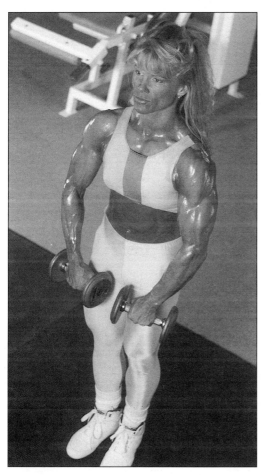

◄Starting Position

1. Stand with back straight, knees slightly bent, and feet slightly less than shoulder-width apart.
2. Grasp the dumbbells using an overhand grip with palms facing downward.
3. Let arms hang straight down at the sides, holding the dumbbells approximately 2-4 inches from upper thigh level.

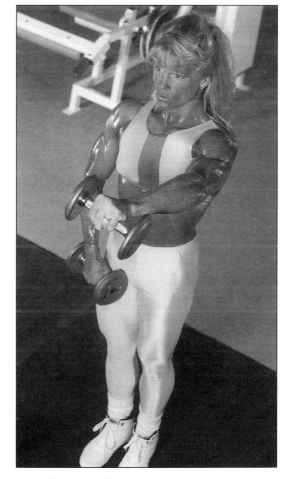

Exercise Technique►

1. Keeping elbows slightly bent throughout the entire movement, raise the left dumbbell from upper thigh level to eye level, and slowly lower dumbbell to starting position.
2. Repeat the movement with the right dumbbell, and continue alternating right and left until the desired number of repetitions is completed.

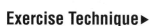

TRAPEZIUS, DELTOID | Seated Front Barbell Press

Primary Muscles Worked
• Anterior Deltoids

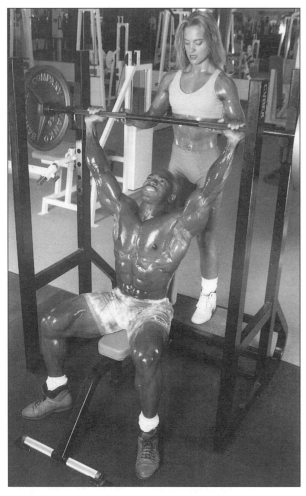

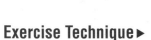

◄Starting Position

1. Sit on the bench with back pressed firmly against the padding for support.
2. Grasp the barbell using an overhand grip, with hands approximately 3-5 inches wider than shoulder-width apart.
3. Have a spotter help you lift the Olympic bar from the standards.
4. At this point, the Olympic bar is held straight above the head, with elbows slightly flexed.

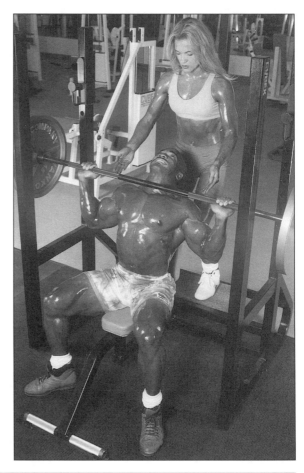

Exercise Technique►

1. Slowly lower the weight down to your anterior deltoids (in front of head), and without bouncing the barbell at the bottom of the movement push it upward to the starting position.
2. Never lock the elbows at the top of the movement.
3. Repeat the movement until the desired number of repetitions is completed.

TRAPEZIUS, DELTOID | Shrugs (Olympic Bar)

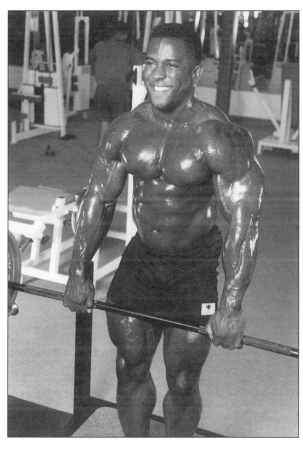

◄Starting Position

1. Keep back erect, knees slightly bent, and a shoulder-width stance throughout the entire movement.
2. Grasp the Olympic bar using an overhand grip with hands slightly wider than shoulder-width apart.
3. At this point, the barbell is held at straight arm's length with a slight bend in the elbows.
4. The Olympic bar is resting at a position across the upper thighs.

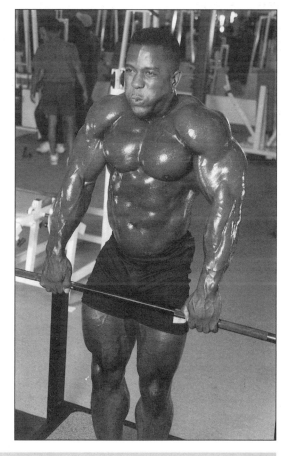

Exercise Technique►

1. To initiate the movement, lift the shoulders toward the ears and hold the contraction for a moment.
2. When the contraction is complete, slowly lower the bar to a point where a comfortable stretch is felt in the working muscles (facilitate maximum range of motion).
3. Repeat the movement until the desired number of repetitions is completed.

TRAPEZIUS, DELTOID | Upright Rows (Olympic Bar)

Primary Muscles Worked
- Trapezius Muscles
- Anterior and Medial Deltoids

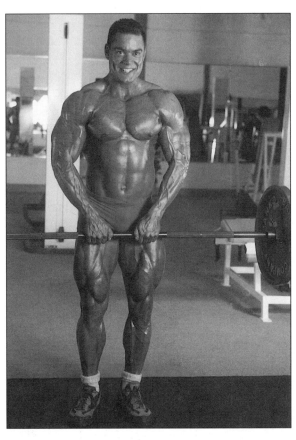

◄Starting Position

1. Keep back erect, knees slightly bent, and a shoulder-width stance throughout the entire movement.
2. Grasp a barbell with an overhand grip with hands approximately two thumb's widths apart.
3. At this point, the barbell is held at straight arm's length with a slight bend in the elbows.
4. The Olympic bar is resting at a position across the upper thighs.

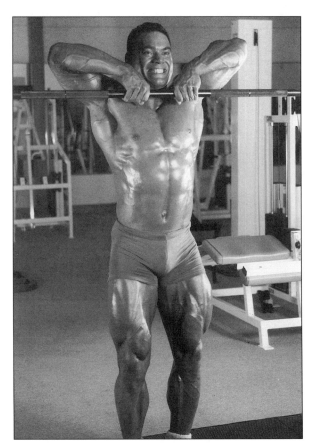

Exercise Technique ►

1. Raise the bar from the extended position to the point where it reaches the chin (raise elbows high), and slowly lower the bar to the starting position.
2. Repeat the movement until the desired number of repetitions is completed.

TRAPEZIUS, DELTOID

Press Behind Neck (Olympic Bar)

Primary Muscles Worked
- Posterior Deltoids
- Upper Trapezius

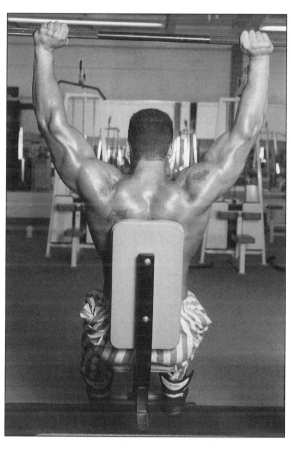

◄ Starting Position

1. Sit on the bench with back pressed firmly against the padding for support.
2. Grasp the Olympic bar using an overhand grip with hands placed 3-5 inches wider than shoulder-width apart.
3. Lift the Olympic bar from the standards and hold it directly above your head, with elbows slightly flexed.

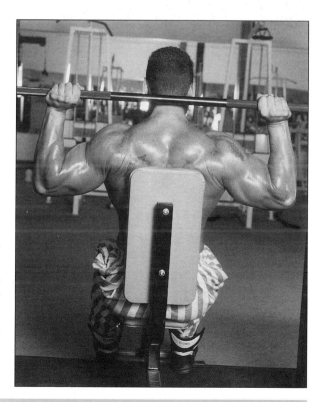

Exercise Technique ►

1. Slowly lower the Olympic bar behind the head to a level slightly below the ears.
2. Without bouncing at the bottom of the movement, push the bar upward to the starting position.
3. Never lock the elbows at the top of the movement.
4. Repeat the movement until the desired number of repetitions is completed.

BICEPS EXERCISES

Biceps Preacher Curls (Olympic Bar)

Primary Muscles Worked
- Biceps Brachii
- Brachialis

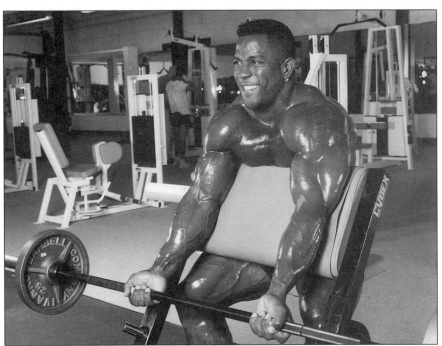

◄ Starting Position

1. Sit on the preacher curl bench.
2. Grasp the Olympic bar using an underhand grip (palms facing upward), with hands shoulder-width apart.
3. Arms are extended (not locked) as triceps are resting over the angled surface of the preacher bench.

Exercise Technique ►

1. Initiate the movement by flexing at the elbows and curling the bar upward toward the shoulders.
2. Triceps always maintain direct contact with the angled surface of the preacher bench.
3. Bar is then slowly lowered to the starting position, and the movement is repeated until the desired number of repetitions is completed.

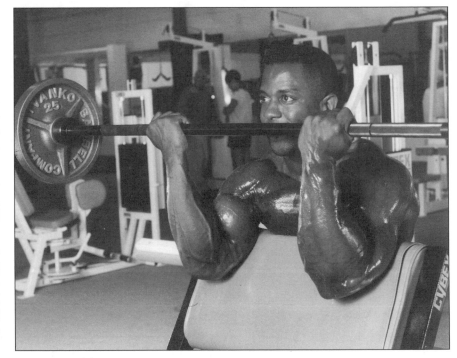

BICEPS EXERCISES

Standing Biceps Curl (Olympic Bar/Narrow Grip)

Primary Muscles Worked
- Biceps Brachii
- Brachialis

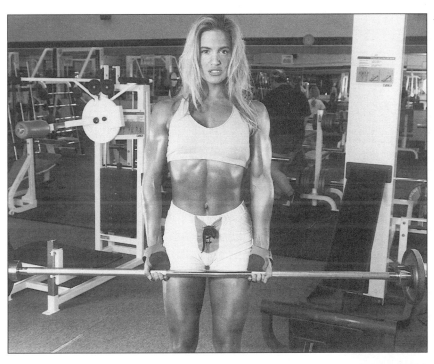

◄Starting Position

1. Grasp the barbell using an underhand grip (palms facing forward) with hands slightly less than shoulder-width apart.
2. Stand with back erect, knees slightly bent, and feet at a shoulder-width stance throughout the entire movement.
3. Arms are fully extended and pressed firmly against the torso.
4. At this point, the bar is resting at a position across the upper thigh.

Exercise Technique ►

1. Initiate the movement by flexing at the elbows, curling the bar toward the shoulders.
2. When the biceps are maximally contracted, slowly lower the bar to the starting position and repeat the movement until the desired number of repetitions is completed.

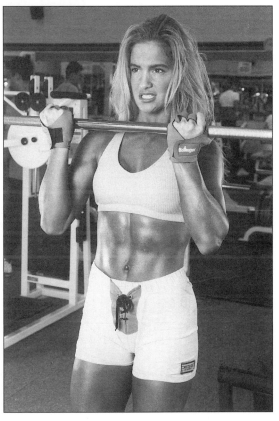

BICEPS EXERCISES — Incline Seated Dumbbell Curls (Alternate)

Primary Muscles Worked
• Biceps Brachii

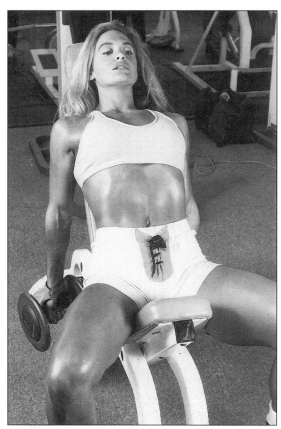

◄ Starting Position

1. Lie on an incline bench with back pressed firmly against the padding and feet flat on the floor.
2. Hang arms down at the sides, holding the dumbbells with an underhand grip (palms facing upward).

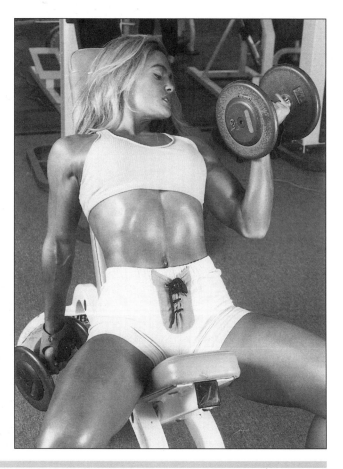

Exercise Technique ►

1. Slowly curl the left dumbbell toward your right shoulder.
2. When maximum biceps contraction occurs, slowly lower the dumbbell to the starting position.
3. Continue alternating right and left arms until the desired number of repetitions is completed.

BICEPS EXERCISES | Standing Dumbbell Curls (Alternate)

Primary Muscles Worked
• Biceps Brachii

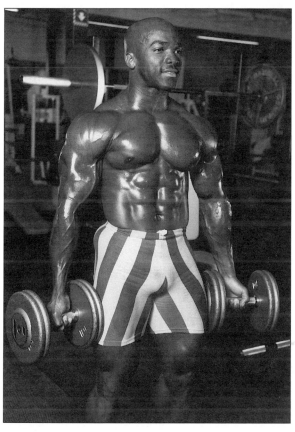

◄ Starting Position

1. Grasp the dumbbells using an underhand grip (palms facing forward).
2. Stand with back erect, knees slightly bent, and feet shoulder-width apart throughout the entire movement.
3. Arms are fully extended and the dumbbells are hanging straight down at the sides.

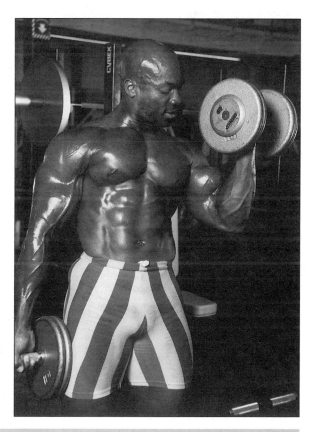

Exercise Technique ►

1. Initiate the movement by flexing at the elbow, curling the left dumbbell up toward the shoulder.
2. The dumbbell is then slowly lowered to the starting position, and the movement repeated with the left arm.
3. Continue alternating until the desired number of repetitions is completed.

BICEPS EXERCISES | Concentration Dumbbell Curls

Primary Muscles Worked
• Biceps Brachii

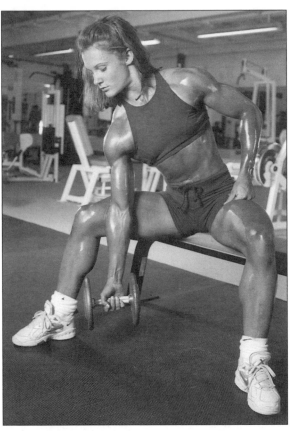

◀ Starting Position

1. Grasp the dumbbell with the right hand, using an underhand grip (palm facing upward), and sit on a flat bench.

2. Legs are spread wide apart.

3. Lean forward at the waist and rest the right elbow on the inside of the right thigh, with the arm in full extension.

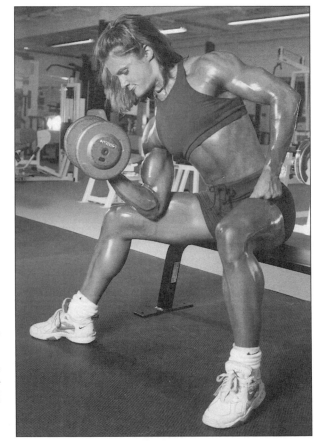

Exercise Technique ▶

1. With the elbow resting on the inside of the thigh, slowly curl the dumbbell toward the shoulder.

2. When maximum biceps contraction occurs, slowly lower the dumbbell to the starting position and repeat the movement until the desired number of repetitions is completed.

3. Repeat for the left hand.

BICEPS EXERCISES | Standing Biceps Curls (Olympic Bar/Wide Grip)

Primary Muscles Worked
- Biceps Brachii
- Brachialis

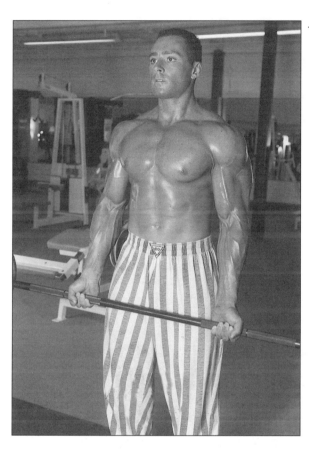

◄Starting Position

1. Grasp the barbell using an underhand grip (palms facing upward), with hands 2-3 inches wider than shoulder-width apart.
2. Stand with back erect, knees slightly bent, and feet slightly wider than shoulder-width apart throughout the entire movement.
3. At this point, arms are fully extended with the bar resting at a position across the upper thigh.

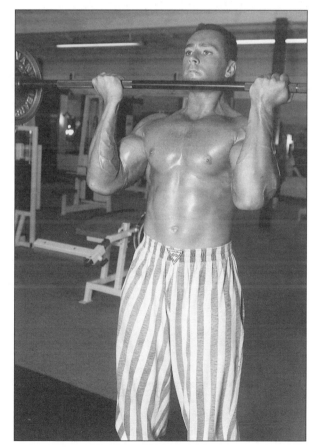

Exercise Technique ▶

1. Initiate the movement by flexing at the elbows, curling the bar up toward the shoulders.
2. When biceps are maximally contracted, slowly lower the bar to the starting position and repeat the movement until the desired number of repetitions is completed.

BICEPS EXERCISES

Standing E-Z Biceps Curls (Wide Grip)

Primary Muscles Worked
- Biceps Brachii
- Brachialis

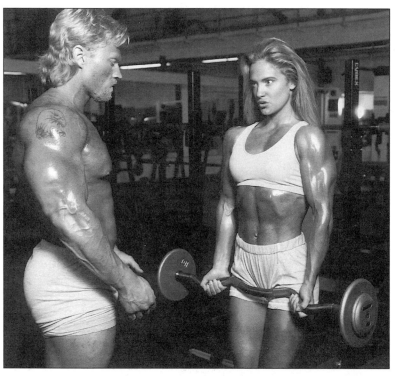

◄Starting Position

1. Stand with back straight, knees slightly bent, and feet slightly less than shoulder-width apart throughout the entire movement.

2. Grasp the E-Z curl bar using an underhand grip (palms facing forward) with hands slightly wider than shoulder-width apart.

3. Arms are fully extended and pressed against the sides of the torso.

Exercise Technique►

1. Initiate the movement by flexing at the elbows and curling the bar up toward the shoulders.

2. When the biceps are maximally contracted, slowly lower the bar to the starting position and repeat the movement until the desired number of repetitions is completed.

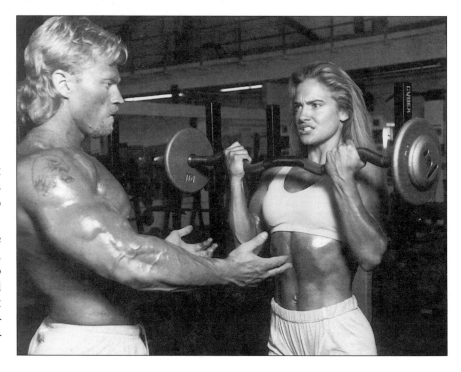

TRICEPS EXERCISES

Decline Triceps Extensions (Olympic Bar)

Primary Muscles Worked
• Outer and Medial Heads of Triceps

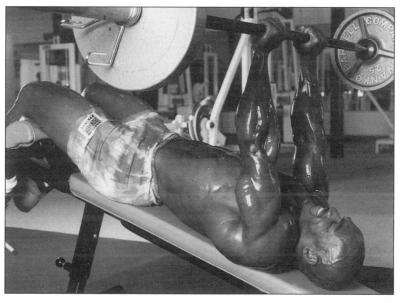

◄Starting Position

1. Grasp the Olympic bar with an overhand grip (palms facing downward) and hands less than shoulder-width apart.

2. Sit on the edge of the decline bench and secure feet and ankles underneath pads.

3. Lie on the decline bench, simultaneously bringing the Olympic bar to a position where you simulate a bench press movement.

4. Once the arms are extended and palms are facing upward, the Olympic bar is held directly over eye level.

Exercise Technique►

1. Keeping the upper arms fixed, slowly flex the elbows and lower the bar to the forehead.

2. Once the bar almost touches the forehead, use the triceps muscle to push the arms back to full extension.

3. Repeat the movement until the desired number of repetitions is completed.

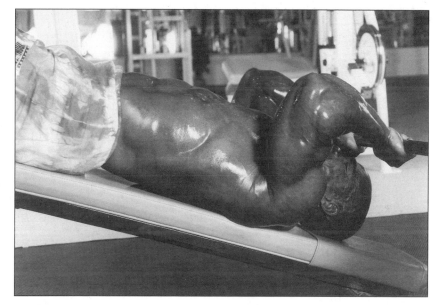

TRICEPS EXERCISES

Triceps Pressdowns (Angled Bar)

Primary Muscles Worked
• Outer and Medial Heads of Triceps

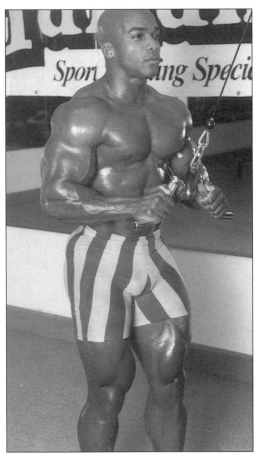

◄Starting Position

1. Attach the angled bar to the overhead pulley.
2. Keep the knees slightly bent, back erect, and feet shoulder-width apart.
3. Facing the overhead pulley, grasp the angled bar using an overhand grip.
4. Pull the bar down far enough to allow the upper arms to rest against the sides of the torso.
5. The elbows should be flexed.

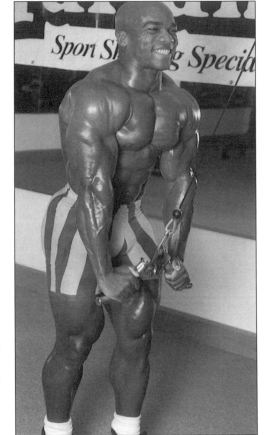

Exercise Technique►

1. Moving only the lower arms, slowly press down on the bar until arms are fully extended.
2. Hold the extended position for a moment and then resist as lower arms return to the starting position.
3. Repeat the movement until the desired number of repetitions is completed.

TRICEPS EXERCISES | Triceps Dip Between Benches

Primary Muscles Worked
• Outer and Medial Heads of Triceps

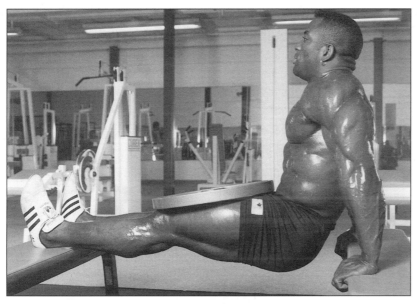

◄Starting Position

1. Stand between two flat benches that are distanced approximately 3 feet apart (this varies depending on the size of the person).

2. Place the hands on the edge of one bench (shoulder-width apart), and feet (heels) on the other bench.

3. Extend the arms completely and hold this position.

Exercise Technique►

1. Initiate the movement by slowly bending the arms until the body is lowered between the benches.

2. Slowly push back up to the starting position by straightening the arms, and repeat the movement until the desired number of repetitions is completed.

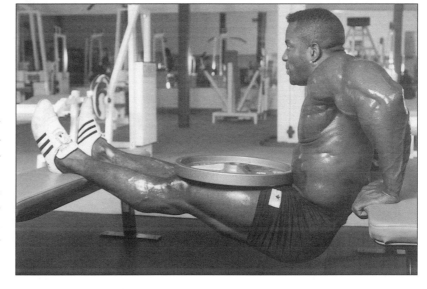

TRICEPS EXERCISES | One-Arm Cable Triceps Extensions

Primary Muscles Worked
• Outer Head of Triceps

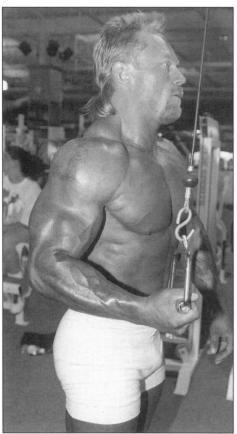

◄ Starting Position

1. Attach a loop handle to the overhead cable pulley.
2. Facing the pulley, grasp the loop handle in the right hand with an underhand grip and step approximately one foot back from the pulley.
3. Pull the handle down far enough to allow the upper arm to rest firmly against the side of the torso.
4. The elbows should be flexed.

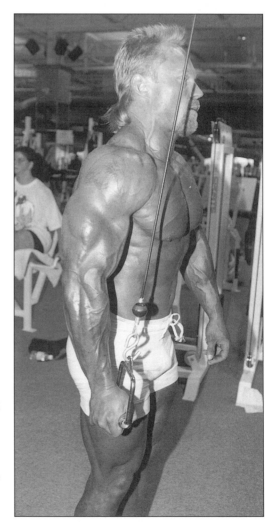

Exercise Technique ►

1. Moving only the lower arm, slowly pull the handle back and downward until the arm is fully extended.
2. Hold the position in full extension for a moment and then resist as lower arm returns to starting position.
3. Repeat the movement until the desired number of repetitions is completed.
4. Repeat for the other hand.

TRICEPS EXERCISES

Overhead Rope Triceps Extensions

Primary Muscles Worked
• All Heads of Triceps

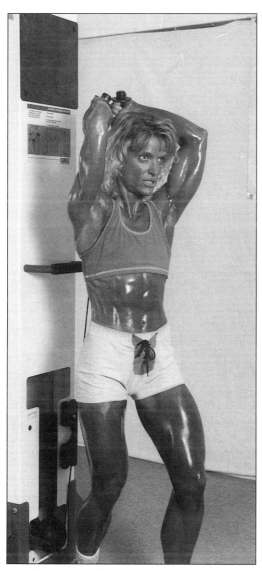

◄Starting Position

1. Attach the rope to the pulley.
2. Stand with back facing the pulley machine.
3. Feet are staggered (one leg in front of the other), forward foot is placed flat on the floor, and the back foot is flexed with only the ball of the foot touching the ground.
4. Grasp the rope with an overhand grip (palms facing each other), and bend slightly forward at the waist.
5. In the starting position, the upper arms follow the ear line.
6. The elbows are completely flexed and the rope is behind the neck.

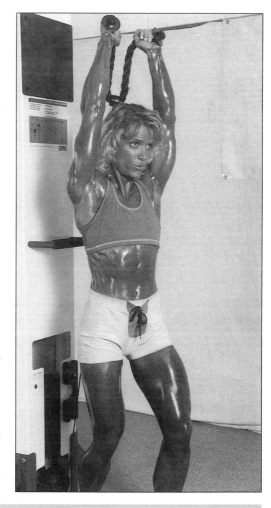

Exercise Technique►

1. Initiate the movement by slowly extending the lower part of the arms.
2. Hold the fully extended position for a moment.
3. Slowly bring the arms back to the starting position.
4. Repeat the movement until the desired number of repetitions is completed.
5. Remember bending only occurs at the elbows. The upper arms remain motionless.

TRICEPS EXERCISES
Seated One-Arm Triceps Extensions (Neutral Grip)

Primary Muscles Worked
• Inner and Medial Heads of Triceps

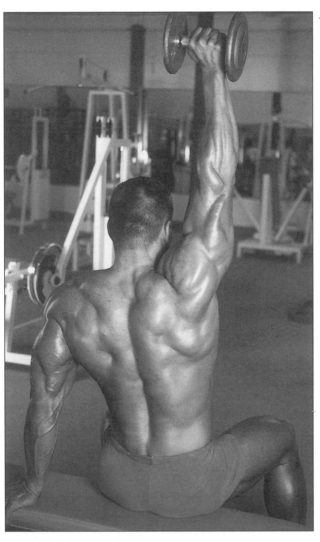

◄Starting Position

1. Sit on a flat bench with feet flat on the floor.
2. Grasp a dumbbell with an overhand grip (palms are facing forward throughout the entire movement).
3. Hold the dumbbell overhead with the arm fully extended.

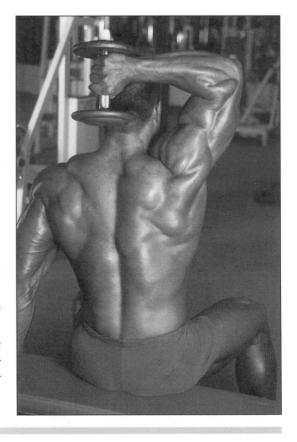

Exercise Technique►

1. Lower the dumbbell until the forearm is parallel to the floor.
2. At this point, the dumbbell is positioned behind the neck (finish of movement).
3. Without bouncing the weight at the bottom of the movement, slowly extend the dumbbell to the starting position and repeat the movement until the desired number of repetitions is completed.
4. Repeat for the other hand.

TRICEPS EXERCISES

Close-Grip Bench Press (Olympic Bar)

Primary Muscles Worked
- All Heads of Triceps   • Anterior Deltoids
- Pectoralis Major (Mid and Lower Chest)

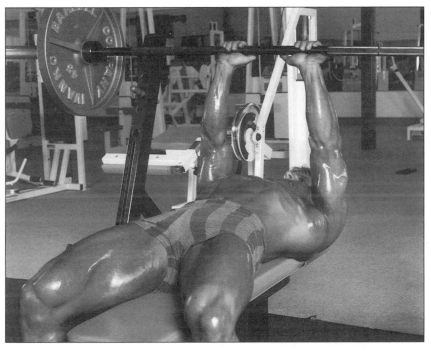

◄Starting Position

1. Lie on a flat bench with back pressed firmly against the padding and feet placed on the floor.

2. Grasp the bar using an overhand grip with hands approximately two thumb's widths apart, and lift bar from the standards.

3. Arms should be fully extended (not locked) and palms facing forward as the bar is held.

Exercise Technique►

1. Bend at the elbows, lowering the bar to the midpoint of the chest.

2. Without bouncing the weight off the chest, use the triceps muscles to press it back to the starting position.

3. Repeat the movement until the desired number of repetitions is completed.

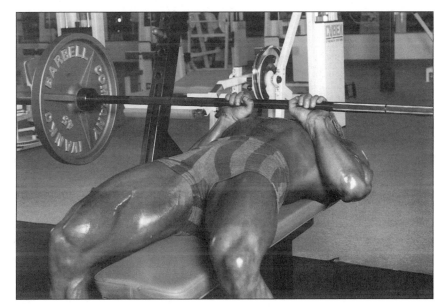

TRICEPS EXERCISES

Dumbbell or Cable Kickbacks

Primary Muscles Worked
• Outer and Medial Heads of Triceps

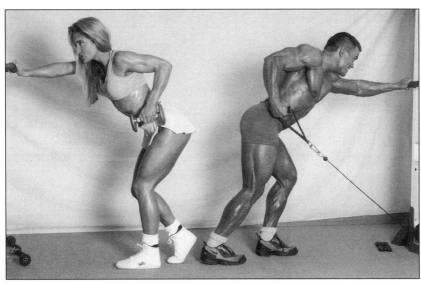

◀Starting Position

1. Grasp a dumbbell or loop handle on the low pulley cable, use an overhand grip (palm facing body with dumbbell, palm facing downward with loop handle).

2. Bend forward at hips and grasp the support handle on the pulley with the non-working arm.

3. Press the upper working arm firmly against the side of the torso (upper arm is now parallel to the floor and lower arm is perpendicular to the floor).

4. Feet should be staggered, one in front of the other.

Exercise Technique▶

1. Initiate the movement by slowly extending the arm fully.

2. Once the arm is fully extended, hold the position for a moment, and then lower the weight to the starting position.

3. Repeat the movement until the desired number of repetitions is completed.

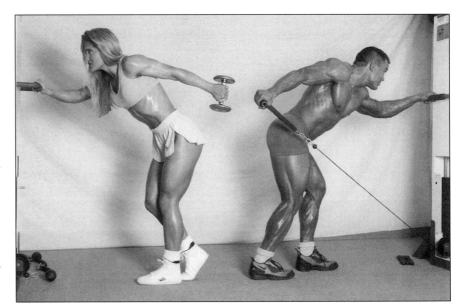

FOREARM EXERCISES

Wrist Curls (Olympic Bar)

Primary Muscles Worked
• Forearm Flexors

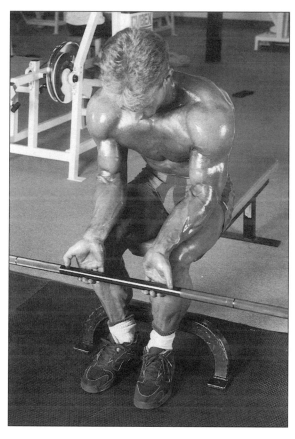

◄Starting Position

1. Grasp the bar with an underhand grip (palms facing upward), and sit on the end of a flat bench.

2. Place feet flat on the floor, with a slightly wider than shoulder-width stance.

3. Lean the torso forward, run the forearms down the thighs until the wrists and hands hang over the ends of the knees.

4. Allow the weight to be lowered until the bar is rolled onto the fingers.

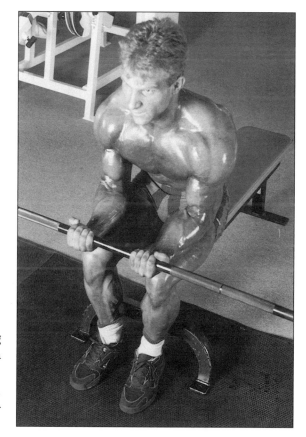

Exercise Technique►

1. Using the forearm muscles, raise the bar by flexing the fingers and curling the wrists to as high a position as possible.

2. Slowly lower the weight to the starting position, and repeat the movement until the desired number of repetitions is completed.

FOREARM EXERCISES | Wrist Extensions (Olympic Bar)

Primary Muscles Worked
• Forearm Flexors

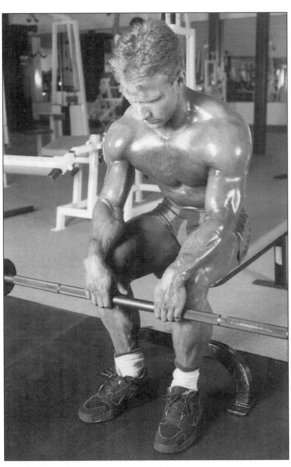

◄Starting Position

1. Grasp the bar with an overhand grip (palms facing downward), and sit on the end of a flat bench.
2. Place feet flat on the floor with a slightly closer than shoulder-width stance.
3. Lean the torso forward, run the forearms down the thighs until the wrists and hands hang over the ends of the knees.
4. Allow the weight to be lowered until the barbell is rolled onto the fingers.

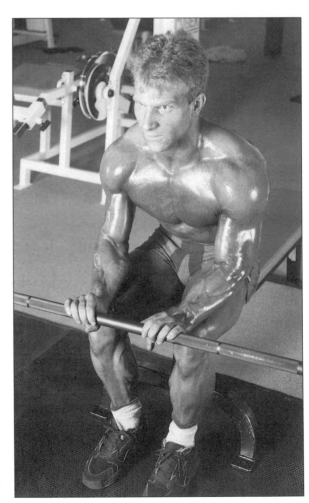

Exercise Technique►

1. Using the forearm muscles, raise the bar by extending the wrists to as high a position as possible.
2. Slowly lower the weight to the starting position, and repeat the movement until the desired number of repetitions is completed.

BACK EXERCISES

Bent-Over Barbell Rows (Olympic Bar)

Primary Muscles Worked
- Latissimus Dorsi
- Biceps, Brachialis
- Trapezius (Mid)

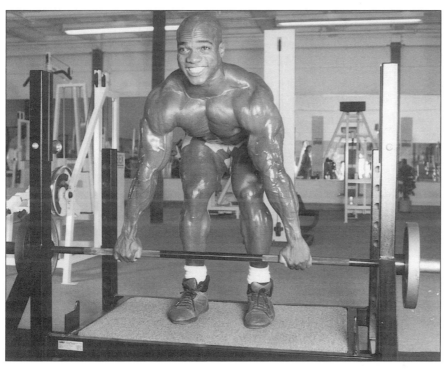

◄Starting Position

1. Grasp the bar using an overhand grip, with hands approximately 4-6 inches wider than shoulder-width apart, and remove the bar from the standards.

2. Take a shoulder-width stance, and keep feet flat on the floor.

3. Slowly bend forward at the hips, keeping back flat, and allowing for a slight bend in the knees.

4. At this point, the torso should be parallel to the ground, with arms fully extended, holding the bar.

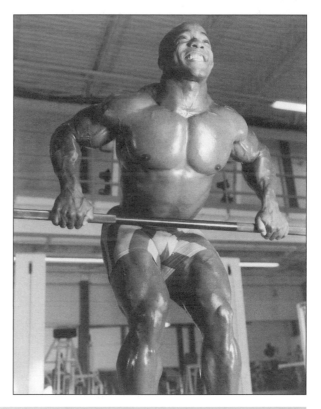

Exercise Technique►

1. Moving only the arms, slowly pull the bar upward allowing it to touch the lower part of the rib cage (torso should not move upward more than 2-4 inches).

2. Lower the weight slowly to the starting position, and repeat the movement until the desired number of repetitions is completed.

BACK EXERCISES

One-Arm Dumbbell Rows (Alternate)

Primary Muscles Worked
- Latissimus Dorsi   • Biceps, Brachialis
- Trapezius (Mid)

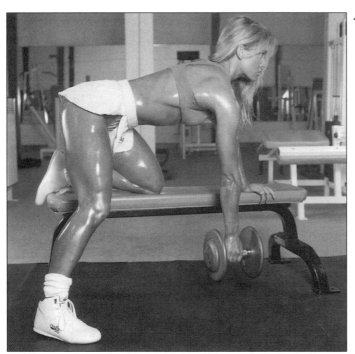

◄Starting Position

1. Grasp a dumbbell with the right hand, using an overhand grip (palms facing the body).
2. Rest the left knee on a flat bench. Right leg should be flexed with the foot flat on the floor.
3. Bend forward at the hips and stabilize the body with a straightened left arm.
4. At this point, the torso should be nearly parallel to the floor.
5. The dumbbell in the right hand is held at full arm's length.

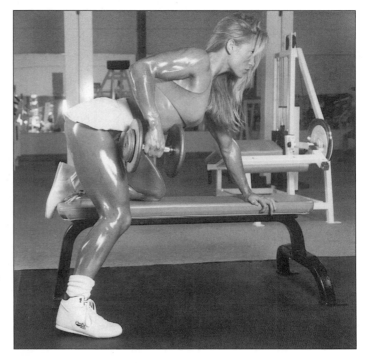

Exercise Technique►

1. Keeping the elbow close to the torso, pull the dumbbell upward in a straight vertical line, allowing it to lightly touch the rib cage.
2. Slowly lower the dumbbell to the starting position, and repeat the movement until the desired number of repetitions is completed.
3. Repeat for the left hand.

BACK EXERCISES

T-Bar Rows

Primary Muscles Worked
- Latissimus Dorsi
- Rhomboids
- Erector Spinae
- Biceps, Brachialis

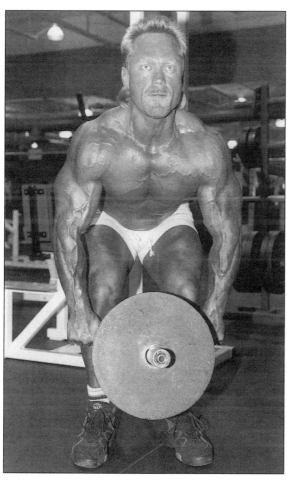

◄Starting Position

1. Bend forward at the hips keeping the back flat and knees bent.
2. Grasp the T-bar handles using an overhand grip (palms facing backward).
3. Raise the torso to a position where it is parallel to the floor.
4. Arms should be fully extended.

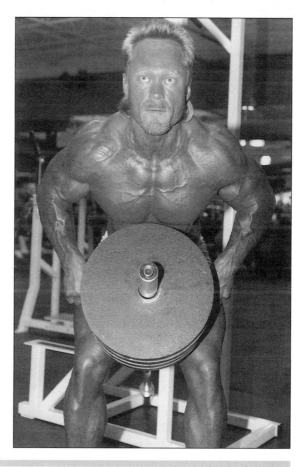

Exercise Technique►

1. Pull hands upward until the weight touches the chest.
2. The torso should not move upward more than 2-4 inches.
3. Slowly return to the starting position, and repeat the movement until the desired number of repetitions is completed.

BACK EXERCISES

Lat Pulldowns to the Front

Primary Muscles Worked
- Latissimus Dorsi
- Rhomboids
- Posterior Deltoids
- Biceps, Brachialis

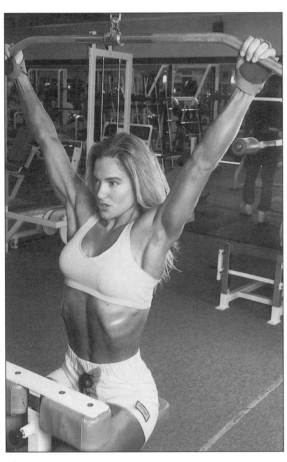

◄Starting Position

1. Stand in front of the lat pulldown machine and grasp the bar using an overhand grip (wide).
2. Sit down with feet flat on the floor, back straight, and thighs secured underneath thigh pads.
3. Arch the torso and lean backward at a 45-degree angle.
4. The torso remains rigid throughout the entire movement.
5. At this point, the arms are fully extended holding the lat bar overhead.

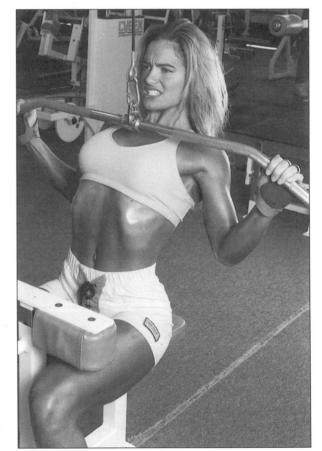

Exercise Technique ►

1. Initiate the movement by pulling the elbows downward and backward.
2. Bring the bar in front of the head until it touches the upper part of the chest and pause.
3. Slowly bring the bar back to the starting position and repeat the movement until the desired number of repetitions is completed.

BACK EXERCISES

Seated Pulley Row

Primary Muscles Worked
- Latissimus Dorsi
- Rhomboids
- Trapezius Muscles
- Erector Spinae

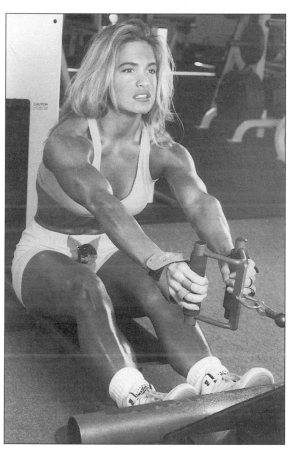

◄ Starting Position

1. Grasp the seated pulley handle with palms facing inward.
2. Straighten the arms, sit on the padding, and place feet on the floor rests at the front end of the machine.
3. Keep a slight bend in the knees throughout the movement.
4. Lean forward, allowing the head to lower between the arms (excellent prestretch for the lats) and keeping the back flat.

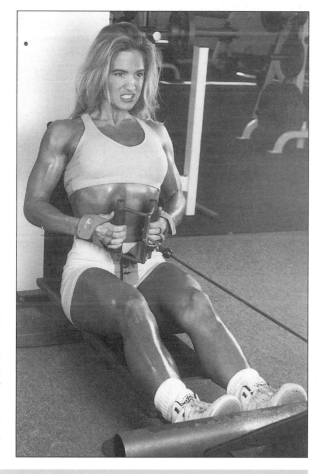

Exercise Technique ►

1. Bring the torso to an erect position pulling the handle toward the abdominals.
2. Remember to slightly arch the back and keep the elbows close to the torso while pulling the handle toward the abdominals, to maximally contract the lats.
3. Return to the starting position, and repeat the movement until the desired number of repetitions is completed.

BACK EXERCISES

Front Chin-Ups

Primary Muscles Worked
- Latissimus Dorsi   • Upper Trapezius
- Biceps Brachii, Brachialis

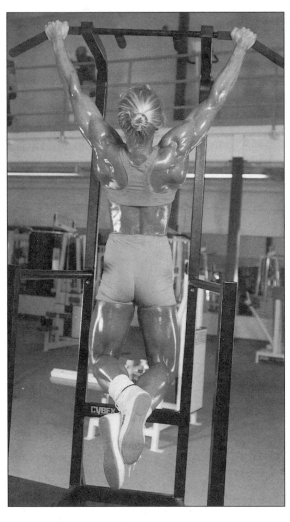

◄Starting Position

1. Grasp a chin-up bar with an overhand grip approximately 3-5 inches wider than shoulder-width apart.
2. Knees are flexed at a 90-degree angle so the ankles can cross over each other.

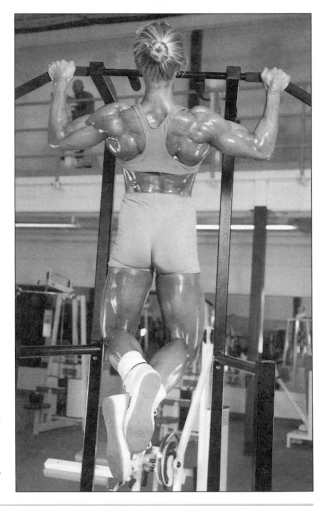

Exercise Technique►

1. Pull the body up in a vertical line until the chin is parallel to the chin-up bar.
2. Slowly lower the body to the starting position, and repeat the movement until the desired number of repetitions is completed.

BACK EXERCISES

Lat Pulldowns Behind the Neck

Primary Muscles Worked
- Latissimus Dorsi
- Posterior Deltoids
- Upper Trapezius
- Biceps Brachii, Brachialis

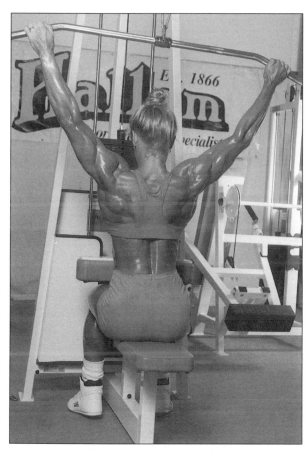

◄Starting Position

1. Stand in front of the lat pulldown machine and grasp the bar with an overhand grip (wide).
2. Sit down with feet flat on the floor, back straight, and thighs secured underneath the thigh pads.
3. At this point, arms are fully extended holding the bar overhead.

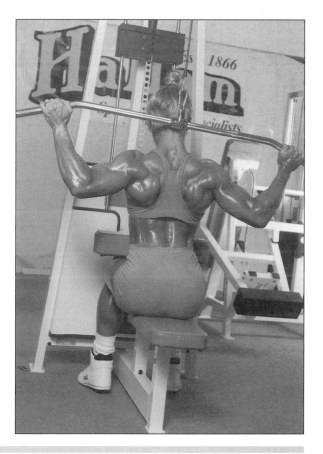

Exercise Technique►

1. Initiate the movement by pulling the elbows downward and backward.
2. As the bar approaches the head, lean slightly forward allowing the bar to touch the top part of the neck.
3. Slowly bring the bar back to the starting position, and repeat the movement until the desired number of repetitions is completed.

BACK EXERCISES

Back Extensions

Primary Muscles Worked
- Erector Spinae
- Gluteal Muscles

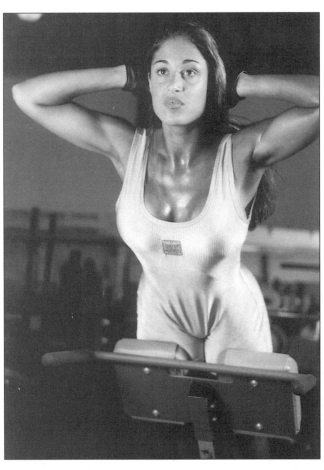

◄ Starting Position

1. Hold the handles of the back extension machine, secure the ankles underneath the small pads and lower your hips onto the larger pads at the front of the apparatus.
2. Keep the legs straight and arms crossed behind the head throughout the entire movement.
3. At this point, the torso should be almost parallel to the floor.

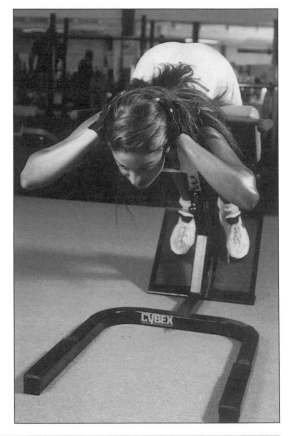

Exercise Technique ►

1. Lower the torso until it is almost perpendicular to the floor.
2. Slowly bring the torso back to the starting position, and repeat the movement until the desired number of repetitions is completed.
3. Remember not to arch upward excessively, for this can cause compression of the vertebrae in the spine.

| THIGH, HIP & GLUTEAL | Safety Squats | **Primary Muscles Worked**
• Vastus Lateralis • Rectus Femoris • Gluteal Muscles
• Vastus Medialis • Vastus Intermedius |

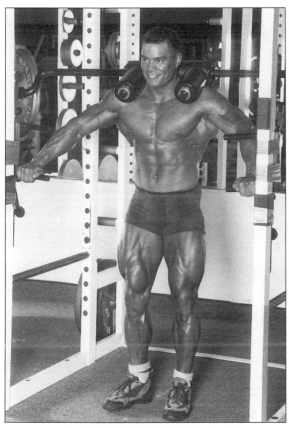

◄Starting Position

1. Rest the pads of the safety squat bar on the trapezius muscles, and lift the safety squat bar off the squatting holders.
2. Feet should be parallel and shoulder-width apart, with knees slightly bent.
3. Keep the safety squat bar steady on the shoulders and place the hands on the rack handles.

Exercise Technique►

1. Keeping the hands on the rack handles throughout the entire movement, slowly lower the glutes toward the floor by bending the knees.
2. When an approximate angle of 90 degrees is reached, push upward with the quadriceps muscles, allowing them maximal muscular activation.
3. Repeat until the desired number of repetitions is completed.

Cue:

The use of the hands during the safety squat helps to balance and maintain strict squatting form, actually allowing you to spot yourself through your sticking point. This will help you to work with heavier loads, without fear of sustaining injuries when exerting force through your weakest point.

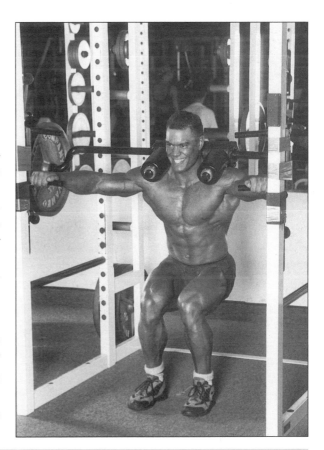

THIG, HIP & GLUTEAL

Seated Leg Extensions (Toes Straight)

Primary Muscles Worked
- Vastus Lateralis
- Rectus Femoris
- Vastus Medialis
- Vastus Intermedius

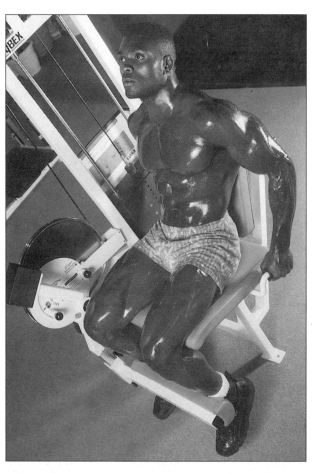

◄Starting Position

1. Sit on a leg extension machine and press the back of the knees firmly against the edge of the seat.
2. Place the front of the ankles under the foot pad and grasp the handles at the sides of the machine.

▼Exercise Technique

1. Moving only the lower legs, lift the desired weight until the quadriceps muscles are fully extended.
2. Hold this position for one second, allowing peak quadriceps contraction to occur.
3. Lower the weight slowly to the starting position and repeat the movement until the desired number of repetitions is completed.

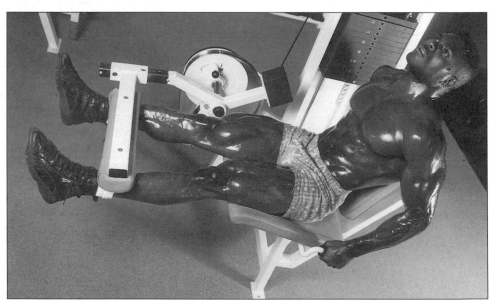

THIGH, HIP & GLUTEAL

Hack Squats

Primary Muscles Worked
- Vastus Lateralis • Rectus Femoris • Gluteal Muscles
- Vastus Medialis • Vastus Intermedius

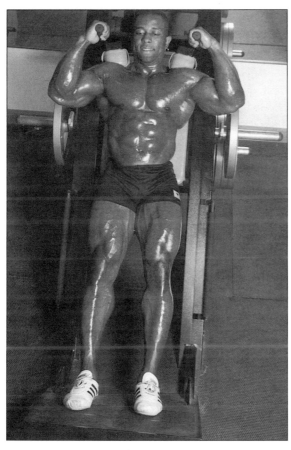

◄Starting Position

1. Position the body on the hack squat machine with trapezius muscles under the shoulder pads, and back pressed firmly against the back rest.

2. Feet are placed on the angled foot rest, with heels approximately 8 inches apart (this varies depending on the individual), and toes angled slightly outward.

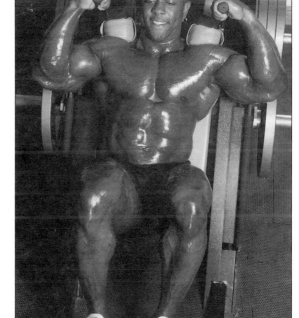

Exercise Technique►

1. Slowly bend at the knees bringing the torso down toward the heels.

2. When the knees are lowered to an approximate 90-degree angle, push upward to return to the starting position.

3. Repeat the movement until the desired number of repetitions is completed.

THIGH, HIP & GLUTEAL

Leg Press

Primary Muscles Worked
- Vastus Lateralis
- Vastus Intermedius
- Vastus Medialis
- Rectus Femoris

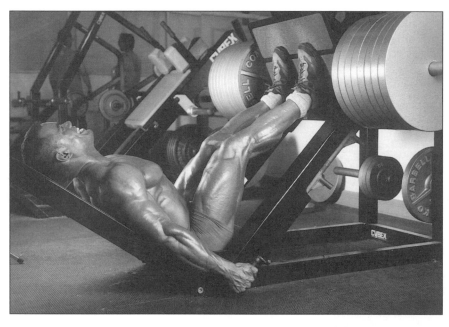

◄Starting Position

1. Lie back on the leg press machine with the buttocks supported on the seat and the back pressed firmly against the back rest pad.

2. Place the feet flat on the platform with a shoulder-width stance, and toes slightly angled outward.

3. Grasp the handles and unlock the weight in preparation to perform the leg press.

Exercise Technique►

1. Slowly bend the legs allowing the knees to travel toward the chest.

2. When the knees have reached an angle slightly greater than 90 degrees (110-115 degrees), slowly straighten the legs to return to the starting position (do not lock the knees at top of movement).

3. Repeat the movement until the desired number of repetitions is completed.

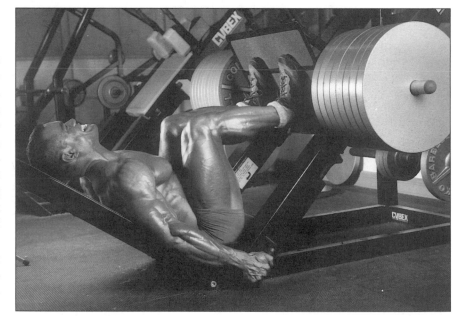

THIGH, HIP & GLUTEAL	Smith Machine Squats	Primary Muscles Worked

Primary Muscles Worked
- Vastus Lateralis
- Vastus Intermedius
- Vastus Medialis
- Rectus Femoris

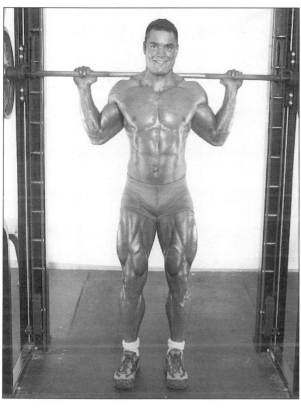

◄Starting Position

1. Position the body underneath the Olympic bar attached to the Smith machine.
2. Grasp the bar with an overhand grip, slightly wider than shoulder-width apart.
3. At this point, the bar is resting comfortably on the trapezius muscles and the feet are shoulder-width stance apart.
4. Unhook the bar from the standards and step forward slightly with both feet.
5. Remember to keep the back erect and look forward throughout the entire movement.

Exercise Technique ►

1. Slowly bend the legs until the knees reach a 90-degree angle.
2. Without bouncing at the bottom of the movement, slowly straighten the legs and return to the starting position.
3. Repeat the movement until the desired number of repetitions is completed.

Cue:

Squatting is an exercise in which technique and balance are of the utmost importance. When squatting inside the Nautilus Smith machine, the element of balance is removed because the Olympic bar is attached to the apparatus. Despite being considered a revolutionary development in the squatting world, Nautilus Smith machine squats might produce too much strain on the lower back and knees. (See *Ironman Magazine*, July 1996, "Safety Squat Bar vs. Smith Machine" by Lorenzo Cornacchia, Tudor O. Bompa, Ph.D., and Vicky Pratt.)

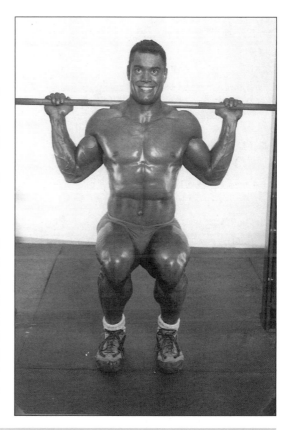

THIGH, HIP & GLUTEAL

Lunges (Dumbbells)

Primary Muscles Worked
- Quadriceps
- Hamstrings
- Gluteal Muscles

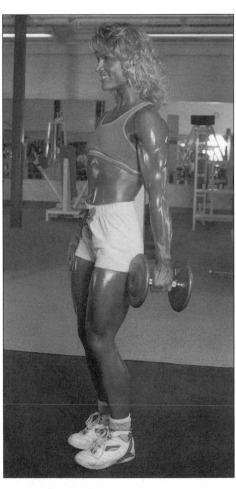

◄Starting Position

1. Grasp a dumbbell with each hand.
2. Hold the dumbbells at the sides of the body with arms fully extended (palms facing your torso).

Exercise Technique►

1. Step forward with the lead leg (stepping leg), keeping the back erect.
2. Bend the knee of lead leg until it has reached a 90-degree angle.
3. At this point, the knee of the back leg should be approximately 2-3 inches from the floor.
4. When fully lowered, push forcefully with the lead leg and return to the starting position.
5. Repeat the exercise with your other leg, and continue to alternate until the desired number of repetitions is completed.
6. Remember that a shorter lead step allows more emphasis to be placed on the quadriceps muscles and a larger step places more emphasis on the gluteal and hamstring muscles.

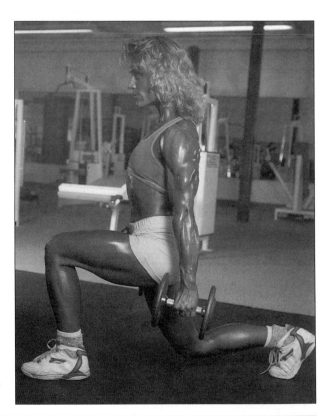

THIGH, HIP & GLUTEAL
Lunges (Olympic Bar)

Primary Muscles Worked
- Quadriceps   • Hamstrings
- Gluteal Muscles

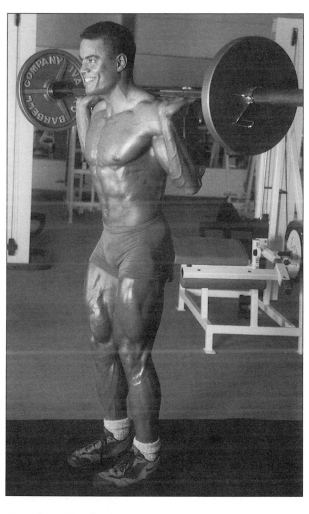

◄Starting Position

1. Position the body underneath the Olympic bar and lift from the standards.
2. The bar should be resting on the trapezius muscles, with the hands grasping the bar slightly wider than shoulder-width apart.
3. Take several steps backward, giving enough clear space to lunge forward.

Exercise Technique►

1. Step forward with the lead leg (stepping leg), keeping the back erect.
2. Bend the knee of the lead leg until it reaches a 90-degree angle.
3. At this point, the knee of the back leg should be approximately 2-3 inches from the floor.
4. When fully lowered, push forcefully with the lead leg and return to the starting position.
5. Repeat with the other leg, and continue to alternate until the desired number of repetitions is completed.
6. Remember that a shorter lead step allows more emphasis to be placed on the quadriceps muscles and a larger step places more emphasis on the gluteal and hamstring muscles.

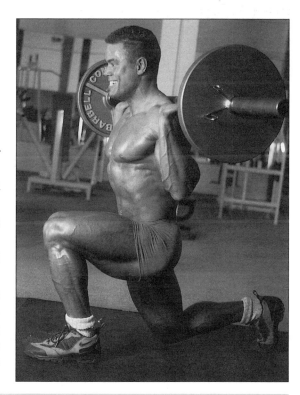

HAMSTRING EXERCISES

Standing Leg Curls

Primary Muscles Worked
- Biceps Femoris
- Semimembranosus
- Semitendinosus

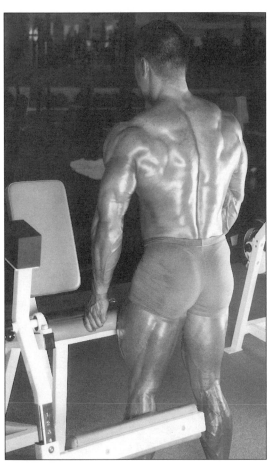

◄Starting Position

1. Standing on the right side of the machine, place the left quad against the thigh pad, and the left heel (calf) under the rectangular ankle pad.
2. With the left hand grasp the pad directly in front, and lean the torso slightly forward.

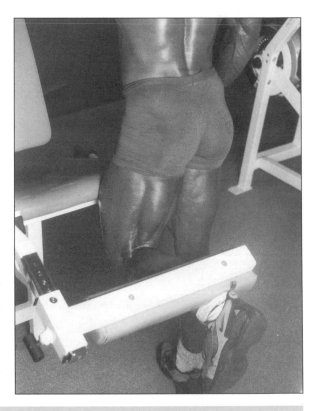

Exercise Technique►

1. Slowly raise the foot toward the buttocks.
2. Go as far upward as possible to allow for maximal contraction.
3. Once the top of the movement is reached, slowly lower the leg while resisting against the weight (do not let the foot touch the floor).
4. Repeat until the desired number of repetitions is completed.
5. Reverse the body position and repeat exercise for the other leg.

HAMSTRING EXERCISES | Lying Leg Curls

Primary Muscles Worked
- Biceps Femoris
- Semimembranosus
- Semitendinosus

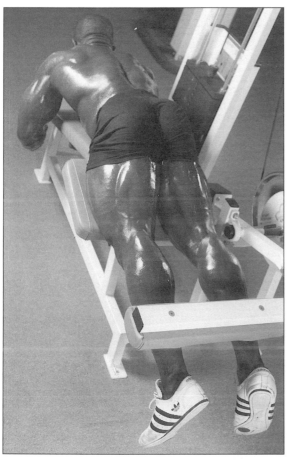

◄Starting Position

1. Lie face down on the hamstring curl machine.
2. Slide the ankles underneath the ankle pads and place the knees at the edge of the bench.
3. Grasp the handles at the top of the machine to keep the body stabilized while performing the set.

Exercise Technique►

1. Raise the heels, bringing them toward the buttocks.
2. Go as far upward as possible to allow for maximal contraction.
3. Once the top of the movement is reached, slowly lower the leg while resisting against the weight (do not let the plates touch—keeping tension on the working muscles).
4. Repeat until the desired number of repetitions is completed.

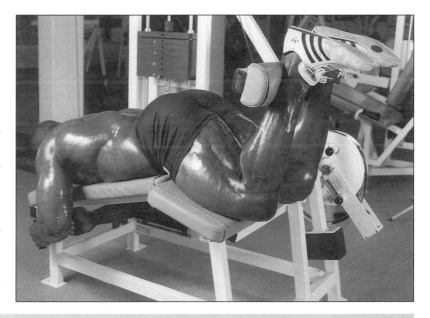

HAMSTRING EXERCISES

Seated Leg Curls

Primary Muscles Worked
- Biceps Femoris
- Semimembranosus
- Semitendinosus

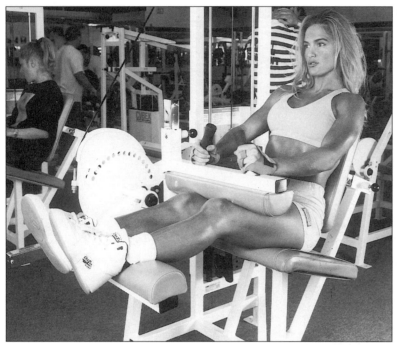

◄Starting Position

1. Sit on the hamstring curl machine with ankles placed on top of the ankle pads.
2. Adjust the thigh pad and lock it down comfortably across the thighs.
3. Keep back pressed firmly against the back support.

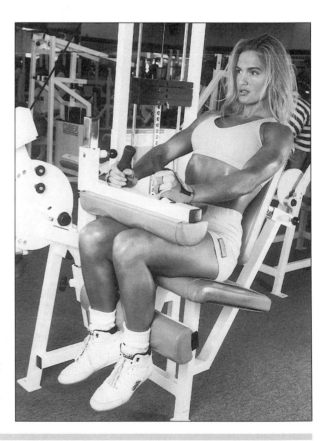

Exercise Technique►

1. Bend the knees bringing the heels under the body and toward the buttocks.
2. Go as far back as possible to allow for maximal contraction.
3. Once the hamstrings are maximally contracted, while resisting, slowly allow the weight to bring the body back to the starting position.
4. Repeat the movement until the desired number of repetitions is completed.

HAMSTRING EXERCISES

Modified Hamstring Deadlifts

Primary Muscles Worked
• Biceps Femoris   • Semimembranosus
• Semitendinosus

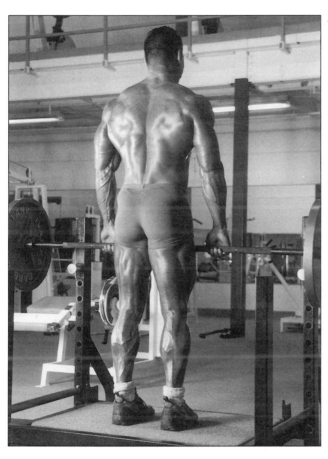

◄Starting Position
1. Grasp an Olympic bar with hands slightly wider than shoulder-width apart.
2. Hold the bar with arms fully extended at thigh level.

Exercise Technique►
1. Keep back flat, buttocks out, and knees slightly bent.
2. Slowly lower the bar past the knees (2-3 inches).
3. At this point, a stretch in the glutes and hamstrings should be felt.
4. Slowly raise the bar by contracting the glutes and hamstrings, and straightening the torso.
5. Repeat until the desired number of repetitions is completed.

Cue:
Most lifters perform this exercise incorrectly by bending too far over. Once the hip muscles are fully flexed, the only way to further lower the bar to the shoes is to hyperflex the spine. When this occurs, the lifter places the lumbar spine in a very vulnerable position (career-ending injury or serious complications could result).

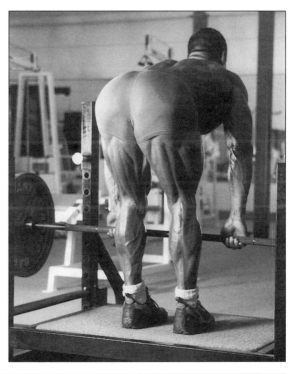

HAMSTRING EXERCISES

Cable Kickback

Primary Muscles Worked
• Gluteus Maximus Muscle Group
• Upper Hamstring Area

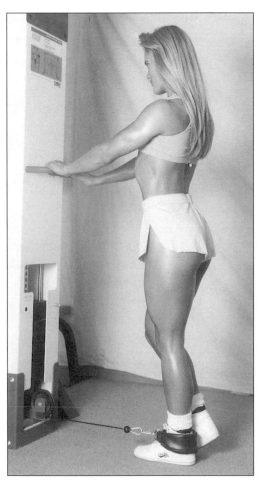

◄Starting Position

1. Attach an ankle strap to the low cable pulley.
2. Facing the pulley, slip the left ankle into the strap and take two steps backward.
3. Grasp the support bar with both hands to stabilize the torso throughout the entire movement.

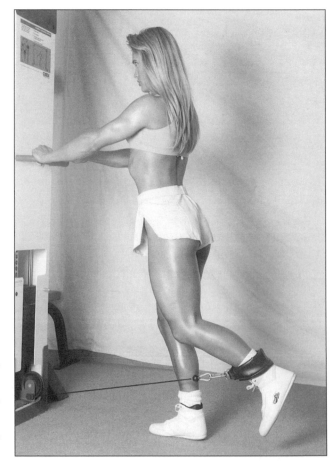

Exercise Technique►

1. Keeping the supporting leg slightly flexed, slowly kick the left leg back from the hips.
2. Hold this contracted position for a moment, and then return the foot to the starting position.
3. Repeat the movement until the desired number of repetitions is completed.
4. Reverse body position and repeat with the right leg.

CALF EXERCISES

Donkey Calf Raises

Primary Muscles Worked
- Gastrocnemius
- Soleus

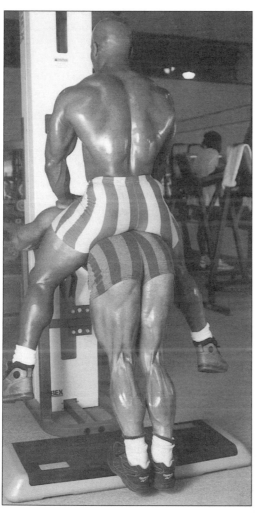

◄Starting Position

1. Stand with toes on the edge of a calf board (approximately 3-5 inches in height).
2. Bend forward at the hips until the torso is parallel to the floor, and stabilize the body by holding onto a piece of equipment (e.g., squat rack).
3. At this point, a partner climbs onto the back and straddles the hips.
4. Allow the heels to drop as far as comfortably possible below the level of the toes.

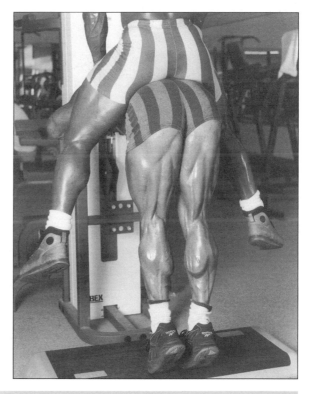

Exercise Technique►

1. Raise the torso as high as possible on the balls of the feet.
2. Once the top of the movement is reached, slowly lower the heels as far below the level of the toes as possible, returning to the starting position.
3. Repeat the movement until the desired number of repetitions is completed.

CALF EXERCISES

Standing One-Leg Calf Raises

Primary Muscles Worked
- Gastrocnemius
- Soleus

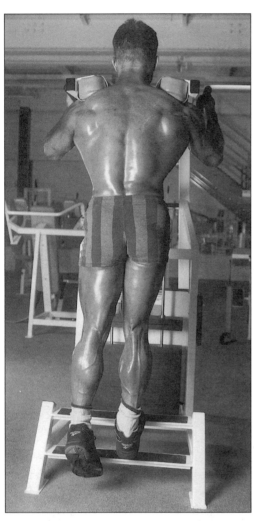

◄Starting Position

1. Stand on a calf machine, with the ball of the right foot at the edge of the platform.
2. Place the hands on top of the shoulder pads to stabilize the body.
3. Allow the heel to drop as far below the level of the toes as possible.

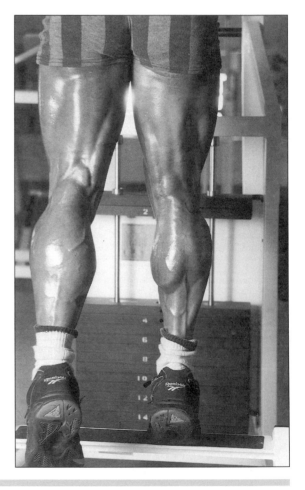

Exercise Technique►

1. Raise the torso as high as possible on the ball of the foot and toes.
2. Once the top of the movement is reached, slowly lower the heel as far below the level of the toes as possible, returning to the starting position.
3. Repeat the movement until the desired number of repetitions is completed.
4. Repeat for the left foot.

CALF EXERCISES

Standing Two-Leg Calf Raises

Primary Muscles Worked
- Gastrocnemius
- Soleus

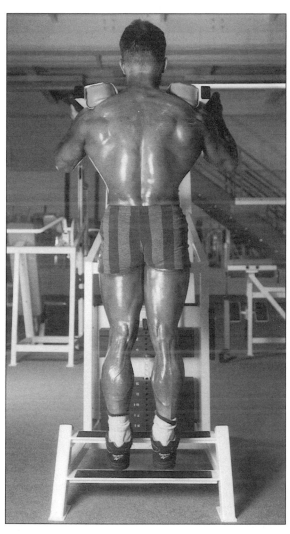

◄Starting Position

1. Stand on a calf machine with the balls of the feet at the edge of the platform.
2. Place the hands on top of the shoulder pads to stabilize the body.
3. Allow the heels to drop as far below the level of the toes as possible.

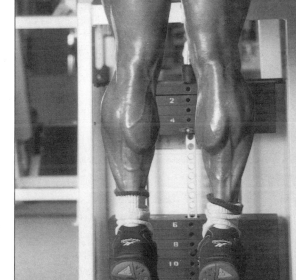

Exercise Technique►

1. Raise the torso as high as possible on the balls of the feet and toes.
2. Once the top of the movement is reached, slowly lower the heels as far below the level of the toes as possible, returning to the starting position.
3. Repeat until the desired number of repetitions is completed.

CALF EXERCISES

Seated Calf Raises

Primary Muscles Worked
- Gastrocnemius
- Soleus

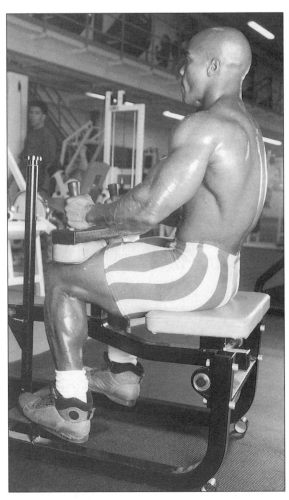

◄Starting Position

1. Sit on the calf machine with the balls of the feet on the edge of the platform.
2. Hook the knees underneath the pads and grasp the handles to stabilize the body.
3. Unhook the safeguard for the weight.
4. Allow the heels to drop as far below the level of the toes as possible.

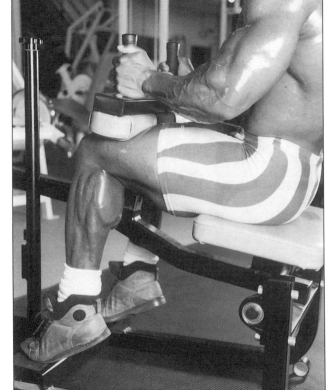

Exercise Technique►

1. Raise the heels until the calves are fully contracted.
2. Once the top of the movement is reached, slowly lower the heels as far below the toes as possible, returning to the starting position.
3. Repeat the movement until the desired number of repetitions is completed.

ABDOMINAL EXERCISES

Nautilus Crunches

Primary Muscles Worked
• Rectus Abdominis (Upper Part)

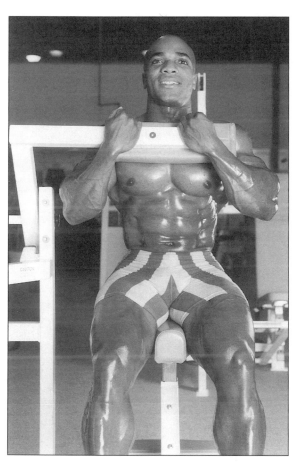

◄Starting Position

1. Sit on the seat of the crunch machine.
2. At this point, a chest pad should be resting firmly against the chest.
3. Place hands across the back of the chest padding for support.

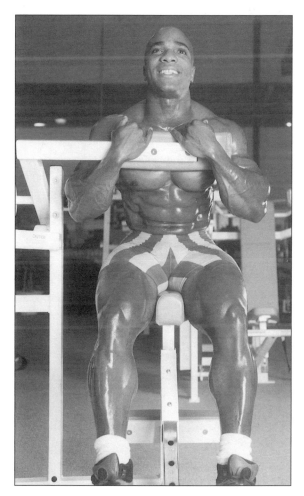

Exercise Technique►

1. Bend the torso forward until the abdominals are maximally contracted.
2. Blow all the air out as the movement is performed.
3. Slowly return to the starting position, never letting the weighted plates make contact (removes tension from the working muscles).
4. Repeat until the desired number of repetitions is completed.

ABDOMINAL EXERCISES

Pulley Crunches

Primary Muscles Worked
- Rectus Abdominis (Upper Part)
- Serratus Anterior   • Intercostals

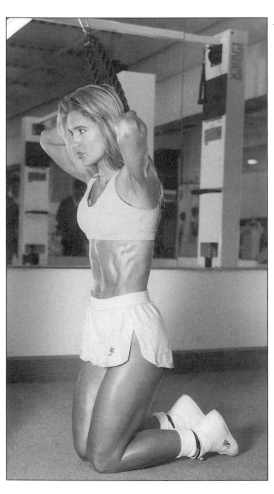

◄Starting Position

1. Attach a rope handle to an overhead pulley and grasp the rope handle with an overhand grip.
2. Hold the rope behind the neck and kneel down (approximately 1 foot from the pulley machine).

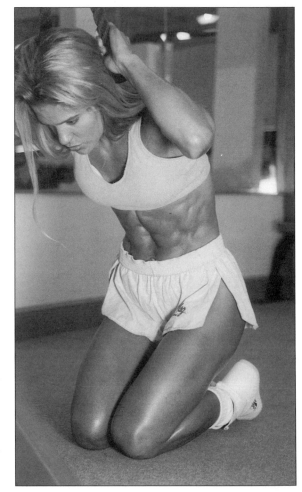

Exercise Technique►

1. Bend over at the waist until the abdominals are maximally contracted.
2. Blow out all of the air as the movement is performed.
3. Repeat the movement until the desired number of repetitions is completed.
4. The objective is to perform the exercise in a controlled manner and to maintain the tension on the working muscles throughout the entire movement.

ABDOMINAL EXERCISES | Knee-Ups (Flat Bench)

Primary Muscles Worked
• Rectus Abdominis (Mainly Lower)

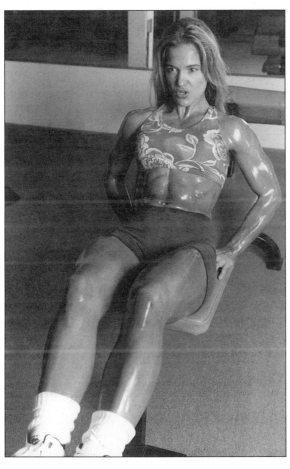

◄Starting Position

1. Sit on the end of a flat bench and place the hands behind you to support the body.
2. Lean back until the torso is approximately at a 45-degree angle to the bench.
3. Extend the legs until they are almost straightened.

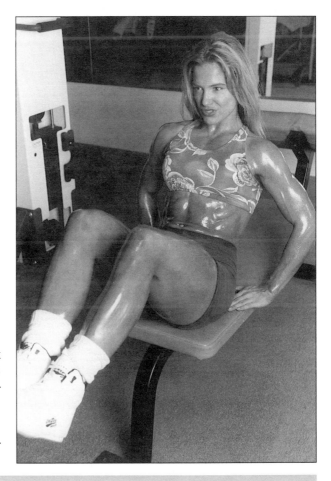

Exercise Technique►

1. Pull the knees toward the chest.
2. As the knees approach the chest, flex the neck allowing the head to curl toward the knees (this will ensure maximal abdominal contraction).
3. Return to the starting position.
4. Repeat the movement until the desired number of repetitions is completed.

ABDOMINAL EXERCISES

Crunches (Flat Abdominal Bench)

Primary Muscles Worked
• Rectus Abdominis (Mainly Upper)

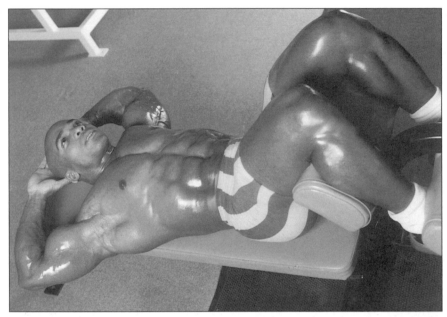

◄Starting Position

1. Lie flat on an abdominal bench with knees bent and feet locked under the ankle pads.
2. Place hands and arms behind the head.

Exercise Technique►

1. Use upper abdominal strength to raise the head and shoulders from the abdominal bench.
2. When rectus abdominis muscles are maximally contracted, pause briefly and return to the starting position.
3. To keep tension on the working muscles, do not allow the torso (upper trapezius and shoulders) to make contact with the bench.
4. Repeat the movement until the desired number of repetitions is completed.

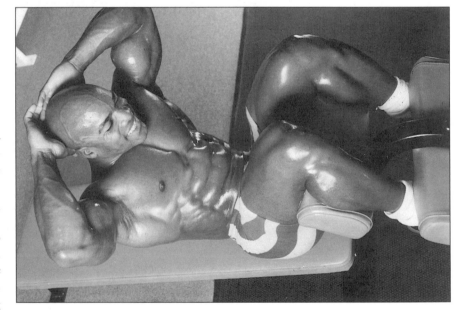

ABDOMINAL EXERCISES

Hanging Leg Raises

Primary Muscles Worked
- Rectus Abdominis (Mainly Lower)
- Serratus Anterior • Intercostals

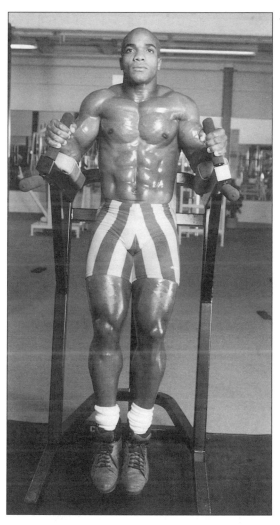

◄Starting Position

1. Grasp handles and support body weight with the arms.
2. Allow the torso to hang down in a straight vertical line.
3. Keep the knees slightly bent throughout the entire movement to remove any unnecessary stress from the lower back.

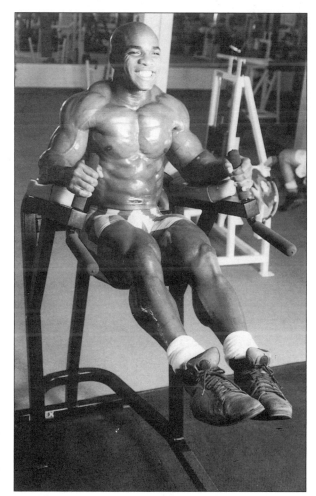

Exercise Technique►

1. Using abdominal strength, slowly raise the legs to the level of the hips.
2. Hold the contraction for a moment then slowly lower the legs to the starting position.
3. Repeat the movement until the desired number of repetitions is completed.

ABDOMINAL EXERCISES

Diagonal Curl-Ups

Primary Muscles Worked
- Rectus Abdominis (Mainly Upper)
- Serratus Anterior   • Intercostals

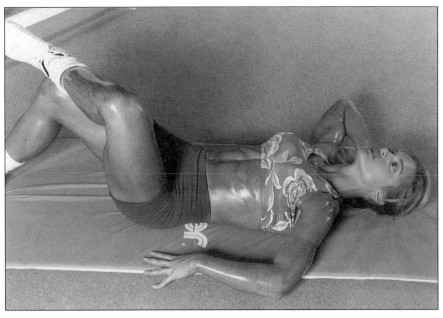

◀Starting Position

1. Lie down on an abdominal board or floor mat with knees bent and feet on the floor.
2. Place the left ankle across the right knee.
3. A triangle should form from their contact.
4. Place the right hand behind the head and place the left hand on the mat for support.

Exercise Technique▶

1. Curl the torso diagonally, bringing the right shoulder up toward the left knee.
2. Once you have reached maximum contraction, pause briefly.
3. Return to the starting position and repeat until the desired number of repetitions has been completed.
4. Reverse body position and repeat for the other side.

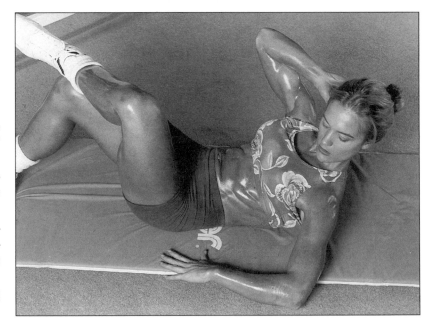

CHAPTER 12

EATING PLANS TO GET RIPPED

Nutrition is a central factor in the life of an athlete, and yet many people are mystified by it. For some athletes, decisions about what foods to eat and when to eat them are overshadowed by how much to eat. When quantity becomes the all-important factor, it can lead to unwanted body fat. Many athletes also suffer through the peaks and valleys of off-season neglect, followed by the rigors of strict dieting and training to force the body back into shape. This cycle causes frustration and places extreme stress on the body. The nutritional needs of serious, dedicated bodybuilders and strength trainers differ from those of the average population and are still quite specific.

Scientific research has helped us to discover exactly what the body needs to build muscle. When we understand the role of nutrients and how the body processes them, we can be selective about food choices. We can combine quantity with quality to provide the body with what it needs to produce energy and build muscle instead of fat. This combination also helps the athlete maintain a muscular, lean look year-round.

Carbohydrates, proteins, and fats are the main energy-producing nutrients. This chapter describes each and how strength trainers and bodybuilders can use these nutrients to enhance their training programs.

Carbohydrates

Carbohydrates act as the body's number one source of energy, and each gram of carbohydrate yields 4 kcal of energy. The body uses adenosine triphosphate (ATP) as its primary energy source. ATP, as blood glucose and muscle glycogen, is produced more quickly from carbohydrates than from fats. The body can synthesize ATP from carbohydrates at a rate of about 1.0 mol/min, and from fats at a rate of about .5 mol/min (Ahlborg, 1967). This means that ATP production occurs at twice the rate from carbohydrates than it does from fat, certainly making carbohydrates the nutrient of choice for energy. When carbohydrate

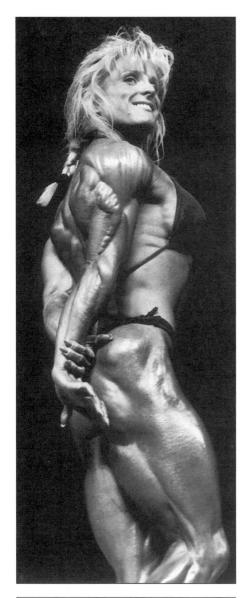

Sue Price shows what happens when diet and training come together perfectly.

sources reach depletion, the body will then turn to its fat stores to produce energy. This plays an important role in contest dieting and the muscle definition phase.

Carbohydrates also play a role in the protection of muscle tissue. Whereas the body uses carbohydrates and fat to produce energy, it uses protein to build and repair muscle tissue. If there are not enough carbohydrates and fat in the diet or in storage to supply the energy demand, the body will then turn to protein use for energy. Under these conditions, the body begins to break down muscle tissue through a process called *gluconeogenesis*, meaning the "production of new glucose." In other words, if carbohydrates are not available, the body breaks muscle tissue down into glucose units for energy (Wardlaw and Insel, 1990). This can sometimes happen as a result of improper or extreme dieting prior to competition. Continual monitoring of carbohydrate, protein, and fat intake is necessary. By keeping a weekly log, you can determine if your carbohydrates should be raised or lowered depending on how you should appear and feel at weekly checkpoints. This ability to fine tune your diet is invaluable and necessary in order to ensure that muscle mass is not sacrificed and energy levels remain at an optimum.

Glucose is the only substrate used by the brain. Anyone who has ever used carbohydrate depletion to prepare for a show will remember feeling light-headed, dizzy, forgetful, irritable, and clumsy. Remember that the brain gets hungry too, so when dieting for a contest, listen to the body and the brain.

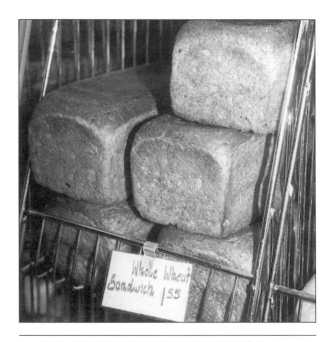

Whole wheat bread is a form of complex carbohydrates.

While a shortage of carbohydrates can create problems, an overabundance can also create problems. When carbohydrate intake is more than the body needs to produce energy, the excess is converted into fat and stored for later use.

The following box illustrates how carbohydrates fall into two categories: simple and complex. Simple sugars include monosaccharides and disaccharides. Polysaccharides make up the complex carbohydrates.

Carbohydrates	
Simple sugars	**Complex carbohydrates**
Monosaccharides	Polysaccharides
Disaccharides	

Simple Sugars

The two most common monosaccharides are glucose, which is blood sugar, and fructose, which is a sugar that comes from fruits. Disaccharides are composed of two monosaccharides. The two most common disaccharides are sucrose, or table sugar, and lactose, which comes from milk.

Once sugar is consumed, the liver either converts most of these simple sugars into glucose for quick energy, or moves them into glycogen or fat storage for use later.

Excessive consumption of this type of carbohydrate might be detrimental to the serious athlete for several reasons.

- Sugary foods typically have low nutritional value in terms of delivering vitamins, minerals, or proteins (Wardlaw and Insel, 1990).
- Unnecessary amounts of sugar are converted into fat.
- Sugary foods cause insulin levels to fluctuate wildly, inhibiting the activity of the glycogen storage enzyme, glycogen synthase, resulting in depressed glycogen storage (Jenkins, 1982).

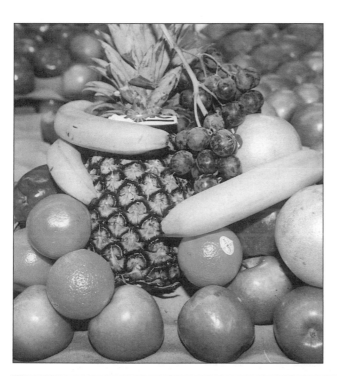

The high sugar content in fruit can add extra calories and cause unwanted fluctuations in the body's insulin levels.

Complex Carbohydrates

As the name suggests, polysaccharides are composed of many (poly) glucose units. They are often referred to as starches, and are found in vegetables,

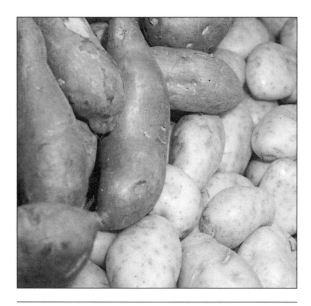

Yams and potatoes—both are great sources of complex carbohydrates.

fruits, and grains. Complex carbohydrates are a source of high energy for every athlete and account for the largest percentage of the diet. These carbohydrates are digested slowly and, therefore, do not cause huge fluctuations in insulin or blood glucose levels (Jenkins, 1982). A frequent intake of complex carbohydrates maintains steady levels of blood sugar and insulin, thus enhancing glycogen synthase activity and increasing glycogen storage.

Glycemic Index

One easy way to ensure that we choose the right carbohydrates is to use the Glycemic Index created by Dr. David Jenkins to help diabetics control insulin levels. Diabetics, like athletes, want to keep blood sugar and insulin levels on an even keel.

The carbohydrates that do not result in large insulin fluctuations because of slow digestion have low glycemic values. The foods that cause rapid changes in blood sugar and insulin levels have high glycemic values. (Jenkins, 1987). Athletes should obviously choose from foods with lower scores, provided that the fat content is also acceptable. (Note: Ice cream does not fall into this category.) Table 12.1 shows the glycemic index for many common foods.

Proteins

Protein is an extremely important part of any diet because it is used to build and repair tissue. Therefore, it is of special significance to bodybuilders and strength trainers. Intense workouts break down muscle tissue, therefore, athletes need larger amounts of protein than normal so the body can repair this damage and increase muscle mass. During periods of intense training, inadequate protein intake may lead to a rate of protein degradation that actually exceeds the rate of protein

Lean fish is an excellent source of protein.

Table 12.1   Glycemic index

Food	Index	Food	Index
Grain and cereal products		**Fruits**	
White bread	100	Raisins	93
Whole wheat bread	99	Banana	79
Brown rice	96	Orange juice	67
White rice	83	Orange	66
White spaghetti	66	Grapes	62
Breakfast cereals		Apple	53
Cornflakes	119	Pear	47
Shredded Wheat	97	Peach	40
All Bran	93	Grapefruit	36
Oatmeal	85	Plum	34
Dairy products		**Vegetables**	
Ice cream	52	Baked potato	135
Yogurt	52	Instant potatoes	116
Whole milk	49	New potatoes	81
Skim milk	46	Yams	74
Sweeteners		Frozen peas	74
Maltose	152	Sweet potato	70
Glucose	138	**Dried legumes**	
Honey	126	Canned baked beans	60
Sucrose	86	Kidney beans	54
Fructose	30	Butter beans	52
		Chickpeas	49
		Lentils	43
		Soybeans	20

Reprinted, by permission, from G.M. Wardlaw and P.M. Insel, 1990, *Perspectives in Nutrition*, (New York: McGraw-Hill), 110.

synthesis, resulting in a loss of tissue protein (U.S. Food and Nutrition Board, 1989). This means that hours of hard training can actually lead to a decrease in muscle size and tone. To prevent this, it is necessary to eat enough protein to allow muscle growth and enough carbohydrates to preserve muscle mass.

Proteins do much more than contribute to the growth and repair of muscle. For instance, proteins are responsible for immune functions—antibodies are proteins. Protein is also necessary for blood-clotting, hormone and enzyme production, vision, fluid balance, and the production of connective tissues (Wardlaw and Insel, 1990).

Amino Acids

Proteins are composed of chains of amino acids (AAs), which are referred to as "the building blocks of protein." There are twenty different AAs, of which the body can synthesize eleven (*nonessential AAs*) from the food we eat, while the remaining nine (*essential AAs*) must be supplied through the diet (see table 12.2). All nine essential AAs must be present in the body for protein synthesis to occur (Wardlaw and Insel, 1990).

Table 12.2 Amino acids	
Nonessential AAs	**Essential AAs**
Can be synthesized by the body	Cannot be synthesized by the body; must be supplied by diet
11 AAs out of 20	9 AAs out of 20

Reprinted, by permission, from G.M. Wardlaw and P.M. Insel, 1990, *Perspectives in Nutrition*, (New York: McGraw-Hill), 159-160.

Complete Proteins Versus Incomplete Proteins

It is extremely important for bodybuilders and strength trainers to consume the right foods so all twenty AAs can work together to form protein. The main concern is to obtain the nine AAs that the body cannot synthesize—the nine essential AAs that must come directly from the diet. The body will take care of the other eleven nonessential AAs. Foods containing all nine of the essential AAs are called *complete proteins*, and these are the athlete's friends. Foods that do not contain all nine of the essential AAs are called *incomplete proteins*. Table 12.3 gives a brief listing of some complete and incomplete proteins and their characteristics.

Vegetarian bodybuilders and strength trainers who rely solely on plant proteins must pay particular attention to their protein intake. While meat eaters can be confident that they are getting all the needed AAs, vegetarians must be more careful. A wide variety of plant proteins must be eaten to provide the

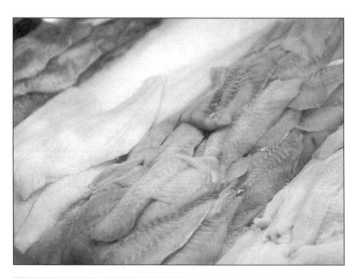

Fish is great for bodybuilders and strength trainers. It is a complete protein and when prepared properly, it is one of the leanest sources of protein.

Table 12.3   Complete proteins and incomplete proteins

	Complete proteins	Incomplete proteins
Definition	Foods that contain all 9 essential AAs	Foods that do not contain all 9 essential AAs
Importance	Can support body growth and maintenance	Cannot support body growth, although some may support body maintenance
Source	Animal proteins	Plant proteins
Foods	Beef, chicken, pork, eggs, fish, milk, cheese, yogurt	Soybeans, legumes, tofu, grains, nuts, seeds, vegetables

Reprinted, by permission, from G.M. Wardlaw and P.M. Insel, 1990, *Perspectives in Nutrition*, (New York: McGraw-Hill), 160-161.

body with all nine essential AAs. Vegetarian athletes will be more likely to get what they need by combining plant proteins.

An example of combining two incomplete protein foods to make a complete package would be to eat bread and peanut butter. In combination they supply the nine essential AAs while alone they do not.

Nutritional Cues:

- Be sure you are eating enough protein for your size. Refer to Nutrition Strategy section of each phase.
- Eat a wide variety of protein foods.

Biological Value of a Protein

The *biological value (BV)* of a protein describes how efficiently body tissue can be created from food protein. According to Wardlaw and Insel (1990), "The BV of a food depends on how closely its amino acid pattern reflects the amino acid pattern in body tissue; and the better the match the more completely food protein turns into body protein." If the AA pattern in a food is very different from human tissue AA patterns, then the food protein is turned into either glucose for use as fuel, or fat for storage, instead of body protein. This explains why egg whites, milk, and animal proteins have the highest biological values and, consequently, the greatest potential to turn into body protein. Humans and other animals have similar AA compositions, while plant AA compositions differ greatly from those of humans. Table 12.4 ranks the BV and *net protein utilization (NPU)* for many of the main staples of an athlete's diet. NPU adjusts the BV of a food to account for its digestibility, and because most proteins are almost completely digested and absorbed, the BV and NPU for most protein foods are similar.

Again, by eating a wide variety of foods we can greatly increase the BV of a meal. This is especially important for vegetarian athletes because, as you can see from table 12.4, the foods with the highest BV are animal proteins.

Table 12.4   Comparative protein quality (biological value and net protein utilization of commonly consumed protein foods)

Food	Biological value	Net protein utilization
Egg	100	94
Cow's milk	93	82
Unpolished rice	86	59
Fish	76	—
Beef	74	67
Soy beans	73	61
Corn	72	36
Oats	65	—
Whole wheat	65	49
Polished rice	64	57
Peas	64	55
Peanuts	55	55

Reprinted, by permission, from G.M. Wardlaw and P.M. Insel, 1990, *Perspectives in Nutrition*, (New York: McGraw-Hill), 167.

How Much Protein Is Enough

There is a lot of confusion surrounding this issue. The RDAs (Recommended Dietary Allowances) promoted by the health care world suggest an intake of .75g-.8g of protein/kg of body weight per day (U.S. Food and Nutrition Board, 1989). Serious bodybuilders and strength trainers, however, are known to consume astounding amounts of protein including meats, beans, and bulk drinks.

RDAs are guidelines for food intake to maintain overall general health, and were not created with the serious athlete in mind. While bodybuilders and strength trainers want to increase size and mass, the average adult usually wants to lose weight or maintain body size. Nevertheless, most people still insist that the RDAs will work for everyone.

Studies that have supposedly taken exercise into account also recommend protein intakes that approximate the RDAs. Peter Lemon points out that these conclusions are often drawn from studies in which the subjects' exercise routines were minimal, and therefore have little correlation to the rigorous workouts of bodybuilders and strength trainers. Some studies have actually taken otherwise sedentary subjects and had them exercise throughout the study. There is no way to compare the intensity of a novice exerciser to the intensity of a serious, seasoned athlete. Information that is useful to bodybuilders and strength trainers must come from sources that study these athletes.

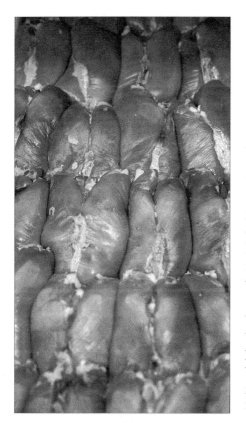

Skinless chicken breast is the cornerstone of the athlete's diet, low in fat and tasty.

Not everyone in the scientific community, however, believes in the protein RDA. Some believe that the surplus amino acids supplied through the consumption of high protein diets might enhance protein synthesis and minimize protein degradation in heavy-resistance training athletes.

Numerous studies involving bodybuilders and strength athletes have found that protein intakes far in excess of the RDA (.8g protein/kg of body weight) are more appropriate. Consolazio et al. (1963) performed a study that compared protein intakes of 350% RDA to intakes of 175% RDA, and found that those athletes consuming 350% RDA of protein experienced greater gains in lean body mass. Similarly, Dragan et al. (1985) found 5% gains in strength and 6% gains in lean body mass when the protein intake of Romanian weightlifters was increased from 275% RDA to 438% RDA.

Not all strength athletes need the same amount of protein. One must take into account size, gender, and type of training. For specific details on exactly how much protein you need, refer to the Nutrition Strategy sections supplied with each training phase. Keep two things in mind. There are good and there are poor protein choices. There is no point in consuming too much protein.

Good Versus Bad Protein Choices

One of the biggest controversies in nutrition today centers on the consumption of meat. On the one hand, we are told that meat is bad for us: it contains too much fat and too much cholesterol, and contributes to cancer and heart disease. On the other hand, we are told that if we follow some basic guidelines, eating meat can be safe and enjoyable. These basic guidelines include the following:

- Avoid fatty meats. See table 12.5.
- Trim all visible fat and, if applicable, always remove the skin before cooking.
- Never fry meat, instead broil, poach, or grill.
- Avoid casseroles since they usually contain ground beef and high-fat sauce.

Problems Associated With Consuming Excessive Protein

The consumption of too much protein can place increased stress on kidney functions (Lemon, 1991). Urea, a major body waste product, results from the breakdown of AAs. The more protein we eat, the more our bodies need to get rid of nitrogen (as urea). Excessive protein ingestion leads to excessive urea production and results in very concentrated urine. One possible consequence of having very concentrated urine is the development of kidney stones—a very painful condition (Wardlaw and Insel, 1990).

Solution: If the diet is high in protein, we must drink lots of water. This will help to flush out the kidneys and dilute urine. If the urine is very yellow and

Table 12.5 Low-fat versus high-fat meat choices

Low-fat meat choices	High-fat meat choices
Chicken breast	Dark chicken meat
Turkey breast	Dark turkey meat (wings, drumsticks, thighs)
Inside round steak	Marbled steaks
Lean fish (snapper, sole, cod, orange roughy, halibut)	Oily fish (mackerel, salmon, sardines)
Tenderloin pork	Most pork products (bacon, ribs, chops, pork roast)
Canned tuna	Canned salmon
Ground turkey or chicken	Ground beef or pork

Reprinted, by permission, from G.M. Wardlaw and P.M. Insel, 1990, *Perspectives in Nutrition*, (New York: McGraw-Hill), chapter 5.

pungent, this could be a sign that urea concentrations are too high, forcing the kidneys to work overtime.

High protein diets might result in increased calcium loss (Allen et al., 1979). Calcium levels that are too low might result in increased blood pressure and osteoporosis (Wardlaw and Insel, 1990). Research indicates, though, that this calcium loss may be prevented by the increased phosphate intake that occurs with increased protein intake (Flynn, A., 1984).

Remember that excess protein means excess calories. When more protein is consumed than the body can use, the excess is stored as fat. While some protein choices may be high in fat, there is a multitude of delicious low-fat protein choices (see table 12.5).

Fats

Of the three energy-producing nutrients (carbohydrates, proteins, and fats), fat is the most calorie dense. Every gram of fat yields 9 kcal of energy, twice the amount of calories found in carbohydrates (4 kcal) and protein (4 kcal). This can be very

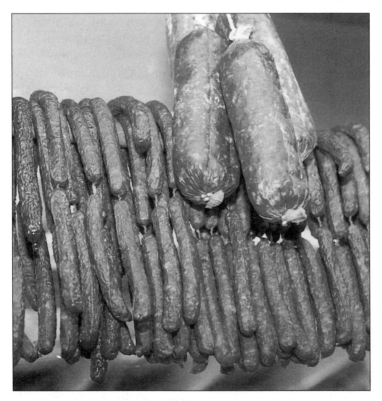

Deli meats are a big no-no! Far too much fat to be a wise protein choice.

deceiving when trying to read food labels. Take for example a food item that contains the following:

carbohydrates	10g
protein	10g
fat	5g

It would seem that this item is quite low in fat. However, when we consider the calorie density, we discover something different:

carbohydrates	**10g x 4 kcal =**	**40 kcal**
protein	**10g x 4 kcal =**	**40 kcal**
fat	**5g x 9 kcal =**	**45 kcal**
	TOTAL	**125 kcal**

The fat content is 36% and accounts for more than 1/3 of the calories, even though the amount of fat is only 1/5 of the 25g serving.

This is of greater significance because consumed fat goes directly into storage, and the body finds it the most difficult nutrient to use as energy. Fat in muscles burns very slowly. While the body can form ATP from carbohydrates at a rate of 1.0 mol/min, the rate of ATP synthesis from fat is only .5 mol/min—twice as slow (Ahlbog et al., 1967). This shows us that while fat yields twice as much energy as carbohydrates, it is harder for the body to use.

The body is extremely efficient and will use carbohydrates to produce energy as long as they are available in muscle or blood glycogen. Only when these stores are depleted, after long bouts of exercise for example, is the body forced to turn to fat stores for energy supply. This is one reason why fat is so hard to lose. The body only uses it as a "last resort."

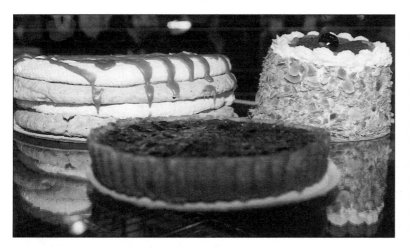

Just say no!

The Sad Fat Facts

During the off season, it is not uncommon for bodybuilders to gain too much weight, and some use contest dieting as a license to overeat. They tell themselves that whatever fat they put on can be taken off again for a show, or that a binge after a contest is compensation for weeks of deprivation. Others, who feel they need to "put on size," believe that the way to increase muscle size is to eat enormous quantities of food during the off season.

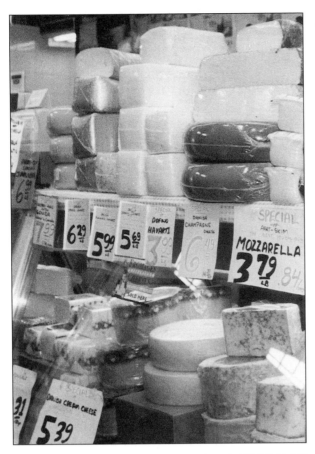

Unless it is the low- or no-fat variety, cheese does not fit into a bodybuilder's diet.

Points to Remember

Fat is not easy to lose, in a long-term sense. When fat weight is gained, the fat goes into the body's fat cells. When these cells cannot hold any more fat, new cells are formed and then filled. While dieting can reduce the fat in the cells, the cells themselves remain. It is hypothesized that because each fat cell needs to contain a certain amount of fat, those individuals with more fat cells will automatically store more fat. Consequently, even though fat might be lost for a contest, the battle against fat could last a lifetime.

When bodybuilders say that they want to "put on size," they want muscle size, not fat size. It is important to realize that while overeating might give some increase in muscle weight, it mainly creates excessive fat.

While some body fat is necessary for the protection of muscles and organs, and for the absorption and storage of fat-soluble vitamins, unnecessary body fat is useless. It does not contribute to force production, nor does it lead to increases in muscle size. If fact, excessive fat is dangerous to our health in terms of cardiovascular disease, diabetes, and joint problems.

Fat cannot and will not turn into muscle. Fat and muscle are two completely different things, and no amount of working out will ever turn fat into muscle. It is possible to build muscle underneath fat, but those precious lines will not show through the extra tissue.

The more fat put on in the off season, the more fat there is to take off in the pre-contest season. The process of gaining and losing large amounts of weight is called *yo-yo dieting*, and it is very stressful for the body.

The Dangers of Yo-Yo Dieting

Each cycle of yo-yo dieting makes it harder for the body to lose weight in subsequent diet attempts. Studies on rats, done by Dr. Eliot Stellar and Dr. Eileen Shrager at the Pennsylvania School of Medicine, revealed that rats forced to repeatedly gain and lose weight took longer to lose weight each time. Another study conducted by Dr. George Blackburn, a Harvard surgeon, found the same results in humans.

Yo-yo dieting might increase the desire for fatty foods. According to the results of animal experiments conducted by psychologist Judith Rodin at Yale, rats chose to eat more fats after dieting than they did before dieting. Bodybuilders can avoid this harmful cycle of yo-yo dieting. The solution is simply to eat intelligently during the off season, look stunning year-round, and eliminate the agony of contest dieting (Wardlaw and Insel, 1990).

Get Ripped: Periodization of Nutrition

Periodization of Nutrition is a brand new concept designed to augment the whole concept of periodized workouts. The training programs we prescribe show athletes how to train their bodies to achieve greater muscle mass, tone, and definition than ever before. Each phase of training is different and therefore places different demands on the body. The nutritional plans will show bodybuilders and strength athletes how to meet the specific nutritional needs of each phase. The greatest results are achieved when training and nutrition work together.

The perfectly sculpted body includes both muscularity and leanness. The proposed nutritional guidelines, therefore, recommend a diet that is lower in fat than the conventional diets of many bodybuilders. There are three basic concepts vital to effective nutrition, and these must be understood before going further into Periodization of Nutrition.

Calorie Cycling

The body continually works to maintain a state of balance (homeostasis). To achieve this, it is constantly adjusting to every change in both the external and internal environments. The body is very expressive about its condition. Some adjustments are experienced immediately, while others become apparent over a period of time. For instance, when the body is cold, we shiver; when it is hot, we sweat; when it is hurt or damaged, we feel pain. These reactions are experienced immediately. The adjustments made in response to food intake, however, are not as quickly discernible. When the body receives the same amount of food every day it regulates the basal metabolic rate (BMR) to use that amount of food energy efficiently. If this changes to a low-calorie diet, the body will initially keep burning the same number of calories as usual, which will result in weight loss over a period of time. Once the body detects disruption in the state of balance, it begins to adjust in order to compensate for the lower amount of food. The BMR drops so less food is used to produce energy and thus prevent starvation, and weight loss stops. This is one reason why crash or fad diets fail. This seemingly insurmountable natural phenomenon poses a problem for bodybuilders and strength trainers. The solution we propose is to establish eating patterns that fluctuate calorie intake more quickly than the body can adapt to the changes. By cycling calories to alternate low-, medium-, and high-calorie days (see figure 12.1), the metabolism rate will remain constant. The nutrition plans in this chapter are organized to provide low-, medium-, and high-calorie days.

Frequent Meals

The premise behind this concept is similar to calorie cycling in that it also prevents the slowing down of the metabolism. It is better to divide the daily calories into five or six small meals and eat frequently throughout the day, than to eat two or three big meals a day with long periods in between. When food intake is infrequent, this also tricks the body into sensing possible starvation, and the response is the same as for lower calorie intake. The metabolism slows, using some nutrients for immediate energy and preserving others as fat storage for use later. On the other

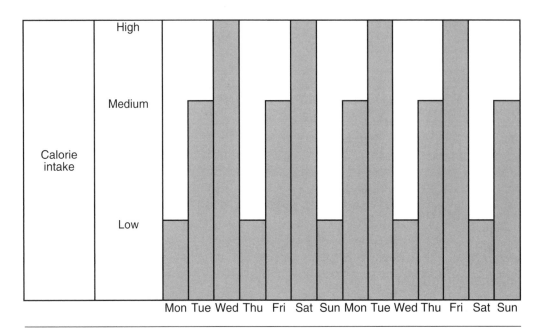

Figure 12.1 Calorie cycling over a 2-week period.

hand, when food intake is often, the body adjusts to this constant supply and continually uses all available nutrients for immediate energy.

The Cheat Day

The term *cheat day* is not uncommon to bodybuilders, although very few really understand the rationale behind it, or how to make a cheat day work for the body. In simple terms, a cheat day is a day planned for eating virtually anything.

The rationale behind cheat days is that they are planned to keep the body off-guard. They also work much the same as calorie cycling (see figure 12.2), in that

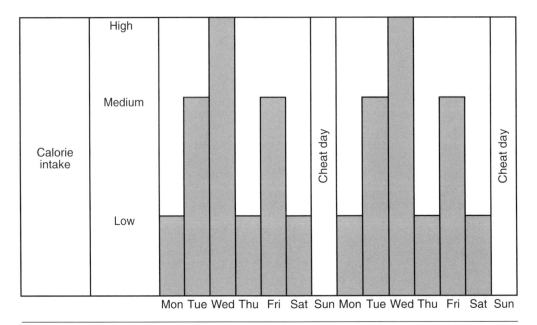

Figure 12.2 Calorie cycling over a 2-week period incorporating "Cheat Days."

they prevent the body from adapting to a specific caloric intake. If clean foods are eaten throughout the week and then suddenly, for one day, fats and sugars are eaten, the body rejects them and reacts by flushing them out of the system. Cheat days can also provide the body with some of the fat-soluble vitamins that might be missing from an ultra low-fat diet and give bodybuilders a psychological lift. In our society, eating is a very social activity and some people virtually abandon this when they become serious athletes. Cheat days restore some of this social activity, such as restaurant dining, popcorn at the theater, or a regular home-cooked meal. They are also a boost for the rest of the week. After a day of sinful eating, it is easier to be strict about the diet throughout the week.

To make cheat days work, some simple but important guidelines must be observed.

- No more than one cheat day per week.
- Clean food must be eaten throughout the rest of the week. No cheese, dessert, fried foods, or other foods of this nature, otherwise every day is a cheat day and this will show, literally!
- Plan the cheat day ahead of time. For example, if it is to be Sunday, make it Sunday every week.
- Maintain some control. A binge is still a binge no matter how you look at it.

Body Fat Testing

A good way to guard against gaining excess adipose tissue is to periodically test your body fat levels. For optimal fitness, experts recommend body fat levels of 12% to 18% for men, and 16% to 25% for women (Wilmore, 1986). For those interested in bodybuilding, even lower values are desirable to make muscle striations visible year-round, and to make contest dieting less traumatic to the body.

Yuhasz Technique of Skinfold Testing

Skinfold testing is an easy and accurate method of measuring the percentage of body fat (BF). Inexpensive skinfold calipers can be purchased in most fitness supply stores. You can also go to a gym where they have staff certified in fitness testing. Generally speaking, the more skinfold sites used during the test, the more representative the results.

The Yuhasz technique is used quite extensively throughout the sports world on many professionals and Olympic sports teams because of its accuracy and reproducible results. Therefore, we recommend it. Use the box to the left to record your findings.

Yuhasz Method of BF Testing				
	Trial 1	Trial 2	Trial 3	Average
Triceps				
Subscapular				
Suprailiac				
Abdomen				
Front thigh				
Chest (men only)				
Rear thigh (women only)				

Testing Sites

The Yuhasz technique uses six sites as opposed to the three or four sites used in many other tests. It measures the "trouble areas" on both men and women—chest for men and rear thigh for women. Other tests that do not include these skinfold sites might underestimate your BF level.

For results to be accurate and meaningful, the testing must be done accurately and precisely. For re-testing purposes, measurements must always be done the same way and taken in the same places. Use the following instructions as a guideline.

1. Firmly grasp a fold of skin between the thumb and forefinger, and lift up.
2. Place the contact surfaces of the caliper about one centimeter from the fingers.
3. Very slightly release the pressure of the fingers so the greater pressure is exerted by the caliper.
4. Release the scissor grip, supporting the weight of the caliper in the hand.
5. When the needle stops, take the reading to the nearest tenth of a millimeter. (Be careful of jaw face slippage on the skin.) (Gledhill, 1987)

Triceps.   The skinfold is located midway on the back of the upper arm. The arm hangs freely and the skinfold is lifted parallel to its long axis.

Subscapular.   The skinfold is lifted vertically and measured below the tip of the scapula.

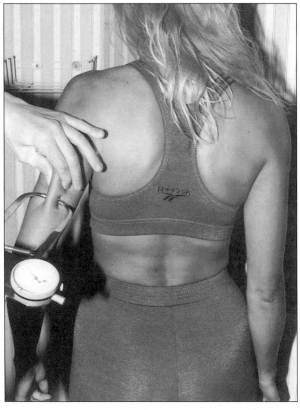

Triceps.

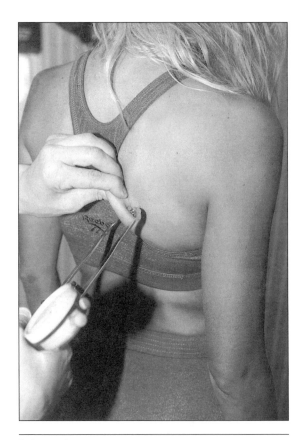

Subscapular.

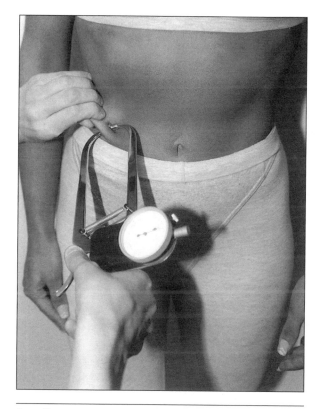

Suprailiac.

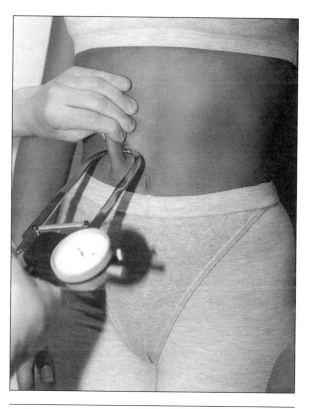

Abdomen.

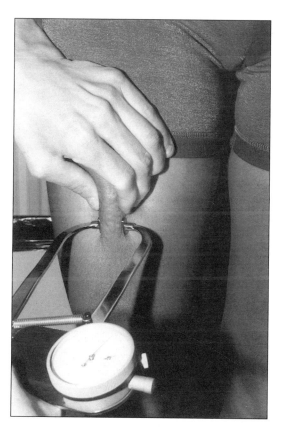

Front thigh.

Suprailiac. The skinfold is located immediately above the crest of the ilium. The fold is lifted at a slight angle to the vertical along the normal fold line.

Abdomen. The skinfold is located to the left of, adjacent to, and in line with the navel. The fold is lifted parallel to the long axis of the body.

Front Thigh. The skinfold is located midway on the front of the upper leg over the quadriceps. The foot is placed on a six-inch step with the knee slightly flexed and muscles relaxed. The fold is lifted parallel to the long axis of the leg.

Chest (Men Only). The site is located above and slightly to the right of the right nipple. The skinfold is taken at a 45-degree angle of the horizontal.

Rear Thigh (Women Only). The skinfold is located midway on the back of the upper leg. The leg is held in the same position as the front thigh measurements. The skinfold is lifted parallel to the axis of the leg.

Yuhasz Calculations

Use the values from the skinfold measurements in the equations that follow to calculate percent body fat.

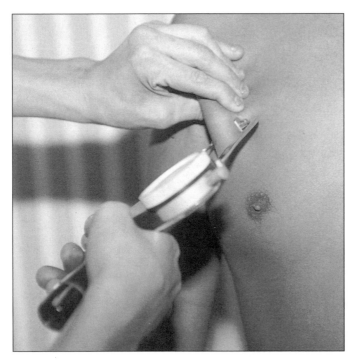

Chest (men only).

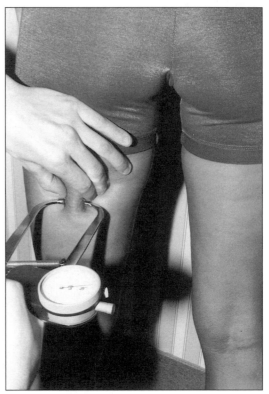

Rear thigh (women only).

Men 16-30 years	**%BF = (sum of 6 skinfolds x .097) + 3.64**
Men 30+ years	**%BF = (sum of 6 skinfolds x .1066) + 4.975**
Women 16-30 years	**%BF = (sum of 6 skinfolds x .217) − 4.47**
Women 30+ years	**%BF = (sum of 6 skinfolds x .224) − 2.8**

Drawbacks With Skinfold Testing

The accuracy of the test depends on the skill of the tester. The tester must pinch the appropriate amount of fat, place the calipers correctly, and pick the correct testing sites on the body. Higher quality calipers will yield more accurate results (Lohman et al., 1984).

Bioelectrical Impedance Analysis

Bioelectrical impedance analysis (BIA) is another method of testing body fat levels. It is based on the fact that the body contains intracellular and extracellular fluids that are capable of conducting electrical currents. It is a known fact that the body's *fat-free mass (FFM)* contains much of the body's water and electrolytes and therefore, is a better conductor of electrical current than fat (Lukaski, 1985).

How BIA Works

An electrode is placed on each hand and foot of the prone subject and an electrical current is applied through these electrodes. Impedance to the current is detected by the electrodes and is used to determine the body's FFM

(Lukaski et al., 1985). FFM is then used to determine the subject's percentage of body fat. This is a completely painless process and no current is felt by the subject.

Drawbacks of BIA

Accuracy depends on many external factors, such as electrode placement, dehydration, food and alcohol consumption, and exercise (Caton et al., 1988). If the tester is inexperienced in BIA testing, or if the testing guidelines are not stringently followed, the measurement will be inaccurate.

Body fat is consistently overestimated in extremely lean subjects, while for obese subjects, percentage of body fat is consistently underestimated (Heyward, 1991).

Hydrostatic Weighing (Underwater Weighing)

Hydrostatic weighing is the most accurate and reliable method for testing %BF. The test involves complicated equipment and must be administered by a skilled technician. Elite testing centers for athletes, such as universities, often provide this service. If it can be arranged, hydrostatic weighing will give you the most accurate reading of your body fat levels available.

How Hydrostatic Weighing Works

To calculate %BF using this method, the technician first determines the subject's dry-land body weight and *residual volume (RV)*. Residual volume is the amount of air remaining in the lungs following a complete exhalation. When these are determined, the subject is submerged in a tank of water and instructed to exhale as much air as possible. Once the subject is motionless, the *underwater weight (UWW)* is recorded. These values are then used in an equation that provides an accurate %BF reading, taking into account dry-land body weight, UWW, RV, water temperature, and weight of the equipment.

The basic premise behind hydrostatic weighing is that since fat is buoyant and weightless under water, the subject's underwater weight will reflect the amount of his or her FFM. Put simply, the heavier you are under water, the leaner you are.

Drawbacks of Hydrostatic Weighing

Three main issues may affect the accuracy of hydrostatic weighing. First, a subject might have a fear of being completely submerged under water. Also, a subject might feel uncomfortable doing a maximal exhalation and holding his or her breath under water. Finally, if the subject is a woman, she might retain more fluid at certain times during her menstrual cycle, causing a change in the amount of her total underwater body weight. This might significantly affect her %BF reading. To correct this, a woman should be tested at a time in her cycle when she is not retaining water (Bunt, Lohman, and Boileau, 1989).

CHAPTER 13

MUSCLE RECOVERY BETWEEN WORKOUTS

Recovery is one of the most important elements of successful training. Athletes who understand this concept will avoid critical fatigue and overtraining.

Recovery From Fatigue

Strength athletes are constantly exposed to various types of training loads, reps, and sets, some of which can often exceed their threshold of tolerance. As a result, the ability to adapt to the desired training load decreases, thus affecting the athlete's overall performance.

When athletes drive themselves beyond their physiological limits, they risk going into a state of fatigue. Basically, the greater the level of fatigue, the greater the training aftereffects, such as low rate of recovery, decreased coordination, and diminished power output. Fatigue experienced in training can often be increased by personal factors, such as stressful conditions in social, school, or work situations.

Muscular fatigue is commonly associated with exercise-induced muscle damage. This is a very complex physiological and psychological phenomenon. Although much research has been devoted to muscular fatigue, neither the exact sites nor the exact causes are well known.

In order to improve muscle size and strength, it is important that training loads be as high as necessary to provide a stimulus for adaptation. In order for the adaptation to take place, training programs must constantly incorporate periods of work with rest, while alternating different levels of intensity. These

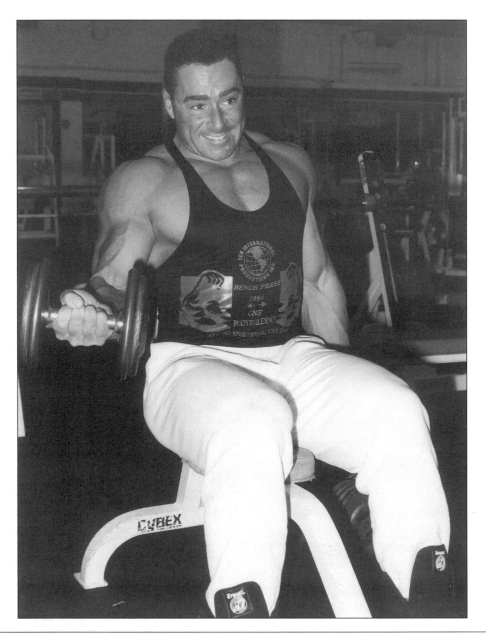

Vito Binetti pushing himself to the limit.

factors will result in a good balance between work and rest. It is important to avoid large increments in training loads. The exposure to heavy loads far beyond an athlete's capacity, or miscalculating necessary rest, will result in decreased ability to adapt to the new load. Failing adaptation triggers biochemical and neural reactions that take an athlete from a state of fatigue to chronic fatigue, and ultimately to the undesirable state of overtraining. Irrespective of its definition, it is certain that fatigue results from physical work that reduces the capacity of the neuromuscular and metabolic systems to continue physical activity.

Researchers have attempted to identify sites of fatigue and, consequently, performance failure, through a conventional simplification of complex phenomenon with many unknown elements. The focus of this section, however, will be on the two main sites, the neuromuscular and metabolic.

Neuromuscular Fatigue

While the general assumption is that fatigue originates in the muscles, clearly the CNS also plays an important role, since incentive, stress, temperature, and other psychological factors can cause fatigue. Increasing evidence suggests that the CNS might be involved in the limitation of performance to a greater extent than once assumed.

The CNS has two basic processes, which are *excitation* and *inhibition*. Excitation is a very favorable, stimulating process for physical activity, while inhibition is a restraining process. Throughout training there is a constant alternation of the two processes. For any stimulation, the CNS sends a nerve impulse to the working muscle causing it to contract and perform work. The speed, power, and frequency of the nerve impulse directly depend on the state of the CNS.

The nerve impulses are most effective when controlled excitation prevails, which is evidenced by a good performance. When the opposite occurs, as a result of fatigue, the nerve cell is in a state of inhibition and the muscle contraction is slower and weaker. The force of contraction relates directly to the electrical activation sent by the CNS and the number of motor units recruited. Therefore, as fatigue increases, the recruitment of motor units decreases.

The nerve cell working capacity cannot be maintained for a very long time. Under the strain of training or competition demands, the working capacity decreases. If high intensity is maintained as a result of fatigue, the nerve cell

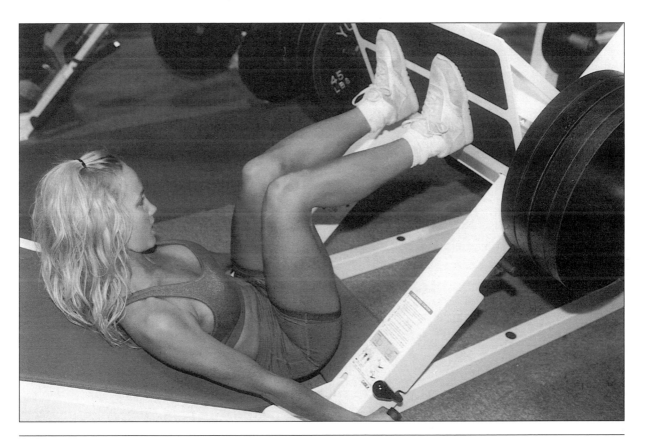

Fitness model Lisa Rutherford.

assumes a state of inhibition to protect itself from external stimuli. Fatigue, therefore, should be seen as the body's way of protecting itself against damage to the contractile mechanism of the muscle.

The skeletal muscle produces force by activating its motor units and regulating their firing frequency, which progressively increases in order to enhance force output. Fatigue that inhibits muscular activity can be neutralized to some degree by a modulating strategy: by responding to fatigue through the ability of the motor units to alter firing frequency. As a result, the muscle can maintain force more effectively under a certain state of fatigue. If the duration of sustained maximum contraction increases, the frequency of the motor units firing decreases, and inhibition will become more prominent (Sherwood, 1993).

Marsden et al. (1971) demonstrated that compared to the start of a 30 second maximum voluntary contraction, the end firing frequency decreased by 80%. Similar findings were reported by Grimby et al. (1992) who stated that, as the duration of contraction increased, activation of large motor units decreased, lowering the firing rate below the threshold level. Any continuation of contraction beyond that level was possible through short bursts (phasical firing), but not appropriate for a constant performance.

The above findings should caution those who promote the theory (especially in football and bodybuilding) that muscle size and strength can only be achieved by performing each set to exhaustion. The fact that as a contraction progresses, the firing frequency decreases, discredits this highly-acclaimed method.

When analyzing the functional capacity of the CNS during fatigue, one must consider the bodybuilder's perceived fatigue and past physical capacity achieved

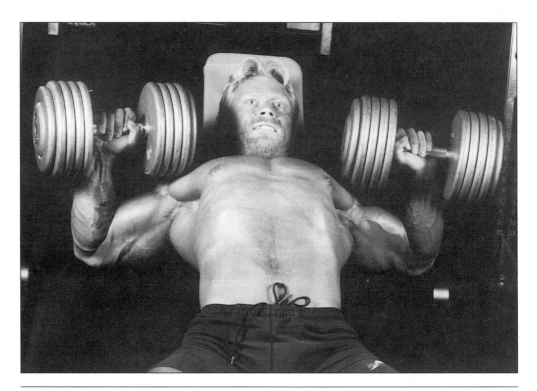

Repping out!

in training. When the athlete's physical capacity is above the level of fatigue experienced in testing or competition, it enhances one's motivation and, as a result, the capacity to overcome fatigue.

Metabolic Sources of Fatigue

Muscle fatigue may be associated with the mechanism of calcium flux in skeletal muscle, although the relationship still remains a mystery. The complex cycle of muscle contraction is triggered by the nerve impulse that depolarizes the surface membrane of the muscle cell, and is then conducted into the muscle fiber. This is followed by a series of events where calcium is bound together with protein filaments (actin and myosin), resulting in contractile tension.

The functional site of fatigue is suggested to be the link between excitation-contraction, which results in either reducing the intensity of these two processes or in decreasing the sensitivity to activation. Changes in the flux of calcium ions affect the operation of excitation-contraction (Sherwood, 1993).

Fatigue Due to Lactic Acid Accumulation

The accumulation of lactic acid in the muscle causes decreased contractile activity in response to stimulation (Fox et al., 1989). As bodybuilders predominantly use anaerobic systems, they rely on anaerobic types of fuels, resulting in increased production and accumulation of lactic acid. The onset of fatigue varies with the type of muscle fiber. Heavy loads cause FT fibers to produce high levels of lactates, which causes these fibers to be affected first.

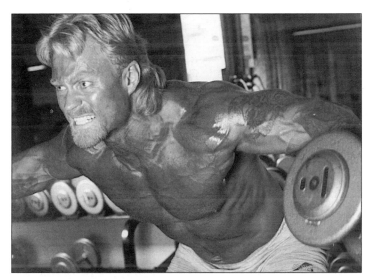

Trevor Butler, desperately trying to fight the onset of lactic acid.

The biochemical exchanges during muscle contraction result in the liberation of hydrogen ions, which in turn produce acidosis (lactate fatigue), which seems to determine the point of exhaustion (Sherwood, 1993).

An increased acidosis also inhibits the binding capacity of calcium through inactivation of troponin, a protein compound. Since troponin is an important contributor to the contraction of the muscle cell, its inactivation might expand the connection between fatigue and exercise. The discomfort produced by acidosis can also be a limiting factor in psychological fatigue (Sherwood, 1993).

Fatigue Due to the Depletion of ATP/CP and Glycogen Stores

The energy system experiences fatigue when the creatine phosphate (CP) is depleted from the working muscle, when muscle glycogen is consumed, or when the carbohydrate store is exhausted (Sahlin, 1986; Sherwood, 1993). The result is obvious. The work performed by the muscle is decreased, possibly because in a glycogen-depleted muscle, the adenosine triphosphate (ATP) is

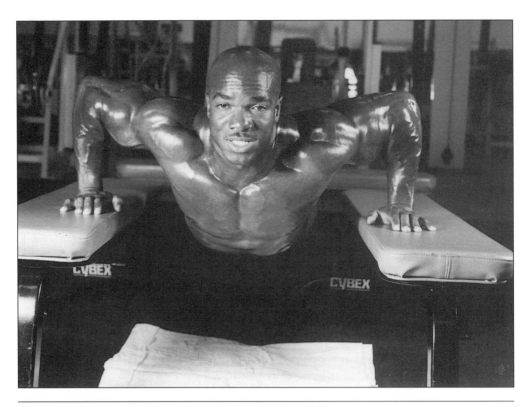

Wesley Mohammed finishing his grueling chest workout.

produced at a lower rate than it is consumed. Several studies show that carbohydrates are essential in the ability of a muscle to maintain high force. Endurance capacity during prolonged moderate- to heavy-bodybuilding activity relates directly to the amount of glycogen in the muscle prior to exercise. This indicates that fatigue occurs as a result of muscle glycogen depletion (Fox et al., 1989). For high-intensity sets, the immediate sources of energy for muscular contraction are ATP and CP. Complete depletion of these stores in the muscle will certainly limit the ability of the muscle to contract (Sherwood, 1993).

With prolonged submaximum work where high reps occur, the fuels used to produce energy are glucose and fatty acids. The availability of oxygen is, therefore, critical throughout this type of training because, in limited quantities, carbohydrates are oxidized instead of free fatty acids. The maximum free fatty acid oxidation will be determined by the inflow of the fatty acids to the working muscle, and by the aerobic training status of the athlete (Sahlin, 1986). The lack of oxygen, the oxygen carrying capacity, and inadequate blood flow all make important contributions to muscular fatigue (Grimby et al., 1992).

Muscle Soreness

There are two basic mechanisms that explain how exercise initiates muscle damage. One is associated with the disturbance of metabolic function, while the other refers to the mechanical disruption of the muscle cell. Whenever muscle soreness occurs, one should immediately alter the training program, because pursuing it at the same level will bring the strength trainer or bodybuilder one step closer to overtraining.

The metabolic mechanism of muscle damage occurs during prolonged submaximum work to exhaustion. Direct loading of the muscle, especially during the eccentric contraction phase, may cause muscle damage, and that metabolic change may aggravate the damage. Disruption of the muscle cell membrane is one of the most noticeable damages.

Eccentric muscle contraction has been known to produce more heat than concentric contraction at the same workload. The increased temperatures can damage structural and functional components within the muscle cell (Armstrong, 1986; Ebbing and Clarkson, 1989).

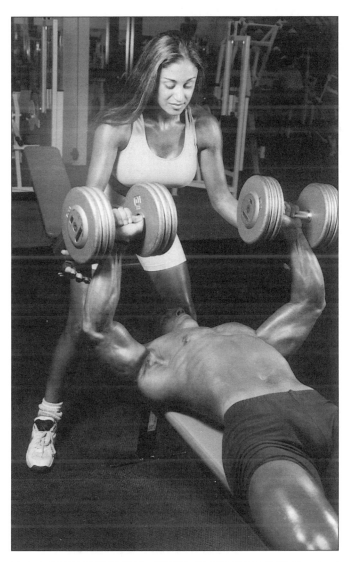

Nino Vojinovic performing eccentric contractions.

Both mechanisms of muscle damage are related to muscle fibers that have been stressed slightly, and when this occurs, they quickly return to normal length without injury. If the stress is severe, the muscle becomes traumatized. Discomfort sets in during the first 24 to 48 hours following the exercise. The sensation of dull aching pain, combined with tenderness and stiffness, tends to diminish within 5-7 days after the initial workout.

For years, lactic acid build-up was considered the main cause of muscle soreness. Research has discovered, however, that the actual cause results from an influx of calcium ions into the muscle cell (Fahey, 1991; Armstrong, 1986; Evans, 1987; Ebbing and Clarkson, 1989).

Calcium is very important in a muscle contraction. It stimulates the fiber to contract, and is rapidly pumped back into the calcium storage area after completion of the contraction. When calcium ions accumulate within the muscle fiber, it causes the release of a substance called *protease* that results in muscle fiber breakdown. The soreness is primarily due to the formation of degraded protein components, or dead tissue. The body initiates a "clean-up" phase to eliminate muscle cells of dead tissue. The muscle starts producing stress protein, which is a protective mechanism to stop further damage. This explains why muscle soreness is not felt every day.

Once a muscle has been traumatized, there is an accumulation of substances, such as histamine, serotonin, potassium, and others, that are responsible for the inflammation occurring to the injured muscle fiber (Prentice, 1990). Once the level of these substances has reached a certain degree, they activate the nerve endings. Perhaps the reason muscle soreness is felt 24 hours later is due to the time required for the damaged muscle cells to accumulate all of these substances (Armstrong, 1986; Ebbing and Clarkson, 1989).

The discomfort and soreness are felt intensely in the region of the muscle-tendon junction. This is because the tendon tissue is less flexible than the muscle tissue, so there is a high chance of injury from intense contraction. As one might expect, during high-intensity training greater damage occurs in the FT fibers than the ST fibers because FT fibers play a greater role in more intense contraction.

The most important preventative technique for the athlete to consider in training is to use the principle of progressive increase of load. Furthermore, applying the concept of Periodization will avoid discomfort, muscle soreness, and any other negative training outcomes.

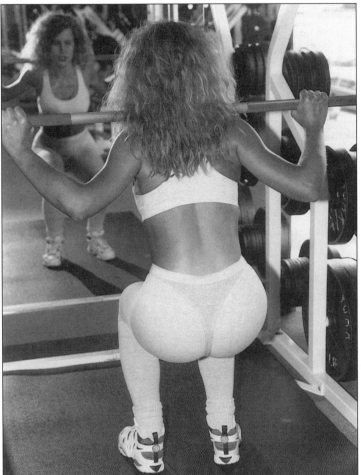

Fitness model Sue Minicucci always warms up.

An extensive overall warm-up will result in better preparation of the body for work. Superficial warm-ups, on the other hand, can easily result in strain and pain. Good stretching sessions at the end of the warm-up, between sets, and at the end of the workout, aid in preventing muscle soreness.

As a result of extensive muscle contraction, typical of strength training, muscles might take up to two hours to reach their resting length. Five to ten minutes of stretching allows the muscle to reach its resting length much faster. This is optimal for biochemical exchanges at the muscle fiber level. At the same time, stretching also seems to ease muscle spasm.

It has been proposed that ingesting 100 milligrams of vitamin C per day may prevent or reduce muscle soreness. Similar benefits seem to result from taking vitamin E. Taking anti-inflammatory medication, such as aspirin, may help combat inflammation of muscle tissue (Sherwood 1993).

Diet is also considered an important element in supplying the athlete with needed nutrition and in aiding the recovery from muscle soreness. Strength trainers and bodybuilders exposed to heavy loads require more protein, carbohydrates, and supplementation in their diets.

Recovery From Strength Training

Whether recovering from fatigue, overtraining, or just an exhausting training session, it is important for an athlete to be aware of the various techniques

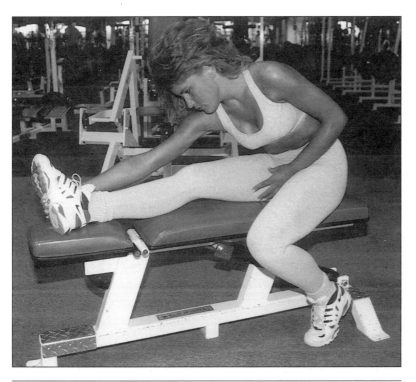

Stretching between sets and at the end of a workout aids in preventing muscle soreness.

available. Understanding the use of these techniques is just as important as knowing how to train effectively. As the athlete continually strives to implement new loads into the training program, the recovery methods are often not adjusted to match these new loads. This situation can harbor potential setbacks with respect to peaking and regeneration following training. Approximately 50% of an athlete's final performance depends on the ability to recover by using recovery techniques. Without the use of proper recovery techniques, adaptation to various training loads might not be achieved.

It is vital for an athlete to be aware of all the factors that contribute to the recovery process, because it is the combination of all these factors in varying degrees that affects the recovery process. The main factors for consideration are listed below:

- The age of the athlete has been shown to affect the rate of recovery. Older athletes generally require longer periods of recuperation than their younger counterparts.

- The better trained, more experienced athlete generally requires less time to recuperate. This is related to a quicker physiological adaptation to a given training stimulus.

- Gender may affect the rate of recovery. Female athletes tend to have a slower rate of recovery. The reason for this is primarily due to differences in the endocrine systems of male and female athletes.

- Environmental factors such as time differences, altitude, and cold climates tend to lessen the affect of the recovery process.

- Replenishment of foodstuff at the cellular level has been shown to affect the recovery process. Proteins, fats, carbohydrates, and ATP/CP restoration within the working muscle cell are constantly required for cellular metabolism, as well as for the production of energy (Fox et al., 1989; Bompa, 1994).

- Negative emotions such as fear, indecisiveness, and lack of willpower, tend to impair the recovery process.

- The recovery process is slow and directly dependent on the magnitude of the load employed in training.

Recovery time depends upon the energy system that is being utilized. Recommended recovery times after exhaustive strength training are presented

Table 13.1 Suggested recovery times after exhaustive training

Recovery process	Recovery time
Restoration of ATP/CP	3–5 minutes
Restoration of muscle glycogen: After prolonged exercise After intermittent exercise (such as strength training)	10–48 hours 24 hours
Removal of lactic acid from muscle and blood	1–2 hours
Restoration of vitamins and enzymes	24 hours
Recovery from high-intensity strength training (both metabolic and CNS to reach overcompensation)	2–3 days
Repayment of the alactacid oxygen debt	5 minutes
Repayment of the lactacid debt	30–60 minutes

in table 13.1. The effectiveness of recovery techniques is greatly dependent on the time they are employed. It is strongly recommended that they be performed during and following each training session (Bompa, 1994; Kuipers and Keizer, 1988; Fry et al., 1991).

Recovery From Short-Term Overtraining

To overcome the effects of short-term overtraining, sessions must be interrupted for 3-5 days. After this rest period, training can be resumed by alternating a training session with a rest day. If overtraining is more severe and the initial rest period is extended, then every week of rest will require roughly two weeks of training to attain the athlete's previous physical condition (Terjung and Hood, 1988).

Repair of damaged muscle tissue falls under the category of short-term overtraining, requiring at least 5-7 days to complete the process, while the regeneration of muscle tissue takes up to 20 days (Ebbing and Clarkson, 1989).

Recovery from muscle damage during the acute phase is best treated with ice, elevation, compression, and active or complete rest, depending upon the extent of the damage. After three days, the coach should begin to introduce other methods of therapy, such as massage. Alternation of hot and cold temperatures can also be an effective way to loosen the stiffness associated with exercise-induced muscle damage (Arnheim, 1988; Prentice, 1990).

According to Fahey (1991), diet may play an important role in muscle tissue recovery. In addition to the obvious need for protein, particularly animal protein, carbohydrates are also required. It has been shown that recovery from muscle injury is delayed when the muscle carbohydrate stores are not adequate. It is vital, therefore, that the athlete pay strict attention to diet from a nutritional basis and from a recovery standpoint.

The use of some vitamin supplements is generally popular when it comes to dealing with muscle damage. Fahey (1991) and Yessis (1990) both feel that vitamins E and C can be of great benefit to the athlete in terms of assisting in the recovery process.

In the case of excitement and sleeping disorders, administration of supportive sedatives might be considered. (Your personal physician can suggest the best sedative for you.) For any injuries, it is important for the bodybuilder or athlete to seek the advice and assistance of qualified physicians and physiotherapists.

Recovery From Injuries

Any serious participant in the sport of bodybuilding and strength training can attest to the wear-and-tear, fatigue, and muscle soreness that can result from a particularly strenuous training session. These aches and pains are caused by microtraumas to the muscle fibers. It is better to treat than to ignore any type of muscle damage, no matter how insignificant it might seem.

Some recovery techniques are very simple and can be done alone, while others might require the help of a friend or even an exercise or physical therapist. We will cover some of the most common and useful recovery and injury prevention techniques.

Flexibility

Flexibility is defined as the ability of a joint to move easily through its entire range of motion (ROM), and it is a very important component of one's overall health and fitness. Good flexibility is known to decrease the incidence of musculotendinous injuries, minimize muscular soreness, promote circulation and relaxation, and improve coordination by allowing increased freedom and ease of movement (Anderson, 1980).

Unfortunately, most bodybuilders either never stretch before or after their workouts, or they stretch incorrectly. This can only be detrimental to their training. If athletes take the time to stretch, before and after each workout, there will be less likelihood of injury. The muscles will also receive the benefit of being strengthened through a greater range of motion, which can lead to greater strength gains.

Where flexibility is concerned, we are dealing with two types of tissue:

- Contractile: These structures include muscles, tendons, and their attachment to bone. They are influenced by the tension placed on them either by contraction or stretching of the muscle.

- Noncontractile: These tissues include joint capsules, ligaments, bursa, cartilage, and all other structures that are noncontractile.

Muscle length is monitored by stretch receptors embedded within the muscle. These receptors monitor information about muscle length and the rate of change that occurs during a movement. This information is then fed to the spinal cord and higher centers, which respond by stimulating protective adjustments that are essential in avoiding muscle injury (Enoka, 1994). When a muscle is lengthened, stretched, or contracted, these receptors fire a signal to the CNS that a change is occurring within the muscle.

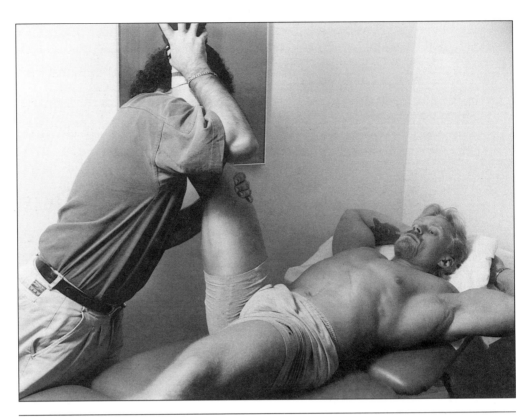

Physiotherapist Lenny Visconti (left) performing a static stretch.

The two receptors involved in muscle activity are the muscle spindle and the golgi tendon organ. The muscle spindles react to the muscle stretch by firing and slowing down the rate of lengthening in the muscle. This is an important mechanism in the prevention of muscle tears caused by exceeding the physiological length of the muscle. Subsequently, the golgi tendon organ responds when the muscle is contracted. The forces that are generated by the contracting muscle fibers pull on the tendons where the golgi tendon organs are located. This results in the firing of the golgi tendon organ that acts to slow down the rate of contraction and maximize the function of the contractile proteins, actin and myosin.

Types of Stretching

Ballistic/dynamic stretching involves bouncing and jerking motions that activate the stretch reflex, causing contraction (not relaxation) of the muscles being stretched (Moore and Hutton, 1980). Ballistic stretching may result in microtraumas to both contractile and noncontractile tissues by forcing the joint beyond its normal ROM. The motions are so fast that tissue tears can occur without the athlete's immediate knowledge; therefore, this type of stretching is not recommended.

Static stretching is a slow, gentle stretch that is held for at least 30 seconds. The joint is taken to the end of its ROM, then gentle pressure is applied to stretch the muscle further. The stretch is held at the point of tightness and should never reach the point of pain. Slow, static stretching is a safer technique than ballistic stretching, because pain would be felt in the muscle fiber before tissue damage could occur.

Warm-Up Cue:

> Temperature greatly affects flexibility. Warming up a joint will increase the extensibility of connective tissue and reduce the risk of muscle strain (Enoka, 1994). It is, therefore, important to warm-up the joints and muscles before stretching. This can be done by performing some light aerobic activity, such as biking, slow jogging, or using the stepping machine for 5 to 10 minutes.

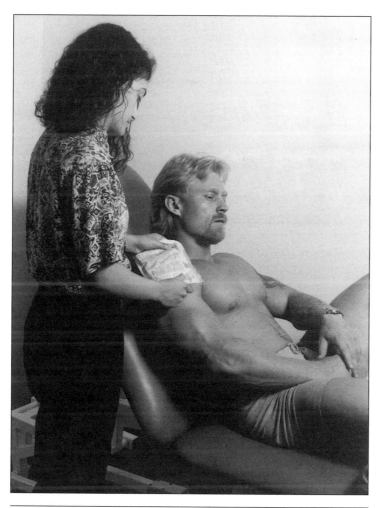

Physiotherapist Shiraz Kapadia (left) applying a cold pack.

Cold Therapy

The therapeutic value of cold therapy (cryotherapy) is often overlooked by bodybuilders and other athletes. The most common forms of cold therapy include ice packs, ice baths, cryogel packs, and ice massage.

Physiological Responses to Cold Therapy

The body responds to cold therapy in many ways. One response is a decrease in swelling.

The key to managing injuries in the acute phase (24 to 48 hours post-injury) is to limit the amount of soft-tissue swelling, because this creates most of the cellular damage, through local tissue hypoxia (deficiency of oxygen) and through the release of chemical mediators (Halvorson, 1990).

The application of cold controls swelling in the following ways:

- It decreases circulation to the injured site by constricting blood vessels in and around the site, which causes blood to become more viscous, or resistant to flow.

- It decreases local fluid accumulation and promotes the absorption of excess fluid.

Cold therapy can also cause a decrease in hemorrhaging. It is thought that the application of cold reflexively controls the bleeding of lacerated blood vessels.

A third benefit of cold therapy can be a decrease in muscle spasm and pain. Studies have shown that the application of cold to an injury decreases the nerve conduction velocity of the gamma motor neurons. These neurons control the spindle muscle fibers and, when activated, provoke the stretch reflex within the muscle (i.e., causes muscle contraction). A reduction in the velocity of gamma motor neurons, therefore, slows down fiber activation and spasticity and consequently helps to relieve pain (Kowal, 1983; Low and Reed, 1990; Wadsworth and Chanmugam, 1983).

Method of Application

The recommended length of time for cold therapy is 10-20 minutes. Depending upon the severity of the injury, it can be applied as often as every hour until swelling is controlled.

Caution

People with peripheral vascular diseases, such as severe blood pressure abnormalities, cardiac abnormalities, or impaired skin sensation, should use cold therapy under the supervision of a physiotherapist or physician.

To avoid frostbite or cold burns, simply place a tissue or thin cloth between the skin and the ice pack.

Cold Therapy and Prevention of Injury

Cold application is highly recommended for bodybuilders following intense training sessions. This will prevent excessive fluid accumulation and muscle soreness that might result from lactic acid build-up or microtearing of the muscle tissue. By treating minor discomforts as they occur, the athlete can better prevent injury and continue with his or her strenuous training.

Heat Therapy

Heat therapy, like cold therapy, is an inexpensive yet effective method of treating injuries. It is administered through the use of hydrocollator (i.e., moist heat) packs, hot compresses, whirlpools, hydrotherapy, electric heating pads, and contrast baths.

Physiological Responses to Heat Therapy

The body responds to heat therapy in many ways.

- Decreased joint stiffness.
- Decreased muscle spasm: heat is thought to relieve muscle spasm by decreasing gamma motor neuron conduction velocity, which in turn decreases muscle spindle activity (contraction).
- Decreased pain: heat also reduces the conduction velocity of the "c" nerve fibers that are responsible for carrying pain messages to the CNS.

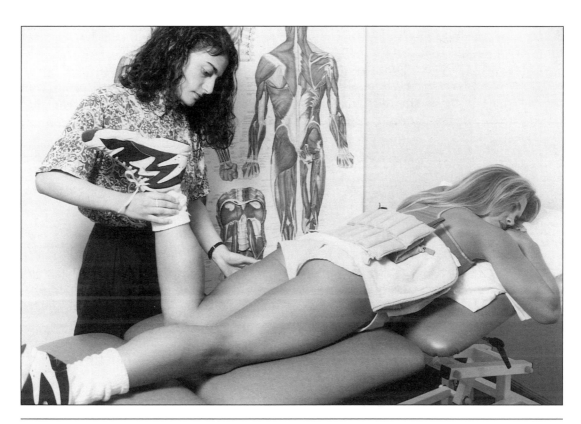

The application of a hot pack seems to increase the blood flow and decrease the pain.

- Increased extensibility of collagen tissue.
- Increased blood flow: heat causes vasodilation and a subsequent increase in the flow of nutrients, antibodies, leukocytes, and oxygen to the tissues, all of which aid in tissue healing.
- Hastened resolution of inflammatory infiltrates, edema, and excessive fluid accumulation (Halvorson, 1990; Low and Reed, 1990; Wadsworth and Chanmugam,1983).

Method of Application

A heat therapy session should last no longer than 20 minutes. The main concern when using heat therapy is the avoidance of burns. When using hydrocollator packs or a heating pad, make sure that there is sufficient toweling between the heat source and the skin. The temperature of whirlpool baths must be closely monitored and should not exceed 108 degrees Fahrenheit (41 degrees Celsius).

Contrast baths use both hot and cold therapies. The injured limb is kept in hot water for one minute and then in cold water for thirty seconds. This cycle can be repeated for 15-20 minutes. The purpose of the contrast bath is to increase local circulation within the injured limb through alternating vasodilation with vasoconstriction. It is probably most useful in the treatment of chronic musculoskeletal injuries that need increased blood flow (Walsh, 1986).

Caution

Take the above precautions to avoid the possibility of burns. Use heat cautiously, or not at all, on subjects with dermatological conditions, open or infected wounds, impaired skin sensation, or gross edema. Do not apply heat to areas affected by circulatory disease.

Heat or Ice?

The physiological effects of heat and cold are quite similar, although the mechanisms are different. The current practice is to use cold therapy on acute soft-tissue injuries and overuse injuries. It is the safest choice when the main concern is the control of swelling and bleeding in the injured tissue. The use of heat is advised once the swelling has subsided and the soft tissues and joints are stiff. By increasing the temperature of the collagen, it is easier to stretch the connective tissue and adhesions.

Rule of thumb: always use cold therapy before heat therapy.

Acupuncture

Acupuncture is used to encourage natural healing, reduce or relieve pain, and improve the function of affected areas of the body. It involves the insertion of very fine needles through the skin and into the tissues at specific points on the body. There is no injection of any substance into the tissues.

Acupuncture points correspond to known neural structures and can be found in the following areas:

- Close to the motor points of muscles
- Along the peripheral nerves
- Where cranial nerves emerge
- In the midline where segmental nerves meet
- At muscle tendon junctions

How Does Acupuncture Work?

Acupuncture stimulates the body to produce its own pain-relieving chemicals called *endorphins*. These chemicals mimic the drug morphine by attaching to opiate receptors found throughout the nervous system. Endorphins help to block the pathways that relay pain messages from the body to the brain, which results in reduced pain. Endorphins also help to regulate the body's biochemical system, which causes a reduction of inflammation and promotes natural healing.

How Safe Is Acupuncture?

There are very few adverse effects or complications from acupuncture therapy. Occasionally, mild bruising, temporary aggravation of symptoms, or syncope

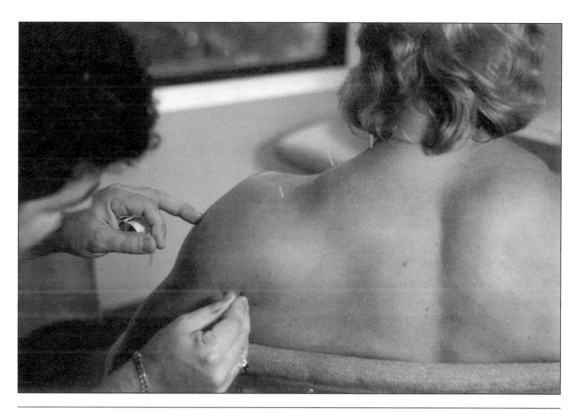

The insertion of acupuncture needles to reduce or relieve pain.

(fainting) may occur with acupuncture. Women in the early stages of pregnancy and hemophiliacs need to be treated with caution.

The average treatment lasts from 15-30 minutes. The number of treatments needed will vary depending upon the individual and the condition being treated. The depth of needle insertion depends on the location of the acupuncture point. The number of needles used normally ranges from 3 to 6.

Due to the heightened awareness of the AIDS virus today, many people fear contact with needles of any sort. The Acupuncture Foundation of Canada Institute (AFCI) recommends the use of only sterile disposable needles, in order to prevent the risk of infection and, in particular, to eliminate any possibility of contracting either the AIDS or the hepatitis virus (AFCI Patient Education Brochure, 1994).

Ultrasound

Ultrasound is probably the most common modality used in the treatment of soft-tissue injuries. It is a form of acoustic vibration, propagated in the form of longitudinal compression waves, at frequencies that are too high to be heard by the human ear (Low and Reed, 1990).

The Effects of Ultrasound

An electrical current is applied to a crystal that is housed in the transducer head, which causes the crystal to vibrate and produce sound waves. This vibration is transmitted to the tissues in the body through a coupling medium,

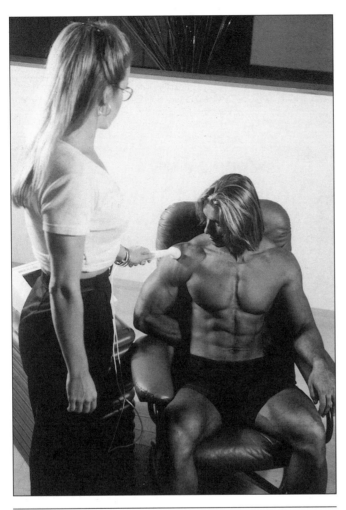

The use of ultrasound to treat soft-tissue injuries.

which is usually a water-soluble gel. The sound waves create a micromassage effect by alternating compression and relaxation of the tissue, and the energy created by the oscillating particles is converted into heat energy (Low and Reed, 1990).

Physiological Effects of Ultrasound

- Micromassage of tissues: the vibration caused by ultrasound causes collagen fiber separation.
- Increase in tissue temperature: the heat caused by ultrasound produces the following effects:
  - Decrease in pain and muscle spasm
  - Increased blood flow and lymphatic flow
  - Increased collagen tissue extensibility
  - Decrease in nerve conduction velocity
- Altering of the permeability of capillaries: by altering capillary permeability, ultrasound helps in the resorption of exudate and adhesions (Low and Reed, 1990; Wadsworth and Chanmugam, 1983).

Ultrasound can be used in all three stages of connective tissue healing.

Acute Stage

During this stage, which occurs 0 to 3 days post trauma, ultrasound causes the release of histamine, which can accelerate the normal resolution of inflammation. This may be due to the agitation of the tissue fluid, which increases the rate of phagocytosis (the engulfing and the destruction of harmful cells and the remnants of white blood cells used to fight the infection) (Low and Reed, 1990).

Granulation Stage

During this stage (3 days to 21 days post trauma), the connective tissue framework for the new blood vessels is laid down by cells known as *fibroblasts*. Ultrasound stimulates the fibroblasts to promote collagen synthesis. It promotes collagen of greater tensile strength, which will reduce the likelihood of reinjury (Enwemcka et al., 1990). Ultrasound also encourages the growth of new capillaries in chronic ischemic tissues (Low and Reed, 1990).

Remodeling Stage

When the body is left to heal on its own, collagen fibers are laid down in a haphazard fashion. The ultrasound aids in the healing process by reorienting the fibers so they properly align, thus promoting healthier, more stable tissue with greater strength and elasticity. The remodeling stage can last from 21 days to 1 year post trauma.

Method of Application

Ultrasound treatments should be administered by a qualified physiotherapist or health professional who will set the specific parameters of the ultrasound unit according to the nature of the injury and desired effects. Most treatments last from 4-6 minutes with only a very mild heat being felt during the treatment.

Caution

If you feel any burning or painful sensation from the ultrasound, immediately inform your therapist. Remember that this is a form of heat therapy and has the potential to burn.

If I've Injured It Once, Will I Always Be Susceptible to Reinjury?

Reinjury generally occurs because most athletes do not aggressively rehabilitate their injuries. If soft tissue injuries are left to recover on their own, they might not regain normal elasticity and tensile strength. Given the amount of force and stress imposed on the tissues during bodybuilding and strength training, reinjury is common in untreated tissue. What is the lesson to be learned from this? Take any and every injury seriously and consult a medical professional or physiotherapist for the best way to rehabilitate your injury.

Electrical Muscle Stimulation

Most electrical muscle stimulation (EMS) units are small battery-operated devices. They transmit electrical currents through lead wires to electrodes that are strategically placed on the body. The electrical stimulation excites the nerves that are responsible for eliciting a muscular contraction.

Uses of Electrical Muscle Stimulation

EMS is primarily used when muscle control is inhibited, or when the athlete cannot contract his or her muscle voluntarily (i.e., after surgery or when swelling inhibits voluntary contraction). Its use can reverse or minimize muscle atrophy due to immobilization, and it maximizes muscle contraction until reinnervation of the peripheral nerve occurs.

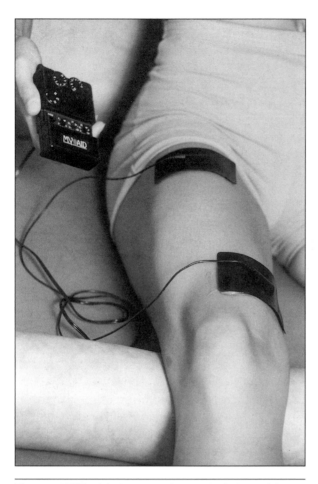

The use of EMS minimizes muscular atrophy during an injury.

The strength gains achieved through EMS can be attributed to several possible neural mechanisms.

1. One theory suggests that there is increased activation of the spinal motor neuron pools that regulate the force of muscle contraction through stimulation of the afferent neurons.

2. There may be an increased sensitivity of synapses as a result of continuous stimulation of input fibers.

3. Other theories point to synchronization of motor unit firing patterns and selective recruitment of large FT fibers over ST fibers (Low and Reed, 1990).

Can EMS Replace Training?

The value of electrical stimulation is very clear in cases of weakened, damaged, or atrophied muscles, where significant gains have been studied and reported (Williams, 1976). The value of using EMS on healthy athletes in an attempt to enhance strength and size development, however, is not so clear. Research in this area seems, for the most part, to indicate that there is little value in using EMS on healthy tissue (Halback, 1980; Massey et al., 1965). Some studies, however, have shown that while EMS alone is not a viable substitute for bodybuilding training, EMS combined with training has led to similar or greater strength gains than training alone (Godfrey et al., 1979; Johnston et al., 1977).

Transcutaneous Electrical Nerve Stimulation

Transcutaneous Electrical Nerve Stimulation (TENS) treats injury through neuromodulation by the application of an electrical stimulus across the skin. This results in a nerve impulse pattern that interferes with the ability of the CNS to perceive and interpret pain.

Theories of TENS Treatment

There are several theories supporting the use of TENS for pain control.

The Gate Control Theory

This theory, proposed in 1965 by Melzack and Wall, puts forward the idea that there is a "gate" that opens and closes within the spinal cord. This gate perceives increases and decreases in pain from the peripheral nerves or the CNS. TENS stimulates the large nerve fibers (A beta) that have a low threshold and a fast conduction velocity. The stimulation of these fibers "closes" the gate to impulses from the small diameter fibers (c fibers) that carry pain messages,

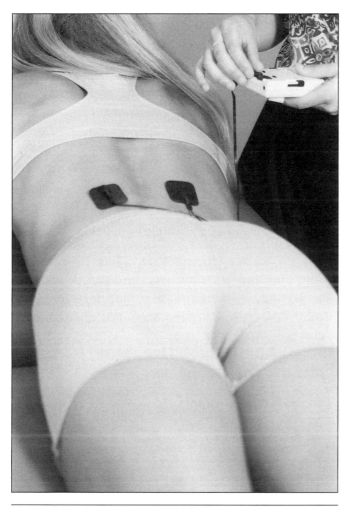

The intensity of the current is increased gradually until a tingling sensation is felt.

thus diminishing the person's perception of pain (Wong and Rapson, 1983).

The Neurotransmitter Theory

According to this theory, TENS stimulates receptors in the muscles that release endorphins in the spinal cord, midbrain, hypothalamus, and pituitary. Beta endorphin is a naturally occurring opiate that has analgesic-type properties (i.e., pain-relieving properties) that decrease the person's perception of pain (Wong and Rapson, 1983).

The Somato-Sympathetic Reflex Theory

This theory proposes that the stimulus from TENS affects the precapillary sphincters, resulting in either capillary or arteriolar vasodilation. There may also be changes in the skeletal muscles by the activation of sympathetic vasodilation. The increased circulation of blood within the muscle hastens removal of waste products and results in less pain (Wong and Rapson, 1983).

Method of Application

Electrodes may be placed on one of the following locations:

- Around the segmentally involved spinal column level.
- On superficial aspects of nerves.
- On acupuncture, motor, and trigger points.

The average length of a TENS treatment is 20-45 minutes. The intensity of the current is increased gradually until a tingling sensation is felt. It should not be painful! TENS can be used for the treatment of acute pain (high frequency 100-200 Hertz/low intensity), or for chronic pain (low frequency 0-4 Hertz/high intensity). A trial of TENS, and instruction regarding the appropriate parameter settings and safe operating procedures, should be carried out in the clinical setting before self-treatments are administered at home.

Caution

Electrodes must not be placed over pacemakers, or over carotid sinus or pharyngeal region. TENS should not be used in cases of impaired skin sensation. During pregnancy certain points should not be used. Consultation with a health care professional is highly recommended.

Laser

Laser is one of the newest methods being used for the treatment of soft-tissue injuries. Laser is an acronym for "Light Amplification by the Stimulated Emission of Radiation," referring to the production of a beam of radiation that displays the characteristics of monochromaticity, coherence, and collimation. The laser releases an almost instantaneous pulse of energy that causes heating when absorbed by the tissues. The most common types of laser are helium-neon and gallium-arsenide.

When and Why Is Laser Therapy Used?

Laser therapy is generally used for pain relief, acute and chronic, as well as tissue healing. Rheumatoid arthritis, osteoarthritis, bursitis, and neurogenic pain also respond well to laser therapy. Young et al. (1989) found that 660, 820, and 870nm wavelengths encouraged macrophages to release factors that stimulate fibroblast proliferation. Acceleration of wound healing by laser might also involve an increase in collagen formation, vasodilation, DNA synthesis, and an increase in RNA production.

Method of Application

Most low- or medium-power laser sources are applied to the skin by a hand-held applicator. Other types of lasers are mounted on a mobile stand and applied about 30 cm away from the patient.

Caution

When using lasers, avoid directing the beam into the eyes. Wear protective goggles for safety reasons. In cases of venous thrombosis, phlebitis, and arterial disease, laser treatment should not be administered.

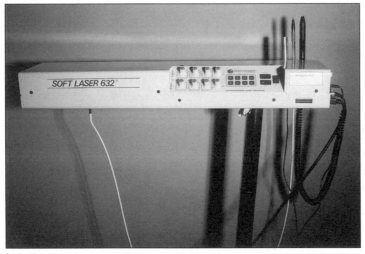 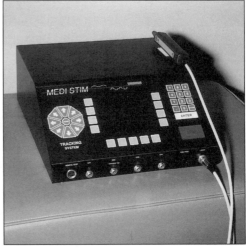

Different types of laser machines.

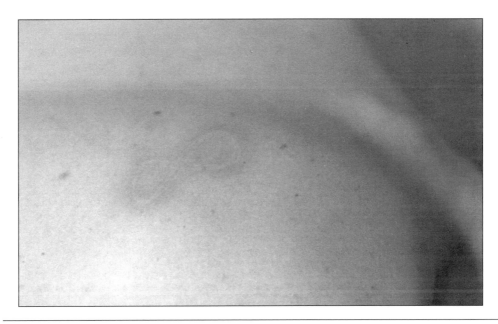

The laser releases an instantaneous pulse of energy, which when absorbed by the tissues causes heating (figure-eight seen on the individual's back).

Massage

Massage is an ancient therapy first referenced as early as 2500 BC in a medical text titled *Nei Ching* (Goats, 1994a). Ancient Indian and Greek texts taught the effectiveness of massage as a therapy for "sport and war injuries" (Goats, 1990).

It is defined as the manipulation of soft tissue structures (i.e., muscle, tendon, ligament, and or fascia) with the hand for purposes of therapeutics (Chamberlain, 1982) and relaxation (Wright et al., 1995).

Physiological Effects of Massage

The numerous physiological effects of massage include: aiding circulation, positive nervous system effects, swelling reduction, muscle spasm reduction, and accelerated connective tissue healing.

Aiding Circulation

Massage has been found to cause vasodilation of the superficial blood vessels, thus enhancing general blood flow to the area being treated (Goats, 1994b). Generally, studies have shown that vigorous massage on healthy adults results in increased local blood flow and cardiac stroke volume (a marker of venous return) (Goats, 1994b). Looking at the effects of massage on blood parameters, Smith et al. (1994) reported that following a 30-minute massage session, creatine kinase (CK) levels (an indirect gauge of muscle damage) had decreased, while serum cortisol and ceutrophil levels (reparative substances) were elevated. It was felt that these changes directly affected the amount of muscle soreness reported by subjects after an eccentric exercise protocol. Athletes who suffer from muscle soreness due to metabolite build-up in the

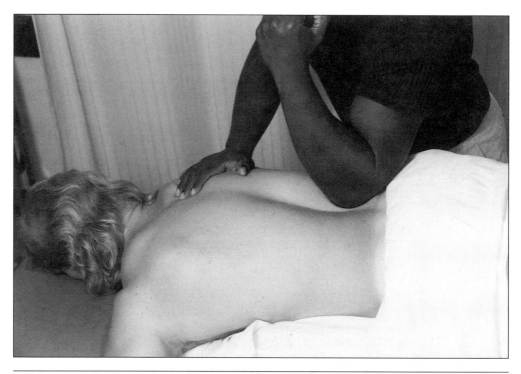

Massage therapy for the purpose of therapeutics and relaxation.

muscles might find massage is the answer. The increased blood flow brings with it a concomitant increase in healing factors transported to the muscles being trained, which will enhance the healing of microtears caused during heavy weight training.

Nervous System Effects

Massage is thought to act as a strong mechanical trigger to reduce pain by activating the pain gate mechanism (Goats, 1990). Some studies have found that athletes generally had a better outlook to their perceived exertion during training after a massage (Cinque, 1989). Many bodybuilders see massage as an important component to rapid recovery of muscle function and energy after a grueling workout or during the stressful period of contest preparation.

Swelling Reduction

Massage is thought to be very effective in reducing edema (swelling). The compression forces created by some of the techniques (i.e., kneading and petrissage) are thought to enhance the opening and closing of valves in the veins and lymph channels, thus aiding drainage of edematous areas (Goats, 1994b).

Caution

Not all types of swelling have been shown to benefit from massage. For example, in cases of acute swelling, massage has been shown to intensify symptoms (Cinque, 1989).

Muscle Spasm Reduction

Massage techniques like petrissage and effleurage are thought to help reduce muscle cramping and spasm by flushing concentrated amounts of lactate acid, one of the metabolites commonly associated with muscle spasms, from the areas involved in heavy training (Goats, 1994b).

Accelerated Connective Tissue Healing

Certain massage techniques such as vigorous friction, improve the mobility of connective tissue while simultaneously producing mild muscle trauma (Chamberlain, 1993; Goats, 1994a, 1994b). The muscle trauma manifests itself as local hyperemia (an inflammatory response), beneficial in restoring adherent or contracted tissue fibers to a more normal alignment through the "remodeling phase of healing" (Goats, 1994a). Massage has also been shown to be an effective pre-event warm-up. Massage, however, should not be substituted for stretching. Rather, it should be used as an adjunct to the athlete's warm-up regime.

Massage Techniques

Effleurage frequently starts and ends a massage treatment. Effleurage is a slow, rhythmic stroke performed along the long axis of the tissue. The stroke can either be superficial or deep, each having its own separate effects. Superficial effleurage is done centripetally and acts to introduce the client to other strokes to follow. When the stroke is progressively deepened, it can improve venous and lymph flow (Callaghan, 1993), thus reducing swelling. The gradual deepening of the stroke helps to reduce the tone in the muscle tissue, thus promoting relaxation and diminishing muscle spasm.

Kneading consists of slow circular compressive movements on the soft tissue against the bony structures below. It enhances fluid flow in the body and produces a reflex vasodilation of the blood vessels. This helps to reduce swelling and subsequently resolves inflammation. More vigorous kneading helps to diminish muscle spasm and lengthens shortened soft-tissue structures (Goats, 1990).

Petrissage is a deeper technique than effleurage and kneading, involving the rolling of folds of skin, subcutaneous tissues, and muscle over the underlying structures with the fingers and thumb in a continuous circular motion. Petrissage helps to stretch contracted and adherent fibrous tissues and also helps to reduce muscle spasm. Since petrissage is a deep technique, it might also help to improve circulation of body fluids and resolve chronic swelling (Goats, 1994a). Variations of the stroke include *wringing*, which is a twisting motion of the soft tissue in opposite directions, and *picking up*, which involves lifting and stretching the soft tissue away from the underlying tissues.

Tapotement is a succession of gentle blows delivered with either a cupped hand (percussion) or the ulnar border of the hand (hacking). This technique causes hyperemia (increased blood flow) in the superficial tissues and also stimulates the body's cutaneous reflexes. Both these effects are beneficial in increasing muscle tone, reducing inflammation, and accelerating the healing process. Other hand variations include *beating,* which employs use of the fingertips, and *pounding,* which employs tightly-closed fists.

The *vibrations* (shaking) technique produces stronger vibrations through the tissue than does tapotement. Vibrations are administered by the trembling of the hands, which are held firmly against the skin. Different from effleurage, vibrations compress swollen tissues, thus aiding in swelling reduction (Goats, 1994a). Vibrations are also believed to help reduce muscle tone and may, therefore, be useful in promoting relaxation.

The *frictions* technique uses transverse movements across the connective tissue surface. These movements imitate the normal forces and mobility of the structures by broadening (not stretching or tearing) healing fibers (Chamberlain, 1982). Frictions is a fairly deep massage technique performed with either the fleshy portion of the thumb or more often the fingertips. It focuses on a specific injury site, either the tendon, ligament, or muscle. The aim of frictions is to maintain mobility of the soft tissues by causing mild tissue destruction, hyperemia, and a subsequent inflammatory response, which acts to realign and lengthen tissue fibers. This ultimately promotes more efficient healing after injury and enhances the strength of the structures. Frictions have also been shown to decrease pain by activating the pain gate mechanism (Goats, 1990).

Massage should be avoided in the following circumstances:

- Over malignancies or open wounds
- With clients suffering from thrombophlebitis
- Over infected tissues
- Over areas of fractures or deep muscle trauma

Common Injuries: Causes and Solutions

There are typical injuries that occur mainly in the knee, lower back, and rotator cuff joint.

Anatomy of the Knee

The knee joint is a hinge joint that permits only a small degree of rotation. Its structure is complicated because it is actually three joints merged into one: an intermediate joint between the patella and the femur, and lateral and medial joints between the femoral and tibial condyles. The bones involved in the knee joint are the femur, tibia, and patella.

The main ligaments of the knee joint include the lateral (fibular) and medial (tibial) collateral ligaments, as well as the anterior and posterior cruciate ligaments. The menisci (cartilage) are C-shaped plates of fibrocartilage between the femoral and tibial plateaus. The patellar tendon is the continuation of the quadriceps femoris tendon and attaches to the tibia (Moore, 1980). Figures 13.1 and 13.2 show the posterior and anterior views of a knee joint.

Common Knee Injuries of Bodybuilders and Strength Trainers

Two very common knee injuries are *patellofemoral pain syndrome* (chondromalacia), which is pain felt behind the kneecap, and *meniscal tears*, which is damage to the cartilage caused by a twisting strain to the knee. The exercise at fault is usually deep knee squatting. Patellofemoral pain syndrome occurs

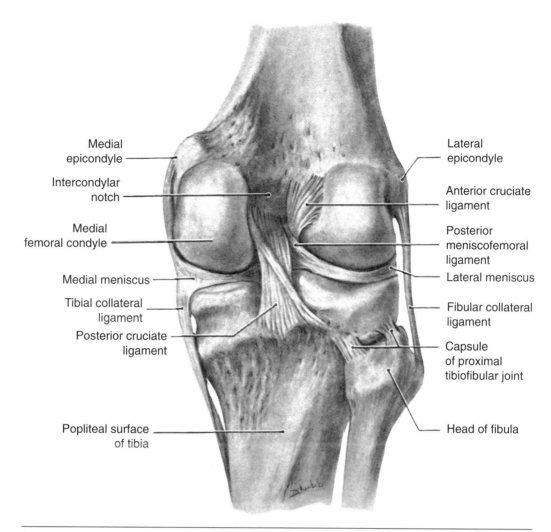

Figure 13.1 Drawing of a posterior view of a dissection of the ligaments of the right knee joint.
Reprinted from Moore 1980.

when pain intensifies during activities that require bending (flexion) of the knee. When the knee is extended (straight), there is no contact between the patella and the underlying femur. As the knee progressively bends, however, there is more and more contact between the patella and the femoral condyles. As patellofemoral forces increase, as occurs during deep squatting, the articular cartilage, or lining of the bone, becomes more susceptible to wear-and-tear changes. This results in painful inflammation experienced behind the knee (Fujikawa, 1983).

Cartilage tears usually occur when a twisting strain is applied to the knee while it is in the flexed position. During a deep knee squat, the knees are flexed and under a great amount of strain. With even a slight twist of the knee, caused by poor balance or fatigue, the meniscus can become wedged between the tibia and the femur, resulting in a meniscal tear.

Injury Prevention

Does this mean we should strike the squat from our training programs? Squatting is arguably the most important exercise for building overall leg

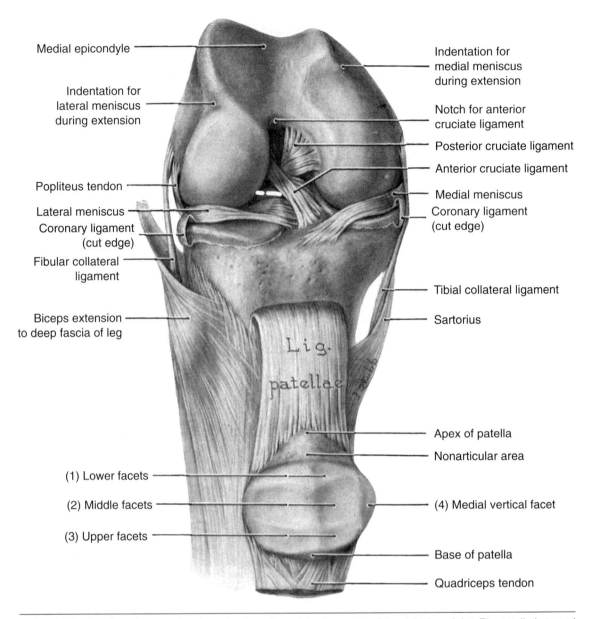

Figure 13.2 Drawing of an anterior view of a dissection of the ligaments of the right knee joint. The patella is turned downward and the joint is flexed. Observe the indentations on the sides of the femoral condyles at the junction of the patellar and tibial articular areas.
Reprinted from Moore 1980.

strength and mass. Most bodybuilders and strength experts feel that it should not be eliminated from routines. We, therefore, recommend using safety squats in place of the traditional squat. The safety squat apparatus is constructed so it can be balanced on the shoulders, leaving the hands free to hold on to the handles mounted on the squat rack. This puts the athlete into an ergonomically safe position for lifting, thus improving his or her balance and creating proper weight distribution. The handles also act as built-in spotters for the athlete. They help the athlete to give him- or herself as much or as little help as necessary during the movement and eliminate the risks associated with having a poor, weak, or distracted spotter. If you are not fortunate enough to belong to a gym that has a safety squat bar, you can still do squats, just be smart about it. Only squat to the 90-degree angle. This will preserve the life of both your knees and your back.

Lower Back Injuries

Low back injuries are feared by all athletes because they can prove to be quite disabling.

Anatomy of the Low Back

The lumbar spine (low back), seen in figure 13.3, consists of five vertebrae. The vertebrae are large bones designed to absorb body weight. Between the vertebrae are the intervertebral discs, seen in figure 13.4, which act as shock absorbers for the spine. The inner core of the discs is a semi-fluid mass called the *nucleus pulposus*. The outer part of the discs is composed of rings of fibrous tissue called the *anulus fibrosus*. The vertebrae are connected by a series of paired joints called *facet joints*. These joints help to control flexion, extension, and rotation of the vertebrae, and also aid in weight bearing (Moore, 1980).

There are numerous ligaments that add stability to the lumbar spine. These include the interspinous ligaments, supraspinous ligaments, posterior and anterior longitudinal ligaments, ligamentum flava, and the capsular ligaments of the facet joints.

For descriptive purposes, the muscles of the low back are divided into layers—superficial, intermediate, and deep. The superficial and intermediate muscles are concerned with movements of the limbs and with respiration, while the deep muscles (figure 13.5) are concerned with movements of the vertebral column. The erector spinae and multifidus muscles are deep muscles that are commonly injured by bodybuilders (Moore, 1980).

The Low Back Culprit

The exercise that is most frequently performed incorrectly and, not surprisingly, is responsible for the majority of low back injuries, is the hamstring deadlift. There are two main problems with this exercise:

- Most athletes tend to perform the hamstring deadlift with a rounded back instead of a straight back.
- Most athletes take the bar too low, stretching the hamstring muscles beyond their physiological limit.

An interesting study by Adams et al. (1980) showed that when one reaches the limit of flexion, the supraspinous and interspinous ligaments sprain first, followed by capsular ligaments and intervertebral discs. They concluded that when the back is rounded and flexed beyond its normal range of motion, it is very easy to suffer ligament damage to the low back. When the back is kept flat during this exercise, the ligaments, muscles, and discs are more mechanically effective at coping with the tensile forces placed on them.

Injury Prevention

Proper lifting technique will always help to minimize injuries to the low back. Proper breathing technique while lifting is very important in the prevention of

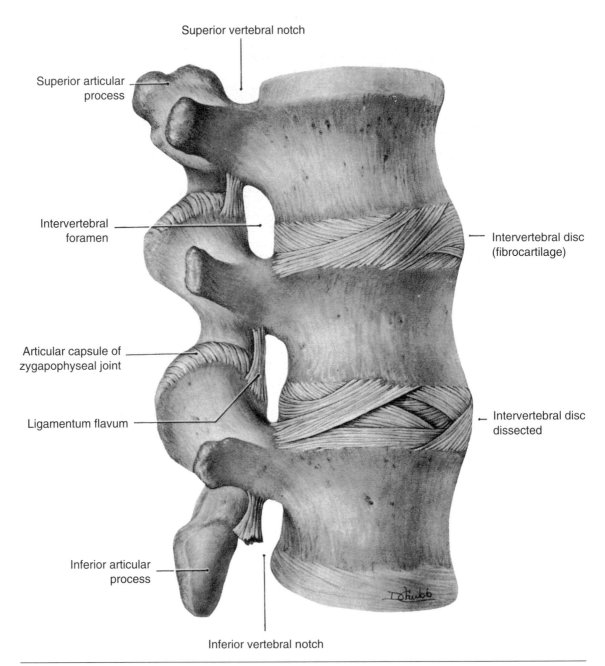

Superior vertebral notch

Superior articular process

Intervertebral foramen

Intervertebral disc (fibrocartilage)

Articular capsule of zygapophyseal joint

Ligamentum flavum

Intervertebral disc dissected

Inferior articular process

Inferior vertebral notch

Figure 13.3   Drawing of a portion of the lumbar region of the vertebral column, lateral view, primarily to show the structure of the anuli fibrosi of the intervertebral discs.
Reprinted from Moore 1980.

injuries. Holding one's breath while pushing the weight is dangerous because it increases intradiscal pressure, which can cause bulging of the disc (commonly referred to as a "slipped disc"). It is important, therefore, to exhale during the pressing action of the exercise and inhale during the relaxation phase.

Many back injuries can be attributed to a weak abdominal musculature. The abdominal muscles protect the low back by helping to stabilize the spinal column and by balancing intradiscal pressures, so don't forget to train your abs!

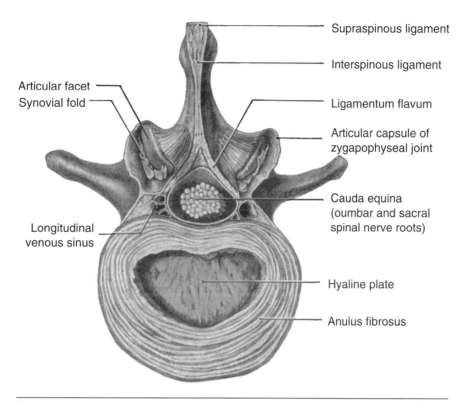

Supraspinous ligament

Interspinous ligament

Ligamentum flavum

Articular capsule of
zygapophyseal joint

Cauda equina
(oumbar and sacral
spinal nerve roots)

Hyaline plate

Anulus fibrosus

Articular facet

Synovial fold

Longitudinal
venous sinus

Figure 13.4 Diagram of a cross-section of an intervertebral disc and the vertebral ligaments. The nucleus pulposus has been scooped out to show the hyaline cartilage plate of the upper surface of the vertebral body.
Reprinted from Moore 1980.

Rotator Cuff Injuries

The rotator cuff is probably the body part most commonly injured by body-builders and strength trainers.

Anatomy of the Rotator Cuff

There are four muscles surrounding the shoulder joint that join the scapula to the humerus: supraspinatus, infraspinatus, teres minor, and subscapularis. The tendons of these muscles blend to form a musculotendinous sheath called the *rotator cuff*, which is attached to the underlying fibrous capsule of the shoulder joint and inserted into the greater and lesser tubercles of the humerus. The rotator cuff protects and stabilizes the shoulder joint by holding the head of the humerus in the glenoid cavity (Moore, 1980). Figures 13.6 and 13.7 provide two views of this injury-prone body part.

Most injuries to the rotator cuff occur to the supraspinatus muscle. This muscle acts to stabilize the shoulder joint, and it abducts and externally rotates the humerus. Together with the deltoid, it helps to elevate the humerus at the shoulder joint. The supraspinatus muscle is vulnerable to injury, especially during activities that involve repetitive use of the arms above the horizontal plane, because of its anatomical position, traveling under the coracoacromial arch to the greater tuberosity of the humerus. In 1972, Neer demonstrated that the functional arc of elevation of the

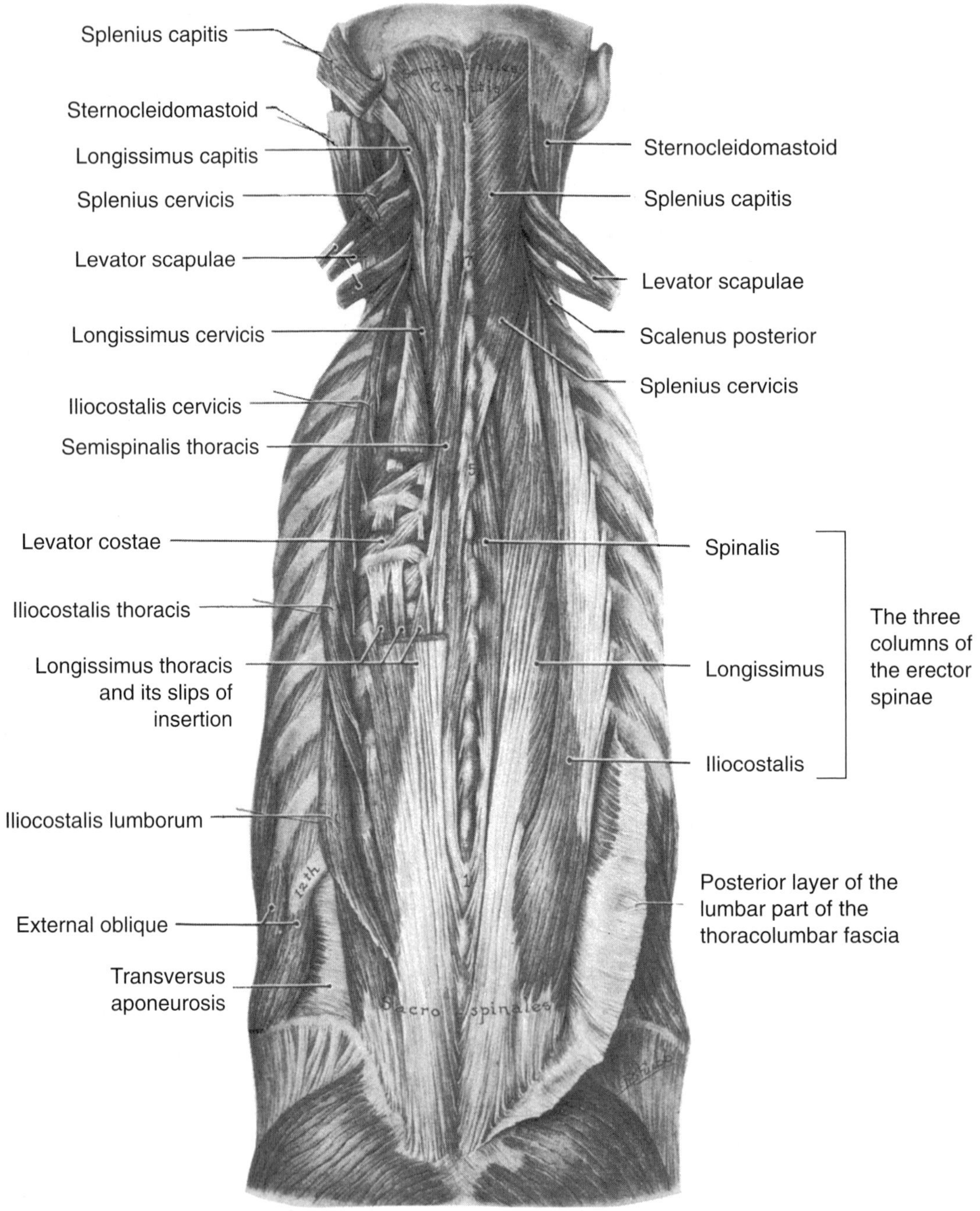

Figure 13.5 Drawing of a dissection illustrating the deep muscles of the back. The superficial layer of deep muscles (splenius capitis and cervicis) is reflected on the left side. The intermediate layer of deep muscles (erector spinae) is intact on the right side, lying between the spinous processes of the vertebrae medially and the angles of the ribs laterally. The deep group are the intrinsic or true muscles of the back.
Reprinted from Moore 1980.

shoulder is forward, not lateral, and that impingement occurs predominantly against the anterior edge of the acromion and the coracoacromial ligament. Impingement tends to occur in the avascular region of the supraspinatus tendon, which over time results in tendinitis (Hawkins et al., 1980).

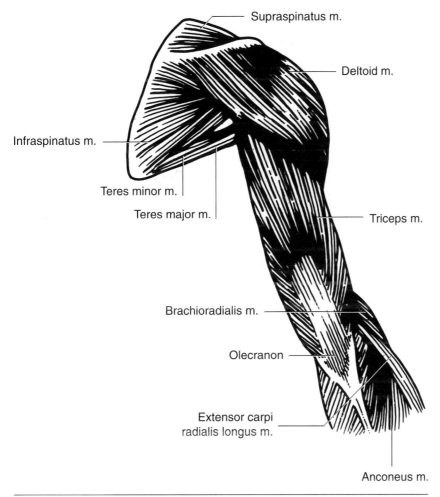

Supraspinatus m.

Deltoid m.

Infraspinatus m.

Teres minor m.

Teres major m.

Triceps m.

Brachioradialis m.

Olecranon

Extensor carpi
radialis longus m.

Anconeus m.

Figure 13.6 Drawing of the muscles of the shoulder joint (posterior view).
Reprinted from Moore 1980.

Two Rotator Cuff Culprits

Two shoulder exercises that can predispose an athlete to rotator cuff injuries are the behind the neck press and the Arnold press.

Behind the Neck Press. The behind the neck press requires a starting position of full lateral rotation with the shoulder in a position of abduction. The second component of the exercise involves pulling the shoulders into a retracted position (pinching the shoulder blades together), while maintaining an externally rotated position. This maneuver tends to lead to shoulder impingement, whereby the rotator cuff becomes jammed under the anteroinferior surface of the acromion, which irritates the tendon and causes it to become inflamed. In addition to the fact that the behind the neck press position is not safe, there are many bodybuilders and strength trainers who just do not have the necessary flexibility to perform the exercise properly. The internal rotators (pectoralis major, teres major, latissimus dorsi, and subscapularis) are usually too inflexible, which prevents full external rotation. As a result, the external rotators must work too hard to compensate and to stabilize the shoulder joint during the pressing motion, leading to mechanical stress that produces injury. Behind the neck pulldowns are equally dangerous to the rotator cuff for the same physiological reasons.

Arnold Press. The Arnold press, named after Arnold Schwarzenegger, involves simultaneous elevation and rotation of the shoulders. It is the rotation component of the exercise that can cause impingement of the rotator cuff muscles. As the shoulder approaches 90 degrees and the shoulders internally rotate, the head of the humerus is forced under the inferior aspect of the acromion. This mechanically pinches the rotator cuff muscles and, with repetition, it is quite likely that overuse tendinitis will occur. While it is true that many professional bodybuilders use the Arnold press, they probably minimize injuries by having excellent technique, strength, and muscular mass.

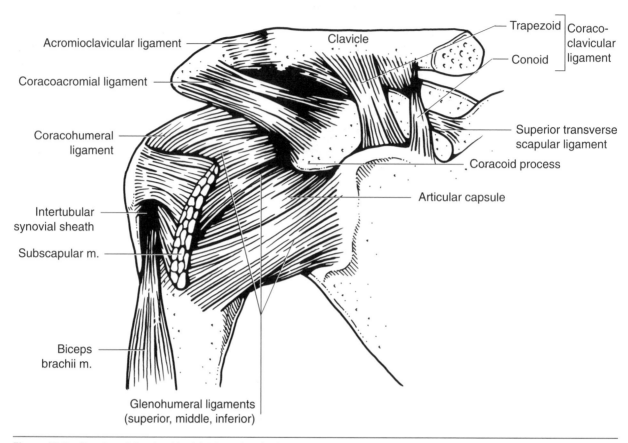

Figure 13.7 Drawing of the shoulder joint (anterior view).
Reprinted from Moore 1980.

Injury Prevention

Almost every bodybuilder and strength athlete will have a shoulder injury at some point in his or her career. The key to remaining injury free is to develop proper flexibility and flawless technique, as well as to avoid the exercises that will wear down your rotator cuff.

CHAPTER 14

DRUG FREE TRAINING

An overwhelming percentage of bodybuilders with competitive aspirations for dramatic increases in size and strength have made the choice to take steroids. The controversy surrounding drug use by bodybuilders has never been greater. Bodybuilders have countless reasons for using these drugs, such as decrease in body fat and increase in muscle mass and strength (Alen and Rahkila, 1988).

According to the research literature, athletes do not administer the recommended therapeutic dosages; they intake doses 10 to 40 times higher (Lamb, 1984). Other research stated that in current users, the mean maximum dosage of oral agents was 173 ± 45 mg a week (mean ± SD), in addition to 202 ± 34 mg a week of injectable steroids, for a total of 375 ± 57 mg a week. The manufacturer's recommended dose of methandrostenolone (Dianabol), an oral anabolic-androgenic steroid, was approximately 35 to 70 mg a week (Strauss et al., 1988). The side effects of steroid use are related to several factors, which include the specific drugs administered, the amount and

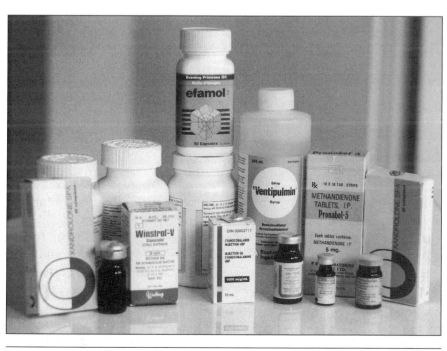

Bodybuilders experiment with a variety of drugs.

frequency of the dosages, the overall length of drug usage, and whether the athlete is administering an injectable or oral steroid (Alen and Rahkila, 1988).

The way steroids work on a cellular level is very complex. Although many bodybuilders use steroids and have a general understanding of the biochemical process that occurs, few truly understand all of the complexities. When a steroid, or group of steroids, is administered either orally or through injection, the main objective is to allow protein synthesis to occur. When a steroid is injected in the muscle it dissipates into the bloodstream; whereas if it is administered orally, it first travels through the gastrointestinal tract to the liver and then dissipates into the bloodstream. Once the steroid has reached the bloodstream, it enters the target cell and binds to its specific receptor. This binding process between the hormone and its specific receptor occurs in the cellular cytosol. The formation of the receptor hormone complex travels to the nucleus of the cell where it binds to specific segments of DNA (deoxyribonucleic acid) and stimulates transcription of the new messenger RNA (ribonucleic acid). This process allows protein synthesis to occur, which is without a doubt the most substantial change in cellular function. The increase in protein synthesis leads to an increase in size and strength of skeletal muscle cells.

It is not uncommon to read books and articles that suggest someone or something is to blame for steroid use. Some people look to the Weiders because they were responsible for the emergence of bodybuilding, which is related to the steroid problem. Nothing could be farther from the truth. Problems are encountered in every sport and nothing is gained by simply laying blame. The answers lie in understanding the problems and finding solutions. Periodization for serious strength training and bodybuilding is our solution—an alternative to steroid use.

Drug Abuse in Bodybuilding

Athletes now make use of a vast arsenal of drugs to improve their performance and appearance (especially in aesthetic or recreational athletes) and to combat some of the side effects of other drugs. In addition to the anabolic steroids, several classes of compounds are used in an attempt to increase muscle mass and strength and improve performance. (See table 14.1.) The list in table 14.1, however, is just the tip of the iceberg. In fact, it might be difficult to find a substance with which some aspiring athlete has not experimented.

Black Market Drugs

The use of anabolic drugs is more prevalent among recreational bodybuilders than competitive athletes. These compounds are used for a more muscular and athletic look rather than for their performance-enhancing effects.

Most physicians feel that prescribing anabolic steroids contributes to the problem of drug use in sports. Many bodybuilders, therefore, obtain anabolic steroids (and other performance-enhancing drugs) from black market dealers, and as prescription sources of anabolic steroids dry up, black market activity increases.

When bodybuilders get both their drugs and drug information from black market and other non-medical sources, they are often encouraged to use a variety of drugs, also easily obtainable from the underground pharmacy. This

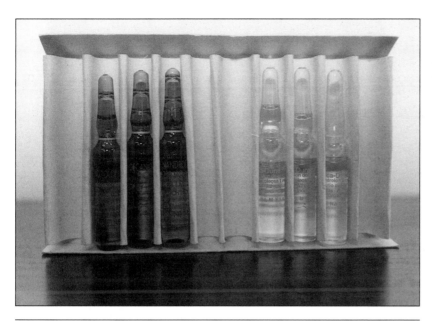

"Real Deca" (right)—"Fake Deca" (left).

unsupervised polypharmacy can result in serious adverse effects.

As dangerous as this polypharmacy is, there is a more sinister side to black market drugs. While black market drugs are easy to obtain, some are of questionable quality and safety. Black market dealers get their supplies wherever they can, sometimes from reputable sources—sometimes not.

The increased awareness of the drug use problem and the legal issues associated with the controlled drug status of anabolic steroids and growth hormones has caused a shortage of "real" drugs on the black market. Thus, more of the black market drugs are coming from makeshift illegal basement laboratories, where counterfeit drugs are produced using whatever materials are at hand. These bogus drugs include pharmaceutical preparations, drugs made in homemade labs, veterinary drugs, vitamins, inert filler compounds, and, in some cases of injectable preparations, just plain oil or water with food coloring.

The dangers of using these counterfeit drugs fall into three categories:

1. If the vial or pill comes from a reputable pharmaceutical company (whether mislabeled or not), there is the danger inherent in the drug itself. Moreover, the bottle or vial might not contain what its label says it contains. For example, some vials containing a combination of testosterone and estrogen, which is used therapeutically to treat the female climacteric, were relabeled as testosterone enanthate, with no mention of the estrogen component.

2. There are the dangers inherent in taking a drug that has been manufactured or constructed in a basement lab. The lack of quality control and, in many cases, the lack of expertise and adequate knowledge of biopharmacology makes black market drugs a high-risk gamble for the athlete. The absence of meticulous protocols and sterile conditions might lead to chemical and biological contamination. Chemical impurities can result in acute or chronic poisoning and damage to the liver and kidneys. Biological impurities can result in bacterial, fungal, and viral infections—possibly even hepatitis and AIDS. There have been several cases of infections in athletes using bogus growth hormone and some injectable anabolic steroids. These infections are both local, in the form of abscesses, and generalized, leading to acute sickness with fevers and joint pain. In some cases, the stoppers used in the vials are reactive or absorptive instead of being inert, and may cause toxic contamination of the contents of the vials.

Table 14.1   Compounds used to increase muscle mass and strength and improve performance

Stimulants	Narcotic analgesics	Growth factors/ peptides	Compounds that increase endogenous androgen	Miscellaneous compounds with putative anabolic or ergogenic effects
Adrenalin	Including agonists, partial agonists, and antagonists	Growth hormone	HCG (human chorionic gonadotropin)	Bee pollen
Adrenergic compounds		GHRH (growth hormone releasing hormone)	Menotropins (Pergonal)	Beta-2 adrenergic agonists such as:
Amphetamines/ amphetamine derivatives		Growth hormone stimulators:	Gonadorelin (Factrel)	Clenbuterol
Arcalion		Ornithine	Cyclofenil	Cimaterol
ATP (Striadyne)		Clonidine	Antiestrogens (clomiphene, tamoxifen)	Fenoterol
Caffeine		L-dopa		Boron
Cocaine		IGF-I (Insulin-like growth factor)		Carnitine
Diet pills		EGF (epithelial growth factor)		Chromium picolinate
Heptaminol		Galanin		Co-enzyme Q
Inosine				Creatine monohydrate
Nicotine				Cyproheptadine
Piraceta				Dibencozide
Sodium succinate				Dimethylglycine
Sydnocarb				Ecdysterone
				GHB-gamma hydroxbutyrate
				Gamma-oryzanol

Other hormones	Anti-inflammatory compounds	Nutritional supplements	Miscellaneous compounds	Miscellaneous compounds with putative anabolic or ergogenic effects
Insulin	Corticosteroids	Vitamins	Alcohol/marijuana	Ginseng
Thyroid hormone (Cytomel, Synthroid, Triacana)	NSAIDs (Nonsteroidal anti-inflammatory drugs	Minerals	Amino acid neurotransmitters (GABA, phenylalanine, tryptophan, glutamine)	Glutathione
	DMSO	B-12 injections		Inosine
		Protein—whole or as individual or branched chain amino acids	Beta-blockers	Ketones
Hypothalamic and pituitary-releasing hormones, such as	Veterinary cartilage based compounds	Medium chain triglycerides	Calcium channel blockers	MCTs
TRH			Cyclobenzaprine	Neurofor
TSH			Diuretics	OKG (ornithine alpha-ketoglutarate)
ACTH			Local anaesthetics	Pangamic acid
ADH or Vasopressin				Pentoxifylline (Trental)
Pitocin				Perchlorates
				Rubranova
				Selegiline (Deprenyl)
				Sitosterol
				Smilax officinalis
				Ubiquinone (Co-enzymeQ10)
				Yohimbine
				Zeranol (Ralgro)

3. Most athletes obtain their anabolic preparations through local gyms and, therefore, there is no medical follow-up. This means that many correctable problems caused by taking the drugs improperly or because of mislabeled or contaminated drugs are missed.

Anabolic Steroids

The anabolic actions of substances produced by the testes have been known for almost a century. Two case reports by Sacchi (1895) and Rowlands and Nicholson (1929) comprise the early evidence of the influence of testicular androgens, specifically testosterone, on growth and musculoskeletal development. Kenyon, in a series of studies extending from 1938 to 1944, investigated and elucidated the metabolic effects of testosterone. He was one of the first to outline possible clinical uses for testosterone (Kenyon et al., 1942).

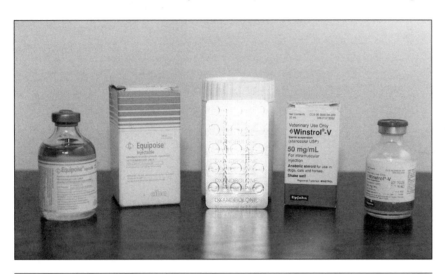

Different liquid and pill forms of anabolic steroids.

The athletic community was quick to realize the performance-enhancing potential of testosterone and put some of the principles outlined by Kenyon and others into practice. By the early 1950s, testosterone and a few analogs, such as methandrostenelone (Dianabol by Ciba), were being used. The East Block athletes were the first users, soon followed by those of most other countries.

Today, anabolic steroids are used by almost all power athletes at some time during their training. This includes those in sports requiring strength or explosive force and, as in bodybuilding, extreme muscularity. Many other athletes use anabolic steroids as well, including those competing in the middle distance and endurance events.

Anabolic steroid use is common among professional athletes and has spread to college and high school athletes (Windsor and Dumitru, 1989) involved in non-Olympic sports such as football, hockey, basketball, and even baseball. Unfortunately, the use of anabolic steroids and other drugs has spread to noncompetitive athletes and even the general public, where they are used for aesthetic measures rather than for increasing competitive athletic performance.

Effects of Androgenic/Anabolic Steroids

The effects produced by testosterone can be subdivided into two somewhat arbitrary categories. These are androgenic, which produce secondary male sexual characteristics, and anabolic, which mainly increase muscle size and strength.

Modifications at any of the 19 carbon groups that make up the testosterone molecule are made for many reasons including altering the anabolic/androgenic ratio or therapeutic index (ideally increasing anabolic and decreasing androgenic effects), increasing the bioavailability of the drug when taken orally, decreasing its absorption time when given parenterally, and increasing the potency of the drug so less drug is used for similar results.

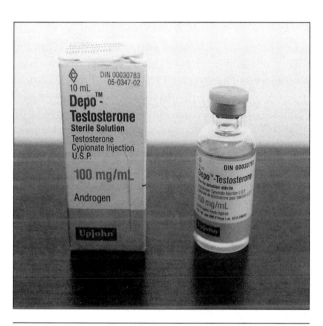

Depo-Testosterone is a widely used anabolic/androgenic steroid.

Do They Work?

While there is some controversy in the literature on the effectiveness of anabolic steroids in enhancing performance, there is no doubt in most athletes' minds that they do work. Athletes worldwide use anabolic steroids and/or exogenous testosterone in an attempt to increase their muscular size and strength.

Acceptance of the ergogenic effects of anabolic steroids began, perhaps, with a review of the literature by Haupt and Rovere (1984). They concluded that if certain criteria were met, such as intensive training, a high protein diet, and specific measurement techniques, then anabolic steroids do seem to enhance athletic performance. Other studies published since this review have shown that anabolic steroids enhance strength, size, and athletic performance (Egginton, 1987) (Griggs et al., 1989).

Adverse Effects

In general, the adverse effects of anabolic steroids can be separated into two groups. One group consists of adverse effects that are an exaggeration of the expected pharmacological properties of the anabolic steroids. Potential hormonally related adverse effects of anabolic steroids in men include gynecomastia, fluid retention, acne, changes in libido, oligospermia, and increased aggressiveness. In women, amenorrhea and other menstrual irregularities commonly occur. There is also a possibility of masculinizing effects from the use of anabolic steroids. Some of these effects, such as coarsening and eventually deepening of the voice, hirsutism, male pattern baldness, reduction of breast size, and clitoral enlargement, may or may not be partially reversible.

In most men, however, once the anabolic steroids are discontinued, the hormonal parameters eventually return to normal, except perhaps in those athletes who have used large amounts of anabolic steroids for prolonged periods of time. In some of these athletes, the serum testosterone might remain depressed for several weeks to months—secondary to testicular atrophy and refractiveness of the hypothalamic-pituitary-testicular axis (Alen et al., 1987). Occasionally, the serum testosterone fails to return to normal and a long-term replacement therapy is necessary.

The other group of adverse effects are those that are not usually thought of as related to either the anabolic or androgenic properties of these compounds. These adverse effects, while controversial as to the role that anabolic steroids have in their genesis and development, result in more than just cosmetic changes. Included in this group are changes in serum cholesterol, cardiovascular disease, prostatic cancer, kidney dysfunction, disturbances in carbohydrate metabolism, emotional disturbances, increased incidence of musculoskeletal injuries, cerebrovascular accidents, hepatic dysfunction (with rare instances of hepatic cirrhosis), hepatocellular carcinoma, and peliosis hepatitis.

We can also separate adverse effects into the short-term and long-term consequences of using anabolic steroids. Many of the short-term consequences are clinically clear, especially those resulting in changes in the female secondary sexual characteristics and in feminization of the male. The long-term consequences, however, are most elusive. There is some speculation that the chronic use of anabolic steroids might, in those genetically susceptible, cause hepatic cirrhosis, peliosis hepatitis, primary hepatoma, atherosclerosis and cardiac disease, diabetes, prostatic cancer, and cerebrovascular accidents.

Growth Hormone

Growth hormone (GH) is one of the hormones produced by the anterior portion of the pituitary gland (situated at the base of the brain under the hypothalamus) under the regulation of the hypothalamic hormones, growth hormone releasing hormone (GHRH), somatostatin, and galanin (Johnston, 1985).

Growth hormone is a species-specific anabolic protein that promotes somatic growth, stimulates protein synthesis, and regulates carbohydrate and lipid metabolism (Isaksson, 1985).

Before 1986, growth hormone was extracted from human pituitaries harvested during postmortems. The natural form of GH, however, like other biological preparations used to treat humans, including blood, have been discovered to contain viral contaminants. For example, a retrovirus contaminant has been implicated in several cases of a fatal neurologic disease, Creutzfeldt-Jakob Disease (CJD, Kuru).

Distribution of all products derived from human pituitaries has been stopped in North America and many other countries because there is no way to screen GH batches to assure their safety. It is still available from some countries. At present, it appears that Russian cadaveric GH is being widely used in North America (Deyssig and Frisch, 1993).

At present, biosynthetic growth hormone

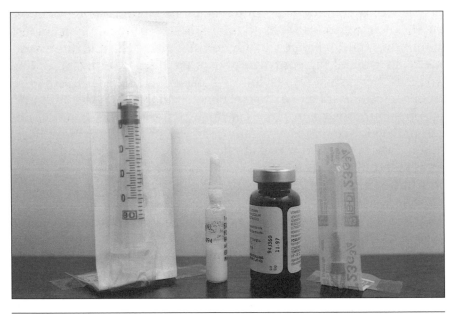

Growth hormone.

produced through recombinant DNA technology using the gene for human growth hormone is used almost exclusively worldwide. It is equal in potency to pituitary human growth hormone (Hintz, 1982).

Adverse Effects of Growth Hormone

The major effect of growth hormone is to promote growth in many different tissues. Receptors for growth hormone exist in the plasma membranes of many types of tissues, particularly in muscle, bone, kidney, liver, intestinal, adipose, and connective tissue. Many of the effects of growth hormone are carried out by insulin-like growth factors I and II. These are growth-hormone-dependent peptides produced in the liver.

Growth hormone increases intracellular amino acid transport, increases nucleic acid synthesis (DNA and RNA), and increases protein synthesis. These functions of growth hormone are similar to the anabolic effects of androgens. It has been found that the presence of growth hormone improves the response of tissues to androgens.

Other effects of growth hormone include stimulation of lipolysis (fat breakdown), increased collagen (or connective tissue) synthesis, and increased calcium and phosphate absorption. Growth hormone increases the available energy supply through fat metabolism. It stimulates the release of fatty acids from adipose tissue and increases the intracellular conversion of fatty acids into acetyl-CoA, thus sparing protein and glucose.

The increased secretion of GH seen during exercise may be of importance due to its anabolic, lipolytic, and glucoregulatory functions.

Growth Hormone Use

GH use by athletes has escalated dramatically in the past five years. In the early 1980s the use of natural GH was not a widespread phenomenon, but with increased availability and the increased tendency to use combinations of anabolic drugs, this has changed.

Along with the increased use of GH also comes an increase in the use of drugs and nutritional substances that may raise endogenous GH levels. Athletes often use combinations of GH stimulators with the hope of increasing GH secretion even further. There is some factual basis for this belief—the synergistic effect of clonidine, propanolol, L-dopa, and others has been documented (Rodriguez et al., 1984). It would appear that the mechanisms by which insulin-induced hypoglycemia, L-dopa, and arginine stimulate GH secretion are all different (Masuda et al., 1990).

Some forms of exercise also increase GH secretion. Intense exercise involving large muscle groups performed for up to one hour seems to result in optimal growth hormone release.

Side Effects.   It is possible that extended use of excessive amounts of exogenous human GH might produce some changes that are normally seen in cases of endogenous GH excess, including acral bony changes, changes in facial features and facial bones, voice changes, glucose intolerance (possibly resulting in relative insulin deficiency and diabetes), hypogonadism, peripheral nerve compression, cardiac enlargement, hypertension, and increased serum cholesterol and triglycerides (Moller et al., 1989).

Diabetes insipidus, a deficiency of vasopressin or ADH from the pituitary, is not a result of growth hormone hypersecretion per se. However, diabetes mellitus, or sugar diabetes (relative insulin deficiency), can result from growth hormone hypersecretion. This is due to the insulin-resistant effect of growth hormone.

There have been scattered reports of an increase in certain cancers in patients receiving GH. Several studies and reviews have concluded that there is a positive correlation between GH therapy and leukemia (Boose et al., 1992).

Growth Factors

Growth factors are the latest cutting-edge drugs being used by pharmacologically advanced bodybuilders. There is also a trickle-down effect to other elite athletes. These drugs have been shown to have potent effects on muscle and connective tissue. In many cases, combinations of these drugs act synergistically, so the combined effect of two or more of them appears significantly greater than the effect of any one of them.

There are a number of growth and trophic agents that have been characterized in the literature. These growth factors promote particular types of cellular growth, differentiation, and migration, and include S100 beta, brain-derived neurotrophic factor (BDNF), neurotrophic 4/5 (NT-4/5), ciliary neurotrophic factor (CNTF), transforming growth factor beta (TGF beta), platelet-derived growth factor-AB (PDGF-AB), leukemia inhibitory factor (CDF/LIF), insulin-like growth factors I and II (IGF), nerve growth factor (NGF), neurotrophin-3 (NT3), epidermal growth factor (EGF), acidic and basic fibroblast growth factors (aFGF, bFGF), endothelins (ET-2), and the heparin-binding growth-associated molecule (HB-GAM).

Insulin-Like Growth Factor I

Insulin-like growth factor I (IGI-I) is being used increasingly by bodybuilders and other athletes. Although IGF-I is used strictly in research, it has become available on the black market. While growth hormone (GH) exerts some direct effects, most of its growth and anabolic effects are mediated by IGF-I and IGF-II. The IGF peptides are bound tightly to plasma proteins (IGFBPs), and because of this binding their activity is extended to several hours as opposed to the 20 to 30 minutes of the unbound forms.

IGF-I is mostly responsible for the anabolic effects of GH. IGF-I is produced in the liver, chondrocytes, kidneys, muscles, pituitary, and gastrointestinal tract. The liver is the main source of circulating IGF-I.

Levels of IGF-I and IGFBP-3 (a GH-dependent protein that binds IGF-I) tie in with GH secretion and increase as GH levels increase. Levels are also age-dependent, with low levels in early childhood, a peak during adolescence, and a decline after age 50. As a consequence of protein binding and thus controlled release, the concentration of IGF-I remains relatively constant throughout the day, in contrast to the fluctuating levels of GH itself.

IGF-I seems to have a split personality in that it exerts both GH and insulin-like actions on skeletal muscles (Fryburg, 1994) by increasing protein synthesis and decreasing protein breakdown. Both GH and IGF-I seem to shift the metabolism to decreasing fat formation and increasing protein synthesis.

It has been shown that IGFs stimulate protein synthesis and inhibit protein degradation at physiological concentrations (Gulve and Dice, 1989). Studies done on normal humans, comparing IGF-I action to insulin action, suggest that insulin-like effects of IGF-I in humans are mediated in part via IGF-I receptors and in part via insulin receptors (Laager et al., 1993).

Only a few studies have looked at the effects of IGF-I on protein synthesis in athletes. One recent study has shown that neither GH nor IGF-I treatments result in increases in the rate of muscle protein synthesis or reduction in the rate of whole body protein breakdown, metabolic alterations that would promote muscle protein anabolism in experienced weightlifters attempting to further increase muscle mass (Yarasheski et al., 1993).

In a new study this year, however, it was reported that larger doses of IGF-I had significant anabolic effects in humans (Mauras and Beaufrere, 1995). This study investigated whether recombinant human insulin-like growth factor I (rhIGF-I) could serve as a protein-sparing nondiabetogenic agent. Twenty-one healthy volunteers were studied in three similar clinical models: rhIGF-I alone, rhIGF-I and prednisone, and prednisone alone. Prednisone, being a potent catabolic agent, was used to determine the anticatabolic effects of IGF-I.

The conclusion drawn from this study is that 100 mcg/kg rhIGF-I, given twice daily (a) has GH-like effects on whole body protein metabolism, (b) markedly diminishes the protein catabolic effect of glucocorticosteriods, and, (c) is nondiabetogenic in prednisone-treated humans. The authors of these studies feel that IGF-I offers promise in the treatment of protein catabolic states. IGF-I could be useful for maximizing the effects of exercise on muscle mass and strength because of its anabolic and anticatabolic effects.

Adverse Effects

Although the growth factors might be useful in a variety of clinical conditions, it has been postulated that several of these factors can have serious health consequences, including promoting asthma, atherosclerosis, and cancer.

In lesions of atherosclerosis, various cytokines and growth factors, which are generally not expressed in the normal artery are upregulated. Several of them, including PDGF, bFGF, HB-EGF, IGF-I, IL-I and TGF-beta, and TNF, play key roles in atherogenesis by stimulating chemotaxis and the proliferation of vascular smooth muscle cells and production of extracellular matrix substances, such as proteoglycans, collagen, and elastic fibers by those cells (Kawakami and Kuroki, 1993).

Epidermal growth factor (EGF), a potent mitogen and tumor promoter, is excreted in urine, permitting it to incubate with urothelial cells (Messing and Murphy-Brooks, 1994). Insulin-like growth factor I (IGF-I) is a potent mitogen for breast cancer cells (Lahti et al., 1994).

A recent study has suggested that stimulants at the EGF receptor (EGF and transforming growth factor alpha) might play a role in the airway smooth-muscle hyperplasia in asthma (Stewart et al., 1994).

Stacking the Hormones

True to form, bodybuilders and other athletes are already stacking IGF-I with a number of other anabolic compounds, including GH, insulin, anabolic steroids, and other growth factors such as EGF and bFGF. Research seems to support this view in that there is often a synergistic effect on protein metabolism when two or more of these compounds are used together.

For example, a combination of GH and IGF-I has been shown to be much more potent in improving nitrogen balance than either one alone (Kupfer et al., 1993). GH/IGF-I treatment also attenuates the hypoglycemia caused by IGF-I alone (Clemmons, 1993).

Interestingly, in the natural state, GH and IGF-I are part of a feedback loop, so that while IGF-I levels may be dependent on GH, elevated IGF-I levels inhibit GH release. Conversely, a decrease in IGF-I, as induced by starvation, leads to a compensatory increase in GH release.

It would appear that in the natural state both peptides are not present together in elevated levels for any significant period of time. Perhaps this is why the use of both compounds together is so effective on protein metabolism, both in decreasing protein breakdown and increasing protein synthesis.

As well as GH/IGF-I combinations, there are other studies supporting combinations of other hormones. In one study, it was reported that GH and insulin separately produced an increase in whole-body and skeletal muscle protein net balance. GH plus insulin was associated with a higher net balance of protein than was insulin alone (Wolf et al., 1992). There thus appears to be a synergistic improvement in whole-body and skeletal muscle protein kinetics when GH and insulin are used together. For example, together they reduce whole-body and skeletal muscle protein loss in cancer patients (Wolf et al., 1992). It has also been shown that insulin and IGH-I have additive effects on protein metabolism (Umpleby et al., 1994).

Studies have shown that without GH and IGH-I, testosterone has limited anabolic effects. The combined use of testosterone and IGF-I, however, results in a synergistic effect on protein metabolism (Donahue et al., 1993). As well, testosterone increases GH secretion partly secondary to its aromatization to estradiol (Weissberger and Ho, 1993).

In summary, while the various growth factors might indeed be anabolic and act synergistically with each other and with other anabolic drugs, such as the anabolic steroids and insulin, they have potentially life-threatening side effects, especially in those individuals who might be genetically susceptible to their atherosclerotic, tumerogenic, and asthmatic effects.

Little is known about the adverse effects of IGF-I or of stacking IGF-I with GH, insulin, anabolic steroids, and other compounds. Mixing and matching all these hormones and other drugs is a fool's game, made all the more dangerous by counterfeit and tainted drugs now on the black market.

Increasing Endogenous Testosterone

There are a number of hormones that stimulate the body's production of testosterone. These endogenous hormones are found in the hypothalamus and the pituitary. Also, there are both synthetic and natural compounds that mimic their effects.

Human Chorionic Gonadotropin

Human chorionic gonadatropin (HCG) is a hormone synthesized by chorionic tissue of the placenta and is extracted and purified from the urine of pregnant women. This hormone, once thought to be produced and excreted only by pregnant women and those with certain tumors, has been found to be produced in a pulsatile fashion by the pituitary in all normal adults (Odell and Griffin, 1987).

HCG produces systemic results similar to luteinizing hormone (LH) when used parenterally. HCG, like LH, stimulates the production of androgens and estrogens in men and women. In men, HCG stimulates Leydig tissue resulting in the secretion of androgens.

HCG acts by directly stimulating the Leydig cells of normal testes. Both single and repeated doses of HCG (dosages varying from 1,500 to 5,000 international units) significantly increase the plasma testosterone in normal men. Single doses increase serum levels of testosterone for several days.

Clinically, HCG is used as one of the compounds to stimulate ovulation in hypogonadotropic women and to stimulate spermatogenesis in men. Although it is frequently used in promoting fat mobilization and aiding weight loss, it is not effective in either of these applications.

Bodybuilders and other athletes are currently using HCG for several reasons. It is used by itself to increase the production of endogenous testosterone. One study reported that plasma testosterone levels, in response to repeated HCG stimulation, were significantly higher in trained than in untrained subjects (Jezova et al., 1987).

HCG is used to prevent testicular atrophy during anabolic steroid usage, and it is effective in doing so. It is used to augment the exogenous intake of anabolic steroids by increasing endogenous production of testosterone and is useful for this purpose. Many studies have documented the plasma testosterone response to injections of HCG even in relatively low doses (Balducci et al., 1987). Using HCG with anabolic steroids does not maintain testicular steroidogenesis since the testicular response to HCG is diminished when anabolic steroids are used concomitantly (Repcekova and Mikulaj, 1977). HCG is also used by athletes to try to decrease testicular atrophy and the negative effects that occur when coming off prolonged dosages of anabolic steroids. Although HCG does stimulate endogenous testosterone production in those athletes who are in a transient hypogonadotropic state secondary to the use of anabolic steroids (Martikainen et al., 1986), it does not help in reestablishing the normal hypothalamic/pituitary/testicular axis, except in cases where depression of testicular steroidogenesis is the main cause of the transient hypogonadotropic state.

HCG may mask the use of testosterone since it increases both endogenous testosterone and epitestosterone production and excretion, thus lowering an elevated testosterone/epitestosterone ratio (Riondino and Strollo, 1981).

Human Menopausal Gonadotropins (HMG)

HMG (Pergonal) is a mixture of FSH (follicle stimulating hormone) and LH extracted and purified from the urine of postmenopausal women. Commercial preparations of HMG, or menotropins, contain 75 international units of FSH and 75 international units of LH, biologically standardized in a lyophilized form. One international unit of HCG is equivalent to 2 international units of LH.

Clinically, HMG is usually used in conjunction with HCG to stimulate ovulation in anovulatory women and to stimulate spermatogenesis in men. It can also be used like HCG to increase endogenous testosterone production in men.

Gonadotropin Releasing Hormone (GnRH)

GnRH, known also as luteinizing hormone releasing hormone (LHRH), is produced in the hypothalamus and controls the pituitary gland's secretion of LH and FSH. Parenteral use of this hormone increases endogenous testosterone production by increasing LH production and secretion, which in turn stimulates the testes. Clinically, it is used for induction of ovulation in women with hypogonadotropic amenorrhea or polycystic ovary syndrome. This substance might be used by athletes as a substitute for HCG.

Antiestrogens

Antiestrogens are compounds that are competitive inhibitors of estrogens, both endogenous and exogenous. We'll describe three: tamoxifen, clomiphene, and cyclofenil.

Tamoxifen (Nolvadex) is a potent nonsteroidal, oral antiestrogen that competes with estrogen at binding sites and has no estrogenic activity. Clomiphene (Clomid) is an analog of chlorotrianisene (Tace), a synthetic estrogen. It is mildly estrogenic and acts as an antiestrogen. Cyclofenil, a nonsteroidal compound, is a weak estrogen related to stilbestrol.

All three compounds elevate endogenous gonadotropin production (both FSH and LH). This effect on the endogenous gonadotropins was once thought to be due to the prevention of a normal check imposed by estrogens on the hypothalamus and pituitary. Recently it has been shown, however, that estrogens act directly on the hypothalamus to increase gonadotropin secretion. Tamoxifen is thought to increase the release of GnRH as well.

These compounds are used by many athletes in an attempt to decrease the feminizing effects of the aromatizable anabolic steroids and to increase HDL cholesterol, thus partially protecting themselves from adverse cardiovascular problems. The use of these compounds has escalated dramatically in the past few years, especially in bodybuilders who feel that Nolvadex makes them "harder."

Clomiphene is useful in the testing of hypothalamic-pituitary reserve in athletes whose serum testosterone remains depressed after the discontinuation of anabolic steroids (Glass, 1988). Clomiphene, along with several other compounds, is useful in treating residual dysfunction in the hypothalamic-pituitary-testicular axis (Di Pasquale, 1990).

Tamoxifen is the antiestrogen of choice among most bodybuilders. However, recent studies have shown that the drug can have the opposite effect on a small number of people. Instead of decreasing estrogen production, it can promote it; instead of acting as an estrogen antagonist, it can act as an agonist.

Tamoxifen might be counterproductive in that it has been shown to decrease testicular steroidogenesis. A recent study reported that tamoxifen reduced the synthesis of testosterone through an inhibition of the 17 alpha-hydroxylase and C17,20-desmolase enzyme systems together with an increased 20 alpha-hydroxysteroid dehydrogenase activity (Vanderstichele et al., 1989).

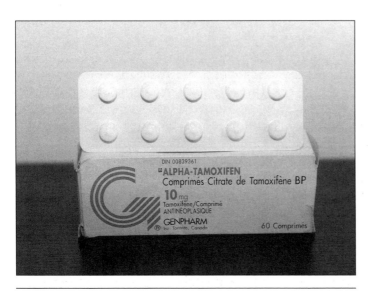

Antiestrogens like tamoxifen inhibit or modify the action of estrogens.

Tamoxifen might also have a negative effect on serum GH. In one study, it was shown that administration of testosterone enanthate significantly increased GHRH-elicited GH release, but this was reverted after estrogen-receptor blockade with tamoxifen (Lima et al., 1989). This likely occurs because testosterone acts on GH release mainly at the suprapituitary level, and this action is secondary to its aromatization to estrogen. Another recent study has shown, however, that tamoxifen increases GH secretion when used with testosterone enanthate (Devesa et al., 1991). More studies must be done to determine the exact effect of tamoxifen on GH release in athletes.

Testolactone

Testolactone (Teslac), an aromatase inhibitor, decreases estrogen production and is used by bodybuilders much like the antiestrogens to counter the feminizing effects of anabolic steroids and testosterone and to elevate LH and free serum testosterone.

Although it is generally felt that testolactone has no appreciable androgenic or anabolic effects, it's quite possible that in addition to competitively binding to the androgen receptor, testolactone also possesses some of the anticatabolic action of androgenic/anabolic hormones. Testolactone has been shown to produce anabolic effects in rats; therefore, the possibility exists that nitrogen, potassium, and phosphorus retention, increase in protein anabolism, and decrease in amino acid catabolism, could also occur in humans.

Testolactone might also have an effect on serum growth hormone (GH). Co-administration of testolactone with testosterone enanthate suppresses the normally observed increase in estradiol following administration of the enanthate, and thus might result in a reduction in serum GH or a reduction in the rise of serum GH with various stimuli.

Insulin

Insulin, insulin-stimulating drugs, insulin-enhancing drugs, and supplements (such as vandium, sulphate, and chromium) meant to augment or increase endogenous insulin, are being used by athletes in an attempt to enhance athletic performance.

Insulin is a polypeptide hormone that regulates carbohydrate metabolism and influences both the synthesis of protein and of RNA and the formation and storage of neutral lipids. Insulin is an anabolic hormone in that it facilitates and increases the transport of glucose and amino acids into muscle and fat cells, increases the synthesis and storage of cellular protein and glycogen in muscle cells and of triglycerides in fat cells, and decreases protein breakdown (May and Buse, 1989).

It appears that long-term exercise, even if mild, improves insulin action in both carbohydrate and lipid metabolism and increases the metabolic clearance rate of insulin (Oshida et al., 1989).

Insulin is used by some athletes (who are not diabetic) for its anabolic effect, usually in combination with anabolic steroids, growth hormone, or both. A recent study has shown that the simultaneous use of insulin and recombinant human growth hormone can have additive anticatabolic effects and thus might be useful for treating cancer cachexia (Wolf et al., 1992). It is possible that insulin and the other anabolic compounds might act synergistically to produce significant anticatabolic and anabolic effects.

Insulin increases the activity of lipoprotein lipase and generally enhances the synthesis of fat; therefore, bodybuilders who use insulin often also use thyroid hormone. The lipolytic effects of the latter may counteract the increased fat synthesis of the former.

Regardless of effects or side effects, the fact is that some bodybuilders are using supraphysiological doses of exogenous insulin and insulogenic agents in order to benefit from insulin's anabolic properties and to combat any glucose intolerance secondary to the use of other anabolic compounds. The use of exogenous insulin has tapered off dramatically after a few bodybuilders had life-threatening hypoglycemic (low blood sugar) attacks resulting in a few cases of hypoglycemic coma. Luckily, there were no deaths.

Insulogenic drugs are being more widely used in the drug regimen of some of the elite bodybuilders. However, they are not innocuous and may cause hypoglycemic attacks and other severe side effects.

Thyroid Hormone

Bodybuilders use thyroid hormone because it helps them get cut and because the use of thyroid hormone is ingrained in the drug arsenal of competing bodybuilders.

Is there some scientific reason why the use of thyroid hormone is so pervasive? Well, in a way yes, since it is true that the thyroid gland slows down when you diet, and can take a nosedive when bodybuilders literally starve themselves to get contest-ready.

Starvation produces a rapid fall in basal metabolic rate (BMR) of 20% or more, mainly due to a fall in triiodothyronine (T3). This mild hypothyroidism may lead to sensations of cold, lethargy, and increased sleep. Starvation impairs thermogenesis (a process whereby excess calories are converted to heat rather than stored as fat) in parallel with the drop in thyroid hormone. During starvation there is also a slowing of the conversion of thyroxine to triiodothyronine.

It is also true that less thyroid is produced with strenuous exercise. As well, alterations in thyroid hormone secretion and serum levels can occur secondarily to the use of both anabolic steroids and growth hormone (Deyssig and Weissel, 1993).

This means that when you are trying to cut up by drastically reducing calories, your thyroid cuts back production of thyroid hormone and so decreases the amount of energy expended and fat burned. This is opposite of what you want. As well, it seems that when we do strenuous exercise, thyroid function decreases (Pakarinen et al., 1991). One way to stop the decrease is to eat more (Loucks and Callister, 1993), hardly an option if, like most bodybuilders, you are trying to cut up by using a high complex-carb, calorie-restricted diet.

All in all, when you seem to need it the most, you get the least. Tossing caution to the wind, bodybuilders decided they needed extra thyroid, especially prior to contests. So, in a way, bodybuilders use thyroid hormone to supplement their own dwindling inner supply, but they usually go beyond just replacement therapy and use too much for too long.

The use of thyroid hormone is not innocuous. The overuse of thyroid hormone results in overall muscle loss, which is explained below. Thus in an attempt to decrease body fat, athletes end up losing a lot of muscle mass that they really can't afford to lose.

By abusing thyroid hormone, some athletes put the brakes on their own natural thyroid production for months, years, and sometimes permanently. While thyroid hormone is being used, the body stops production of its own thyroid hormones. The thyroid stops producing both T3 and T4, and the pituitary and the hypothalamus stop producing their respective releasing hormones that normally control the production of thyroid hormones by the thyroid gland.

In addition to the adverse physiological effects of large amounts of thyroid hormone (with associated neurological and cardiovascular complications), the significant muscle loss, and the suppression of the hypothalamic-pituitary-thyroid axis, there has been some evidence that both hyperthyroidism and thyroxine replacement therapy might be associated with subclinical liver damage (Beckett et al., 1985).

As you can see, thyroid hormone can be compared to the bowls of porridge in the story of Goldilocks and the Three Bears. There is a level that is just right. Too little (cold) or too much (hot) thyroid hormone causes havoc in the body.

How does thyroid affect muscle protein and body fat?

Thyroid hormones exert most of their effects by increasing the basal metabolic rate, controlling protein synthesis, and enhancing the lipolytic response of fat cells to other hormones.

Thyroxine and triiodothyronine can affect muscle mass because they stimulate both protein synthesis and degradation depending on dosage and the presence and levels of other hormones and regulators. In physiological concentrations, thyroid hormones stimulate the synthesis as well as the degradation of proteins, whereas in higher or supraphysiological doses, protein catabolism (breakdown) predominates—as part of the overall hypermetabolism that occurs.

Thus in hyperthyroidism or with the use of high doses of thyroid hormone, the net effect is muscle wasting (with an increase in the turnover of body protein) rather than hypertrophy. Prolonged use of large doses of thyroid might result in extensive muscular wasting. In contrast, an excess in thyroid hormone can produce cardiac muscle hypertrophy (Muller and Seitz, 1984).

Clenbuterol and Other Beta-2 Andrenergic Agonists

Clenbuterol, a drug used in asthma and in labor, is used by bodybuilders and other athletes because of its stimulant and anabolic properties. This compound, like other third generation beta-2-selective adrenergic agonists, has increased beta-2 selectivity; and thus they are more specific bronchodilators, with fewer cardiovascular and neuromuscular side effects (Whitsett et al., 1981).

Of the newer beta agonists, the ones most often used are carbuterol, clenbuterol, fenoterol, mabuterol, procaterol, reproteral, rimiterol, salbutamol, terbutaline, and tolbuterol. These agents are taken in different ways, namely by mouth, injection, and inhalation (except for clenbuterol, which is only effective orally).

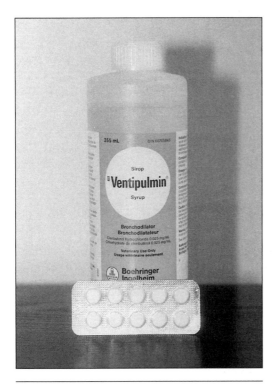

One of the beta-2 andrenergic agonists.

Studies in animals have shown that beta-adrenergic agonists have potent growth-promoting effects, resulting in measurable increases in lean muscle mass and loss of body fat. Not all beta agonists, however, have anabolic properties, and it appears that various compounds have different anabolic and antilipogenic actions (Reeds et al., 1988). Of those tested, clenbuterol, cimaterol, and, to a lesser extent, fenoterol influence muscle growth via beta-adrenoceptor stimulation, resulting in increases in muscle mass, body weight, and muscle protein synthesis rate.

Clenbuterol has been shown to prevent muscle atrophy (Babij and Booth, 1988), decrease myofibrillar protein breakdown (Benson et al., 1991), and cause a significant increase in protein synthesis and skeletal and cardiac muscle growth (mainly type II muscle fiber types), a decrease in subcutaneous and total body fat, and an increase in energy expenditure. In one study, the chronic administration of clenbuterol caused hypertrophy of histochemically identified fast- but not slow-twitch fibers within the soleus, suggesting that the role of beta-2 receptors lies in regulating muscle fiber type composition as well as growth (Zeman et al., 1988). Other studies have shown that clenbuterol decreases subcutaneous fat by increasing lipolysis and depressing lipogenesis (Miller et al., 1989). It also appears that the anabolic effect might be independent of other anabolic hormones, including the sex hormones (Yang and McElligott, 1989).

Side effects with clenbuterol appear minimal, although there is some evidence that clenbuterol treatment induces pressor effects in normotensive animals under stress (Gutkind et al., 1989). In humans, the most common adverse effects—headaches, nervousness, and inability to sleep (usually seen at the higher doses)—are common to most other sympathomimetic amines such as the amphetamines, ephedrine, and propanolamine.

Although several studies of animals have documented clenbuterol's anabolic effects, no human studies have as yet been done to determine its effects on athletic performance. As is often the case, effects seen in vitro or in animals under controlled conditions do not translate fully when the same compound is used in humans. In practice, clenbuterol is not the anabolic wonder drug that the literature makes it out to be.

You Can Do It Without Drugs

The four most important factors to consider when trying to maximize lean body mass are lifestyle, exercise, diet, and supplements. By maximizing all four, you can achieve a state where diet, training strategy, workload capacity, recovery capacity, and anabolic drive are all working in harmony. This, in turn, will maximize the effects of the endogenous hormones in order to achieve maximum growth as quickly as is genetically possible.

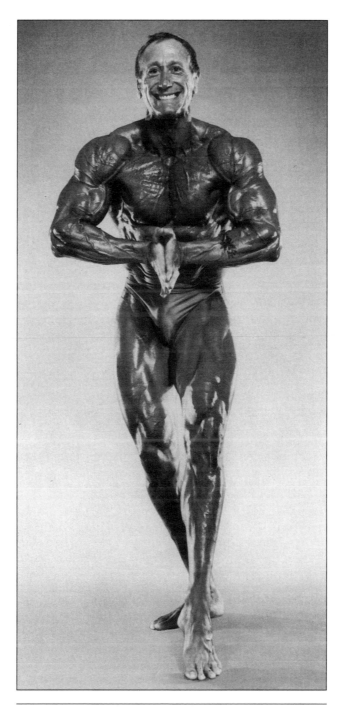

The drug-free physique of André Elie.

By manipulating your diet, exercise, lifestyle, and supplements, you can fine-tune your hormonal systems and achieve an increased anabolic drive that can take the place of drugs. All athletes could benefit from this manipulation, especially those involved in sports where strength and lean body mass are of primary importance for athletic success (Hakkinen, 1989).

You can do it without drugs and avoid the myriad health and financial problems that plague drug-using athletes.

APPENDIX 1

Table A.1 Training log

Enter: Exercise
Load and number of repetitions per set (i.e., 180·6)

No.	Exercise	Sets									
		1	2	3	4	5	6	7	8	9	10

Reprinted from Bompa 1996.

APPENDIX 2

Table A.2	Maximum lift based on repetitions					
% of 1 RM **Reps**	**100** **1**	**95** **2**	**90** **4**	**85** **6**	**80** **8**	**75** **10**
Lbs. lifted	700.00	665.00	630.00	595.00	560.00	525.00
	695.00	660.25	625.50	590.75	556.00	521.25
	690.00	655.50	621.00	586.50	552.00	517.50
	685.00	650.75	616.50	582.25	548.00	513.75
	680.00	646.00	612.00	578.00	544.00	510.00
	675.00	641.25	607.50	573.75	540.00	507.00
	670.00	636.50	603.00	569.50	536.00	502.50
	665.00	631.75	598.50	565.25	532.00	498.75
	660.00	627.00	594.00	561.00	528.00	495.00
	655.00	622.25	589.50	556.75	524.00	491.25
	650.00	617.50	585.00	552.50	520.00	487.50
	645.00	612.76	580.50	548.25	516.00	483.75
	640.00	608.00	576.00	544.00	512.00	480.00
	635.00	603.25	571.50	539.75	508.00	476.25
	630.00	598.50	567.00	535.50	504.00	472.50
	625.00	593.75	562.50	531.25	500.00	468.75
	620.00	589.00	558.00	527.00	496.00	465.00
	615.00	584.25	553.50	522.75	492.00	461.25
	610.00	579.50	549.00	518.50	488.00	457.50
	605.00	574.75	544.50	514.25	484.00	453.75
	600.00	570.00	540.00	510.00	480.00	450.00
	595.00	565.25	535.50	505.75	476.00	446.25
	590.00	560.50	531.00	501.50	472.00	442.50
	585.00	555.75	526.50	497.25	468.00	438.75
	580.00	551.00	522.00	493.00	464.00	435.00
	575.00	546.25	517.50	488.75	460.00	431.25
	570.00	541.50	513.00	484.50	456.00	427.50
	565.00	536.75	508.50	480.25	452.00	423.75
	560.00	532.00	504.00	476.00	448.00	420.00
	555.00	527.50	499.50	471.75	444.00	416.25
	550.00	522.50	495.00	467.50	440.00	412.50
	545.00	517.75	490.50	463.25	436.00	408.75

(continued)

Table A.2   *(continued)*

% of 1 RM Reps	100 1	95 2	90 4	85 6	80 8	75 10
Lbs. lifted	540.00	513.00	486.00	459.00	432.00	405.00
	535.00	508.25	481.50	454.75	428.00	401.25
	530.00	503.50	477.00	450.50	424.00	397.50
	525.00	498.75	472.50	446.25	420.00	393.75
	520.00	494.00	468.00	442.00	416.00	390.00
	515.00	489.25	463.50	437.75	412.00	386.25
	510.00	484.50	459.00	433.50	408.00	382.50
	505.00	479.75	454.50	429.25	404.00	378.75
	500.00	475.00	450.00	425.00	400.00	375.00
	495.00	470.25	445.50	420.75	396.00	371.25
	490.00	465.50	441.00	416.50	392.00	367.50
	485.00	460.75	436.50	412.25	388.00	363.75
	480.00	456.00	432.00	408.50	384.00	360.00
	475.00	451.25	427.50	403.75	380.00	356.25
	470.00	446.50	423.00	399.50	376.00	352.50
	465.00	441.75	418.50	395.25	372.00	348.75
	460.00	437.00	414.00	391.00	368.00	345.00
	455.00	432.75	409.50	386.75	364.00	341.25
	450.00	427.50	405.00	382.50	360.00	337.50
	445.00	422.75	400.50	378.25	356.00	333.75
	440.00	418.00	396.00	374.00	352.00	330.00
	435.00	413.25	391.50	369.75	348.00	326.25
	430.00	408.50	387.00	365.50	344.00	322.50
	425.00	403.75	382.00	361.25	340.00	318.75
	420.00	399.00	378.00	357.00	336.00	315.00
	415.00	394.25	373.50	352.75	332.00	311.25
	410.00	389.50	369.00	348.50	328.00	307.50
	405.00	384.75	364.50	344.25	324.00	303.75
	400.00	380.00	360.00	340.00	320.00	300.00
	395.00	375.25	355.50	335.75	316.00	296.25
	390.00	370.50	351.00	331.50	312.00	292.50
	385.00	365.76	346.50	327.25	308.00	288.75
	380.00	361.00	342.00	323.00	304.00	285.00
	375.00	356.25	337.50	318.75	300.00	281.25
	370.00	351.50	330.00	314.50	296.00	277.50
	365.00	346.75	328.50	310.25	292.00	273.75
	360.00	342.00	324.00	306.00	288.00	270.00
	355.00	337.25	319.50	301.75	284.00	266.25
	350.00	332.50	315.00	297.50	280.00	262.50
	345.00	327.75	310.50	293.25	276.00	258.75
	340.00	323.00	306.00	289.00	272.00	255.00
	335.00	318.25	301.50	284.75	268.00	251.25
	330.00	313.50	297.00	280.50	264.00	247.50
	325.00	308.75	292.50	276.25	260.00	243.75
	320.00	304.00	288.00	272.00	256.00	240.00
	315.00	299.25	283.50	267.75	252.00	236.25

% of 1 RM Reps	100 1	95 2	90 4	85 6	80 8	75 10
Lbs. lifted	310.00	294.50	279.00	263.50	248.00	232.50
	305.00	289.75	274.50	259.25	244.00	228.75
	300.00	285.00	270.00	255.00	240.00	225.00
	295.00	280.25	265.50	250.75	236.00	221.25
	290.00	275.50	261.00	246.50	232.00	217.50
	285.00	270.75	256.50	242.25	228.00	213.75
	280.00	266.00	252.00	238.00	224.00	210.00
	275.00	261.25	247.50	233.75	220.00	206.25
	270.00	256.50	243.00	229.50	216.00	202.50
	265.00	251.75	238.50	225.25	212.00	198.75
	260.00	247.00	234.00	221.00	208.00	195.00
	255.00	242.25	229.50	216.75	204.00	191.25
	250.00	237.50	225.00	212.50	200.00	187.50
	245.00	232.75	220.50	208.25	196.00	183.75
	240.00	228.00	216.00	204.00	192.00	180.00
	235.00	223.25	211.50	199.75	188.00	176.25
	230.00	218.50	207.00	195.50	184.00	172.50
	225.00	213.75	202.50	191.25	180.00	168.75
	220.00	209.00	198.00	187.00	176.00	165.00
	215.00	204.25	193.50	182.75	172.00	161.25
	210.00	199.50	189.00	178.50	168.00	157.50
	205.00	194.75	184.50	174.25	164.00	153.75
	200.00	190.00	180.00	170.00	160.00	150.00
	195.00	185.25	175.50	165.75	156.00	146.25
	190.00	180.50	171.00	161.50	152.00	142.50
	185.00	175.75	166.50	157.25	148.00	138.75
	180.00	171.00	162.00	153.00	144.00	135.00
	175.00	166.25	157.50	148.75	140.00	131.25
	170.00	161.50	153.00	144.50	136.00	127.50
	165.00	156.75	148.50	140.25	132.00	123.75
	160.00	152.00	144.00	136.00	128.00	120.00
	155.00	147.25	139.50	131.75	124.00	116.25
	150.00	142.50	135.00	127.50	120.00	112.50
	145.00	137.75	130.50	123.24	116.00	108.75
	140.00	133.00	126.00	119.00	112.00	105.00
	135.00	128.25	121.50	114.75	108.00	101.25
	130.00	123.50	117.00	110.50	104.00	97.50
	125.00	118.75	112.50	106.25	100.00	93.75
	120.00	114.00	108.00	102.00	96.00	90.00
	115.00	109.25	103.50	97.75	92.00	86.25
	110.00	104.50	99.00	93.50	88.00	82.50
	105.00	99.75	94.50	89.25	84.00	78.75

Reprinted from Bompa 1996.

APPENDIX 3

If for any reason (such as the equipment available), an athlete cannot lift the load necessary to calculate 1RM, but only 3, 4, or 5RM, one can still figure out his or her 1RM by using the chart below. In order to calculate 1RM, perform the maximum number of repetitions with the load available (say 4 repetitions with 250 lbs), and then:

1. Choose from the top of the chart the column headed "4"—the number of repetitions you did.
2. Find the row with "250 lbs"—the maximum load you had available.
3. Find the number where column "4" and row "250" meet.
4. This number is your 1RM at that given time.

Table A.3 Maximum weight chart

Lbs.	10	9	8	7	6	5	4	3	2
5	7	6	6	6	6	6	6	5	5
10	13	13	13	12	12	11	11	11	11
15	20	19	19	18	18	17	17	16	16
20	27	26	25	24	24	23	22	22	21
25	33	32	31	30	29	29	28	27	26
30	40	39	38	36	35	34	33	32	32
35	47	45	44	42	41	40	39	38	37
40	53	52	50	48	47	46	44	43	42
45	60	58	56	55	53	51	50	49	47
50	67	65	63	61	59	57	56	54	53
55	73	71	69	67	65	63	61	59	58
60	80	77	75	73	71	69	67	65	63
65	87	84	81	79	76	74	72	70	68
70	93	90	88	85	82	80	78	76	74
75	100	97	94	91	88	86	83	81	79
80	107	103	100	97	94	91	89	86	84
85	113	110	106	103	100	97	94	92	89
90	120	116	113	109	106	103	100	97	95
95	127	123	119	115	112	109	106	103	100
100	133	129	125	121	118	114	111	108	105
105	140	135	131	127	124	120	117	114	111

(continued)

Table A.3   (continued)

Lbs.	10	9	8	7	6	5	4	3	2
110	147	142	138	133	129	126	122	119	116
115	153	148	144	139	135	131	128	124	121
120	160	155	150	145	141	137	133	130	126
125	167	161	156	152	147	143	139	135	132
130	173	168	163	158	153	149	144	141	137
135	180	174	169	164	159	154	150	146	142
140	187	181	175	170	165	160	156	151	147
145	193	187	181	176	171	166	161	157	153
150	200	194	188	182	176	171	167	162	158
155	207	200	194	188	182	177	172	168	163
160	213	206	200	194	188	183	178	173	168
165	220	213	206	200	194	189	183	178	174
170	227	219	213	206	200	194	189	184	179
175	233	226	219	212	206	200	194	189	184
180	240	232	225	218	212	206	200	195	189
185	247	239	231	224	218	211	206	200	195
190	253	245	238	230	224	217	211	205	200
195	260	252	244	236	229	223	217	211	205
200	267	258	250	242	235	229	222	216	211
205	273	265	256	248	241	234	228	222	216
210	280	271	263	255	247	240	233	227	221
215	287	277	269	261	253	246	239	232	226
220	293	284	275	267	259	251	244	238	232
225	300	290	281	273	265	257	250·	243	237
230	307	297	288	279	271	263	256	249	242
235	313	303	294	285	276	269	261	254	247
240	320	310	300	291	282	274	267	259	253
245	327	316	306	297	288	280	272	265	258
250	333	323	313	303	294	286	278	270	263
255	340	329	319	309	300	291	283	276	268
260	347	335	325	315	306	297	289	281	274
265	353	342	331	321	312	303	294	286	279
270	360	348	338	327	318	309	300	292	284
275	367	355	344	333	324	314	306	297	289
280	373	361	350	339	329	320	311	303	295
285	380	368	356	345	335	326	317	308	300
290	387	374	363	352	341	331	322	314	305
295	393	381	369	358	347	337	328	319	311
300	400	387	375	364	353	343	333	324	316
305	407	394	381	370	359	349	339	330	321
310	413	400	388	376	365	354	344	335	326
315	420	406	394	382	371	360	350	341	332
320	427	413	400	388	376	366	356	346	337
325	433	419	406	394	382	371	361	351	342
330	440	426	413	400	388	377	367	357	347
335	447	432	419	406	394	383	372	362	353
340	453	439	425	412	400	389	378	368	358
345	460	445	431	418	406	394	383	373	363
350	467	452	438	424	412	400	389	378	368

Lbs.	10	9	8	7	6	5	4	3	2
355	473	458	444	430	418	406	394	384	374
360	480	465	450	436	424	411	400	389	379
365	487	471	456	442	429	417	406	395	384
370	493	477	463	448	435	423	411	400	389
375	500	484	469	455	441	429	417	405	395
380	507	490	475	461	447	434	422	411	400
385	513	497	481	467	453	440	428	416	405
390	520	503	488	473	459	446	433	422	411
395	527	510	494	479	465	451	439	427	416
400	533	516	500	485	471	457	444	432	421
405	540	523	506	491	476	463	450	438	426
410	547	529	513	497	482	469	456	443	432
415	553	535	519	503	488	474	461	449	437
420		542	525	509	494	480	467	454	442
425		548	531	515	500	486	472	459	447
430		555	538	521	506	491	478	465	453
435		561	544	527	512	497	483	470	458
440		568	550	533	518	503	489	476	463
445		574	556	539	524	509	494	481	468
450		581	563	545	529	514	500	486	474
455		587	569	552	535	520	506	492	479
460		594	575	558	541	526	511	497	484
465		600	581	564	547	531	517	503	489
470		606	588	570	553	537	522	508	495
475		613	594	576	559	543	528	514	500
480		619	600	582	565	549	532	519	505
485		626	606	588	571	554	539	524	511
490		632	613	594	576	560	544	530	516
495		639	619	600	582	566	550	535	521
500		645	625	606	588	571	556	541	526
505		652	631	612	594	577	561	546	532
510		658	638	618	600	583	567	551	537
515		665	644	624	606	589	572	557	542
520		671	650	630	612	594	578	562	547
525		677	656	636	618	600	583	569	553
530		684	663	642	624	606	589	573	558
535		690	669	648	629	611	594	578	563
540		697	675	655	635	617	600	584	568
545		703	681	661	641	623	606	589	574
550		710	688	667	647	629	611	595	579
555		716	694	673	653	634	617	600	584
560		723	700	679	659	640	622	605	589
565		729	706	685	665	646	628	611	595
570		735	713	691	671	651	633	616	600
575		742	719	697	676	657	639	622	605
580		748	725	703	682	663	644	627	611
585		755	731	709	688	669	650	632	616
590		761	738	715	694	674	656	638	621
595		768	744	721	700	680	661	643	626

(continued)

Table A.3   *(continued)*

Lbs.	10	9	8	7	6	5	4	3	2
600		774	750	727	706	686	667	649	632
605		781	756	733	712	691	672	654	637
610		787	763	739	718	697	678	659	642
615		794	769	745	724	703	683	665	647
620		800	775	752	729	709	689	670	653
625		806	781	758	735	714	694	676	658
630		813	788	764	741	720	700	681	663
635		819	794	770	747	726	706	686	668
640		826	800	776	753	731	711	692	674
645		832	806	782	759	737	717	697	679
650		839	813	788	765	743	722	703	684
655		845	819	794	771	749	728	708	689
660		852	825	800	776	754	733	714	695
665		858	831	806	782	760	739	719	700
670		865	838	812	788	766	644	724	705
675		871	844	818	794	771	750	730	711
680		877	850	824	800	777	756	735	716
685		884	856	830	806	783	761	741	721
690		890	863	836	812	789	767	746	726
695		897	869	842	818	794	772	751	732
700		903	875	848	824	800	778	757	737
705		910	881	855	829	806	783	762	742
710		916	888	861	835	811	789	768	747
715		923	894	868	841	817	794	773	753
720		929	900	873	847	823	800	778	758
725		935	906	879	853	829	806	784	763
730		942	913	885	859	834	811	789	768
735		948	919	891	865	840	817	795	774
740		955	925	897	871	846	822	800	779
745		961	931	903	876	851	828	805	784
750		968	938	909	882	857	833	811	789
755		974	944	915	888	863	839	816	795
760		981	950	921	894	869	844	822	800
765		987	956	927	900	874	850	827	805
770		994	963	933	906	880	856	832	811
775		1,000	969	939	912	886	861	838	816
780		1,006	975	945	918	891	867	843	821
785		1,013	981	952	924	897	872	849	826
790		1,019	988	958	929	903	878	854	832
795		1,026	994	964	935	908	883	859	837
800		1,032	1,000	970	941	914	889	865	842
820		1,058	1,025	994	965	937	911	886	863
840		1,084	1,050	1,018	988	960	933	908	884
860		1,110	1,075	1,042	1,012	983	956	930	905
880		1,135	1,100	1,067	1,035	1,006	978	951	926
900		1,161	1,125	1,091	1,059	1,029	1,000	973	947
920		1,187	1,150	1,115	1,082	1,051	1,022	995	968

Reprinted from Bompa 1996.

GLOSSARY OF TERMS

Actin: a protein involved in muscular activity.

Adaptation: persistent changes in structure or function of a muscle as a direct response to progressively increased training loads.

Adaptation Threshold: the level of adaptation an individual reaches as a result of training in a given training phase. To surpass the threshold, one has to increase the stimulation (loading) level.

Agonistic Muscle: a muscle directly engaged in a muscular contraction, and working in opposition to the action of other muscles.

All-or-None Law: a stimulated muscle or nerve fiber contracts or propagates a nerve impulse either completely, or not at all (i.e., a minimal stimulus causes a maximum response).

Amino Acid (AA): basic unit of structure in proteins.

Anabolic: protein building.

Androgenic: a substance that possesses masculinizing properties.

Antagonistic Muscle: a muscle that has an opposite effect on a mover, or agonistic muscle, by opposing its contraction.

ATP Deficiency Theory: the disturbance in the equilibrium between consumption and manufacturing of ATP. The constant taxation of ATP apparently results in increased muscle hypertrophy.

Atrophy: a gradual shrinking of the muscle tissue as a result of disuse or disease.

Ballistic: dynamic muscular movements.

Bioelectrical Impedance Analysis (BIA): a method of measuring body fat. An electrical current is transmitted through the body, and the resistance or impedance to the current is measured. Because the body's fat free mass contains much of the body's water and electrolytes and is therefore a better conductor of electrical current, impedance to the current gives us information about the person's percentage of body fat.

Biological Value (BV): describes how efficiently body tissue can be created from food proteins.

Calorie Cycling: the practice of alternating low-, medium-, and high-calorie days to prevent the body from adapting to any particular amount of food intake. Helps to keep the metabolism from slowing down during periods of dieting.

Carbohydrate: any of a group of chemical compounds, including sugars, starches, and cellulose, containing carbon, hydrogen, and oxygen only. One of the basic food stuffs.

Cardiac Stroke Volume (or Stroke Volume): the amount of blood pumped out of each ventricle per beat. The normal amount is approximately 70 ml/beat in a resting man of average size, tested in a supine position.

Catabolic: increases the degradation of protein.

Ceiling of Adaptation: a certain level of adaptation an individual has reached during training. The scope of training is to break the ceiling of adaptation in order to increase it, and as a result, to improve performance.

Central Nervous System (CNS): the spinal cord and the brain.

Cheat Day: a planned day used during periods of dieting to help prevent the body from adapting to specific caloric intakes.

Chronic Hypertrophy: the long-lasting hypertrophy resulting from structural changes at the muscle level following the employment of heavy loads (over 80% 1RM).

Complete Proteins: proteins that contain all of the nine essential amino acids. They are found in animal protein sources.

Complex Carbohydrates: also known as polysaccharides or starches. They are composed of many glucose units and are found in vegetables, fruits, and grains.

Creatine Kinase (CK): a soluble muscle protein that when found in the circulatory system is indicative of muscle damage. Specific isomers of creatine kinase are used to differentiate between damage to skeletal muscle and cardiac muscle.

Creatine Phosphate (CP): a high-energy compound stored in muscles; it supplies energy for high-intensity activities that last less than 30 seconds.

Cross-Bridges: extensions of myosin, a contractile protein. Cross-bridges play a major role in muscle contraction.

Cryotherapy: the use of cold to treat or prevent injuries.

Detraining: reversal of adaptation to exercise. Effects of detraining occur more rapidly than training gains, with significant reduction of strength (and work) capacity within two weeks from cessation of training.

Disaccharides: simple sugars composed of two monosaccharides. The most common are sucrose (table sugar) and lactose (found in milk).

Double Pyramid Load Pattern: pertaining to increasing the load from the bottom up, and decreasing it again to the initial level.

Dynamic Flexibility: the performance of a motion requiring flexible muscles in an active manner (as opposed to static). Often called *ballistic flexibility*.

Eccentric Contraction: a muscle action that produces a lengthening of muscle fibers as it develops tension.

Edema: a local or generalized condition in which the body tissues contain an excessive amount of tissue fluid. Acute swelling/edema refers to the rapid onset of tissue fluid build-up in an area that lasts for a short course of time (i.e., not chronic).

Effleurage: a slow, rhythmic stroke, either superficial or deep, performed along the long axis of the body's tissue and utilized during massage therapy.

Electromyography (EMG): measurement of the electrical activity of the excitable membranes of the muscle or muscle group.

Endorphin: powerful opioid peptide manufactured in the brain that regulates pain perception. Responsible for the euphoric sensations experienced during vigorous exercise, such as the runner's high, second wind, and so on. A member of the morphine family.

Essential Amino Acids: amino acids that cannot be synthesized by the body, and therefore must be supplied by the diet.

Excitation: ability to react to a stimulus.

Fasciculus (fasciculi pl.): a group or bundle of skeletal muscle fibers held together by a connective tissue call the *perimysium*.

Fast-Twitch Fiber (FT): a muscle fiber characterized by fast contraction time, high anaerobic capacity, and low aerobic capacity, all making the fiber suited for high power output activities.

Fat: a compound containing glycerol and fatty acids. One of the major basic foodstuffs.

Fat Free Mass (FFM): the weight of the body, minus the fat.

Fixators: muscles that are stimulated to act in order to stabilize the position of a bone to perform a motion. Also know as *stabilizers*.

Flat Pyramid Load Pattern: a loading pattern, which after the warm-up lift, stabilizes the load for the entire duration of strength training.

Flexibility: the range of motion about a joint (static flexibility); opposition or resistance of a joint to motion (dynamic flexibility).

Frictions (Cyriax's deep frictions massage): a technique that uses transverse movements across the connective tissue surface of either muscles, tendons, or ligaments to initiate and restore the normal forces and mobility of the structures.

Glycemic Index: a chart that was created to help diabetics control their insulin levels. Foods are given a glycemic value that tells whether or not they are digested slowly or quickly (i.e., whether or not they will cause harmful insulin fluctuations). Bodybuilders have found this to be a useful tool for dieting purposes.

Glycogen: the form in which carbohydrates (glucose) are stored in the muscles and liver.

Glycolysis: the incomplete chemical breakdown of glycogen into pyruvic acid (through aerobic glycolysis) or lactic acid (through anaerobic glycolysis).

Growth Hormone (GH): a hormone secreted by the anterior lobe of the pituitary gland that stimulates growth and development.

Heavy Load: a load using a percentage over 80-85% of the maximum.

Hemorrhage: bleeding.

Homeostasis: the maintenance of a relatively stable internal physiological condition. As the stress of exercise causes changes in the internal environment, the body is constantly working to restore balance, or achieve homeostasis.

Hydrostatic Weighing: an accurate technique used to measure body fat, whereby the subject is submerged in a water tank and weighed. This value, along with the dry-land weight, residual volume, and water temperature, are used to calculate percentage of body fat.

Hyperemia: an increase in the quantity of blood flowing through any part of the body. This is often experienced as a "pump" or the feeling of blood-engorged muscles after weight training.

Hyperplasia: an increase in the number of cells in a tissue or organ.

Hypertrophy: an increase in the size of a tissue or organ due to increased cell size, rather than increased cell number.

Incomplete Proteins: proteins that do not contain all of the nine essential amino acids. They are found in plant proteins.

Inhibition: to repress or slow down the stimulating (excitation) effect of the CNS (by decreasing the electrical activity).

Intensity: refers to the qualitative element of training. In bodybuilding training, intensity is expressed as a percentage of 1RM.

Isokinetic Contraction: a contraction in which tension is developed, but there is no change in the length of the muscle.

Isotonic Contraction: a contraction in which the muscle shortens while lifting a constant load. Also know as a *concentric* or *dynamic contraction*.

Joint: junction of two or more bones in the human body, in which the bones are joined in a functional relationship.

Kneading: a circular compressive massage technique done on the soft tissue against the bony structures below. This technique enhances the flow of tissue fluid in the body, reduces swelling and inflammation, decreases muscle spasm, and lengthens shortened soft-tissue structures.

Lactic Acid (LA): a fatiguing metabolite of the lactic acid (anaerobic) system resulting from the incomplete breakdown of glucose.

Lactic Acid System: an anaerobic energy system in which ATP is manufactured through the breakdown of glucose, in the absence of oxygen, to lactic acid. Used in high-intensity work over a short duration (less than 2 minutes).

Ligament: a strong band of fibrous tissue used to connect bones to each other.

Limiting Amino Acid: the essential amino acid that is in shortest supply in the body and that is consequently responsible for the cessation of protein synthesis.

Line of Pull: the line of action of the tension developed by a muscle.

Lipotropin: a trophic hormone secreted by the anterior lobe of the pituitary gland. Its physiological function is unclear, but its amino acid sequence is similar to that of endorphins and enkepahlins (another endogenous morphine-like substance) and hence is also believed to produce analgesia.

Low Load: pertaining to loads between 0-49% of one's maximum.

Macrocycle: a phase of training of 2-6 weeks in duration.

Maximum Load: refers to a load of 90-100% of one's maximum.

Medium Load: pertaining to loads between 50-89% of one's maximum.

Membrane: a structural barrier composed of lipids and proteins.

Microcycle: a phase of training of approximately 1 week in duration.

Microtears: small tears found in muscle, ligaments, and/or tendons.

Monosaccharides: simple sugars. The two most common are glucose (blood sugar) and fructose (found in fruit).

Motor Neuron: a nerve cell, which when stimulated, effects muscular contraction. Most motor neurons innervate skeletal muscle.

Motor Unit: an individual motor nerve and all the muscle fibers it innervates.

Myofibril: the part of a muscle fiber containing two protein filaments—myosin and actin.

Myosin: a protein involved in muscular contraction.

Negative Calorie Balance: a state in which the body is burning off more calories than it is consuming. This is necessary if weight loss is to occur.

Net Protein Utilization (NPU): adjusts the biological value of a protein to account for its digestibility.

Neural Adaptation: an increase in the nervous coordination of a group of muscles involved in contraction. Often gains in strength during prepuberty are the result of improved neural adaptation.

Neuromuscular Junction: the union of a muscle and its nerve.

Neuron: a nerve cell. A cell specialized to initiate, integrate, and conduct electric signals.

Nonessential Amino Acids: amino acids that can be synthesized by the body and therefore do not need to be supplied by the diet.

One Repetition Maximum (1RM): the maximum amount of weight that a person can lift once; 100% of one's lifting capacity.

Overcompensation: often called *supercompensation*, refers to the relationship between work and regeneration as a biological base for physical and psychological arousal before a heavy workout.

Overloading: an increase of work in training with the scope to bring about improvements in strength.

Periodization of Bodybuilding: the methodological structure of training phases intended to bring about the best improvements in muscle size, tone, and definition.

Periodization of Nutrition: the structure of nutritional and training supplement needs in order to match training phases as per the periodization of strength for bodybuilding.

Petrissage: a deep massage technique that consists of rolling folds of skin, subcutaneous tissue, and muscle over the underlying structures between the fingers and thumb in a continuous circular motion. Petrissage helps to reduce muscle spasm and stretch contracted and adherent fibrous tissues.

Phase Specific: pertaining to a particular training phase (i.e., hypertrophy phase, muscle definition phase, etc.).

Plantar Flexion: movement of the foot forward and downward.

Plateau: period during training when no observable progress is made.

Polysaccharides: see *complex carbohydrate*.

Prime Movers: the muscles primarily responsible for the performance of a technical movement.

Proprioceptive Neuromuscular Facilitation (PNF): flexibility technique designed to enhance the relaxation and contraction of a body part, based on neurophysiological principles.

Protein: a substance that is composed of amino acid chains. It is used for tissue growth and repair, as opposed to fuel for the body.

Pump: the thick, full feeling during weight training, which is the result of blood engorging the muscles being trained.

Pyramid Load Pattern: a method of load patterning, whereby the load for an exercise starts low, gradually increases with each set, hits a high point, and then decreases.

Receptor: specific protein-binding site in plasma membrane or interior of target cell.

Recommended Dietary Allowance (RDA): a guideline of food intake for the general population. RDA values may not be appropriate for serious bodybuilders because of the heightened demands placed on the body.

Sensory Neuron: a nerve cell that conveys impulses from a receptor to the CNS. Examples of sensory neurons are those excited by sound, pain, light, and taste.

Skewed Pyramid Load Pattern: a pyramid in which the load is constantly increased throughout the session, with exception being made for the last set, when the load is lowered.

Slow-Twitch Fiber (ST): a muscle fiber characterized by slow contraction time, low anaerobic capacity, and high aerobic capacity, all making the fiber suited for low power output activities.

Specificity Training: principle underlying construction of a training program for a specific activity or skill.

Spotter: an individual who watches and/or assists a lifter while a set is being performed.

Stabilizers (Fixators): muscles that are stimulated to act, to anchor, or to stabilize the position of a limb.

Standard Loading: a load that remains at the same level for a certain period of time.

Static Flexibility: passively stretching an antagonistic muscle by placing it in a maximal stretch position and holding it in place.

Step-Loading Principle: pertaining to increasing the load from week to week, normally for three weeks, followed by a week of unloading so the body can regenerate before a new increase.

Stretch or Myotatic Reflex: a reflex that responds to the rate of muscle stretch. This reflex has the fastest known response to a stimulus (in this case, the rate of muscle stretch). The stretch reflex elicits a contraction of the muscle being stretched and the synergistic muscles, while inhibiting the antagonistic muscles, when it senses that a stretch is being performed too quickly or rigorously.

Summation: an increase in muscle tension or contractile strength, in response to rapid, repetitive stimulation relative to single twitch.

Supermaximum Load: a load that exceeds 100% of one's 1RM (1 repetition maximum). These weights should only be used by experienced lifters, especially in the maximum strength phase of training.

Synergist Muscles: muscles that actively provide an additive contribution to the agonist muscle during a muscle contraction.

Tapotement: a massage technique that uses a succession of gentle blows delivered with either a cupped hand (percussion) or the ulnar border of the hand (hacking) onto the body to increase blood flow, stimulate cutaneous reflexes, increase muscle tone, reduce inflammation and accelerate the healing process.

Tendon: collagen fiber bundle that connects muscle to bone and transmits muscle contractile force to the bone.

Testosterone: the male sex hormone produced in the testes; responsible for secondary male sexual characteristics.

Transient Hypertrophy: temporary enlargement of the muscles due to water accumulation in the muscles, and not due to permanent tissue growth. This occurs during and shortly after an intense weight-training session, and subsides after a short time when the body returns to its normal state (homeostasis).

Twitch: a brief period of contraction followed by relaxation in the response of a motor unit to a stimulus (nerve impulse).

Unloading: the decrease of load, often for the purpose of allowing the body and mind to regenerate and refresh itself before a new loading phase.

Urea: a major body waste product formed from the breakdown of amino acids.

Valsalva Maneuver: expiration against a closed glottis, resulting in an increase in intrathoracic and blood pressure. Occurs during weightlifting when the breath is held during an exercise, instead of maintaining a regular breathing pattern. This may be dangerous to those with cardiovascular disorders.

Vasodilation: expansion of the blood vessels, especially the arteries and their branches.

Vibrations (Shaking): a massage technique administered by trembling of the hands against the skin firmly to compress swollen tissues and reduce swelling, to reduce muscle tone, and to promote relaxation.

Viscous: the property of a fluid that makes it resist flow.

Yo-Yo Dieting: the process of repeatedly gaining and losing large amounts of body weight.

BIBLIOGRAPHY

Acupuncture Foundation of Canada Institute. (1994), Patient Education Brochure. Toronto.

Adams, M.A., W.C. Hutton and J.R.R. Stott. (1980), "The Resistance to Flexion of the Lumbar Intervertebral Joint." *Spine*, 5(3 May/June):245-253.

Ahlborg, B., et al. (1967), "Muscle Glycogen and electrolytes during prolonged physical exercise." *Acta Physiol Scand*, 70:129-142.

Alen, M. and P. Rahkila. (1988). Anabolic-androgenic steroid effects on endocrinology and lipid metabolism in athletes. *Sports Medicine Journal*. 6:327-332.

Alen, M., P. Rahkila, M. Reinila, and R. Vihko. (1987), "Androgenic-anabolic steroid effects on serum thyroid pituitary and steroid hormones in athletes." *American Journal of Sports Medicine*, 15(4):357-361.

Allen, L.H., E.A. Oddoye, and S. Margen. (1979), "Protein-induced hypercalciuria: A longer term study." *American Journal of Clinical Nutrition*, 32:741-749.

Anderson, B. (1980), *Stretching*, New York, N.Y.: Shelter Publications.

Anon. (1985), "Human GH withdrawn." *Pharm. Journal*, 234:625.

Appell, H.J. (1990), "Muscular atrophy following immobilization: A review." *Sports Medicine*, 10(1):42-58.

Armstrong, R.B. (1986). Muscle damage and endurance events. *Sports Medicine*. Vol 3: 370-381.

Arnheim, D. Modern principles of athletic training. 7th edition. (1989). *Times Mirror/Mosby College Publishing*. St Louis, MO.

Asmussen, E. and K. Mazin. (1978). A central nervous component in local muscular fatigue. *European Journal of Applied Physiology*. 38:9-15.

Babij, P. and F.W. Booth. (1988), "Clenbuterol prevents or inhibits loss of specific mRNAs in atrophying rat skeletal muscle." *American Journal of Physiology*, 254:657-60.

Balducci, R., V. Toscano, D. Casilli, et al. (1987), "Testicular responsiveness following chronic administration of HCG (1500 IU every six days) in untreated hypogonadotropic hypogonadism." *Horm Metab. Res.*, 19(5):216-221.

Baroga, L. (1978). Contemporary tendencies in the methodology of strength development. *Educatia Fizica si Sport*. 6:22-36.

Beckett, G.J., H.A. Kellett, S.M. Gow, et al. (1985), "Raised plasma glutathione S-transferase values in hyperthyroidism and in hypothyroid patients receiving thyroxine replacement: Evidence for hepatic damage." *Br. Med. Journal*, 291:427-431.

Benson, D.W., T. Foley-Nelson, W.T. Chance, et al. (1991), "Decreased myofibrillar protein breakdown following treatment with clenbuterol." *Journal Surg. Res.*, 50(1):1-5.

Bigland-Ritchie, R. Johansson, O.C.J. Lipold, and J.J. Woods. (1983). Contractile speed and EMG changes during fatigue of sustained maximal voluntary contractions. *Journal of Neurophysiology.* 50(1):313-324.

Bompa, T.O. (1994), *Theory and Methodology of Training.* Dubuque, Iowa: Kendall/Hunt Publishing Inc.

Bompa, T.O. (1993), *Power Training: Plyometrics For Maximum Power Development.* Oakville-New York-London: Mosaic Press/Coaching Association of Canada.

Bompa, T.O., M. Hebbelinck, and B. Van Gheluwe. (1978), *A Biochemical Analysis Of The Rowing Stroke Employing Two Different Oar Grips.* Brasilia, Brazil: The XXI World Congress in Sports Medicine.

Boose, A.R., R. Peters, H.A. Delemarre Van de Wall, and A.J. Veerman (1992), "Growth hormone therapy and leukemia (Review)." *Tijdschrift voor Kindergeneeskunde,* 60(1):1-6.

Bunt, J.C., T.G. Lohman, and R.A. Boileau. (1989), "Impact of total body water fluctuations on estimation of body fat from body density." *Medicine and Science in Sports and Exercise,* 21:96-100.

Callaghan, M.J. (1993). The role of massage in the management of the athlete: a review. *Br. J. Sports Med.* 27(1): 28-33.

Caton, J.R., P.A. Mole, W.C. Adams, and D.S. Heutis. (1988), "Body composition analysis by bioelectrical impedance: Effects of skin temperature." *Medicine and Science in Sports and Exercise,* 20:489-491.

Chamberlain, G.J. (1982). Cyriax's friction massage: a review. *The Journal of Orthopedic and Sports Physical Therapy.* 4:16-22.

Cinque, C. (1989). Massage for cyclists: the winning touch. *Phys Sports Med.* 17: 167-170.

Clemmons, D.R. (1993), "Use of growth hormone and insulin-like growth factor I in catabolism that is induced by negative energy balance." *Horm Res.,* 40(1-3):62-67.

Conlee, R.K. (1987). Muscle glycogen and exercise endurance: a twenty year perspective. *Exercise and Sport Sciences Review.* 15:1-28.

Consolazio, C.F., R.A. Nelson, L.O. Matoush, R.S. Harding, and J.E. Canham. (1963), "Nitrogen excretion in sweat and its relation to nitrogen balance experiments." *Journal of Nutrition,* 79:399-406.

DeLuca, C.J., R.S. LeFever, M.P. McCue, and A.P. Xenakis. (1982), "Behaviour of human motor units in different muscles during lineally varying contractions" *Journal Physiology* (Lond), 329:113-128.

Denny-Brown, D. (1949), "Interpretation of the electromyogram." *Arch Noural Psychiat,* 61:99-128.

Devesa, J., N. Lois, V. Arce, et al. (1991), "The role of sexual steroids in the modulation of growth hormone (GH) secretion in humans." *Journal of Steroid Biochem. Mol. Biol.,* 40(1-3):165-173.

Deyssig, R. and M. Weissel. (1993), "Ingestion of androgenic-anabolic steroids induces mild thyroidal impairment in male body builders." *Journal of Clin.Endocrinol. Metab.,* 76(4):1069-1071.

Deyssig, R. and H. Frisch. (1993), "Self-administration of cadaveric growth hormone in power athletes." *Lancet,* 341(8847):768-769.

DiPasquale, M.G. (1990), *Anabolic Steroid Side Effects - Fact, Fiction and Treatment*. Warkworth, Ontario: MGD Press.

Donahue, L.R., G. Watson and W.G. Beamer. (1993), "Regulation of metabolic water and protein compartments by insulin-like growth factor-I and testosterone in growth hormone-deficient lit/lit mice." *Journal of Endocrinology*, 139(3):431-439.

Dragan, G.I., A. Vasiliu, and E. Georgescu. (1985), "Effects of increased supply of protein on elite weight lifters." In *Milk Proteins* 1984, T.E. Galeshoot and B.J. Tinbergen (Eds.), Wageningen, The Netherlands: Pudoc, 99-103.

Ebbing, C. and P. Clarkson. (1989). Exercise-induced muscle damage and adaptation. *Sports Medicine*. Vol 7: 207-234.

Edgerton, R.V. (1976), "Neuromuscular adaptation to power and endurance work." *Canadian Journal of Applied Sports Sciences*, 1:49-58.

Egginton, S. (1987), "Effects of an anabolic hormone on striated muscle growth and performance." *Pflugers Arch*, 410(4-5):649-55.

Enoka, R. (1994), *Neuromechanical Basis of Kinesiology*. Second Edition, USA Library of Congress Cataloging-in-Publishing Data. Champaign, IL: Human Kinetics.

Enwemcka, C.S., O. Rodriqiez and S. Mendosa. (1990), "The Biochemical Effects of Low-intensity Ultrasound on Healing Tendons." *Ultrasound in Medicine and Biology,* 16(8).

Evans, W.J. (1987). Exercise-induced skeletal muscle damage. *The Physician and Sports Medicine*. Vol 15(1): 89-100.

Fahey, T.D. (1991). How to cope with muscle soreness. *Power Research.*

Flynn, A. (1984), "Milk proteins in the diets of those of intermediate years." In *Milk Proteins* 1984, T.E. Galehoot and B.J. Tinbergen (Eds.) Wageningen, The Netherlands: Pudoc, 154-159.

Fox, E.L., R.W. Bowes, and M.L. Foss. (1989), *The Physiological Basis of Physical Education and Athletics*. Dubuque, Iowa: Wm. C. Brown Publishers.

Fry, R.W., R. Morton, and D. Keast. (1991), "Overtraining in athletics." *Sports Medicine*, 2(1):32-65.

Fryburg, D.A. (1994), "Insulin-like growth factor I exerts growth hormone-and insulin-like actions on human muscle protein metabolism." *American Journal of Physiology*, 267:E331-E336.

Fujikawa, K., B.B. Seedham and V. Wright. (1983), "Biomechanics of the Patello-Femoral Joint-Part 1: A Study of the Contact and the Congruity of the Patello-Femoral Compartment and Movement of the Patella." *Engineering in Medicine,* 12(1):3-11.

Glass, A.R. (1988), "Pituitary-testicular reserve in men with low serum testosterone and normal serum luteinizing hormone." *Journal of Androl*, 9(3):224-230.

Gledhill, N. (1987). *Fitness Assessment*. pp 1-40.

Goats, G.C. (1990). Interferential current therapy. *Br. J. Sports Med.* 24:87-90.

Goats, G.C. (1994a). Massage—the scientific basis of an ancient art: part 1, the technique. *Br. J. Sports Med.* 28(3): 149-151.

Goats, G.C. (1994b). Massage—the scientific basis of an ancient art: part 2, physiological and therapeutic effects. *Br. J. Sports Med.* 28(3):153-156.

Godfrey, C.M., H. Jayawardena, T.A. Quance, et al. (1979), "Comparison of Electrostimulation and Isometric Exercise in Strengthening the Quadriceps Muscle." *Physiotherapy Canada*, 31:265-267.

Goldber, L.J. and B. Derflier. (1977), "Relationship among recruitment order, spike amplitude, and twitch tension of single motor units in human masseter muscle." *Journal of Neurophysiology*, 40:879-890.

Goldberg, A.L., J.D. Etlinger, D.F. Goldspink, and C. Jablecki. (1975), "Mechanism of work-induced hypertrophy of skeletal muscles." *Medicine and Science in Sports and Exercise*, 7:185-198.

Gollhofer, A., P.A. Fujitsuka, N. and M. Miyashita. (1987), "Fatigue during stretch-shortening cycle exercises: Changes in Neuro-muscular activation patterns of human skeletal muscle." *Journal of Sports Medicine*, 8:30-47.

Griggs, R.C., W. Kingston, R.F. Jozefowicz, et al. (1989), "Effect of testosterone on muscle mass and muscle protein synthesis." *Journal of Applied Physiology*, 66(1):498-503.

Grimby, G. (1992), *Strength and Power is Sport*. Komi, P.V. (Ed.), Oxford: Blackwell Scientific Publications.

Gulve, E.A. and J.F. Dice. (1989), "Regulation of protein synthesis and degradation in L8 myotubes: Effects of serum, insulin and insulin-like growth factors." *Biochemical Journal*, 260(2):377-8.

Gutkind, J.S., M.G. Kazanietz, I. Armando, et al. (1989), "Pressor response induced by clenbuterol treatment in immobilized normotensive rats." *Journal of Cardiovascular Pharmacology,* 13(5):793-8.

Hainaut, K. and J. Duchatteau. (1989). Muscle fatigue: effects of training and disuse. *Muscle and Nerve*. 12:660-669.

Hakkinen, K. (1989), "Neuromuscular and hormonal adaptations during strength and power training." *A Review of Sports Medicine Physical Fitness*, 29(1):9-26.

Hakkinen, K. (1991), *Personal Communications on "Maximum Strength Development for Sports"*. Madrid.

Halback, J.W. (1980), "Comparison of Electro-myo-stimulation to Isokinetic Training in Increasing Power of the Knee Extensor Mechanism." *Journal of Orthopaedic and Sports Physical Therapy,* 2:20-24.

Halvorson, G. (1990), "Therapeutic Heat and Cold for Athlete Injuries." *The Physician and Sports Medicine,* 18(5):87-94.

Hartman, J.H. and H. Tünneman. (1988), *Fitness and Strength Training*. Berlin: Sportsverlag.

Haupt, H.A. and G.D. Rovere. (1984), "Anabolic steroids: A review of the literature." The *American Journal of Sports Medicine*, 12(6):464-484.

Hawkins, R.J. and J.C. Kennedy. (1980), "Impingement Syndrome in Athletes." *The American Journal of Sports Medicine,* 8(3):151-158.

Heyward, Vivian H. (1991), *Advanced Fitness Assessment and Exercise Prescription*. Champaign, IL: Human Kinetics Publishers, Inc.

Hintz, R.L. (1982), "Clinical comparison of natural and recombinant HGH." *Lancet*, 1:276.

Houmard, J.A. (1991), "Impact of reduced training of performance in endurance athletes." *Sports Medicine*, 12(6):380-393.

Isaksson, O.G.P. (1985), "Review of biological effects." *Ann. Rev. of Physiology,* 47:483-499.

Israel, S. (1972), "The acute syndrome of detraining." *Berlin: GDR National Olympic Committee,* 2:30-35.

Ivy, J.L. (1991), "Muscle glycogen synthesis before and after exercise." *Sports Medicine,* 11:6-19.

Jenkins, D.J.A. et al. (1987), "Metabolic effects of a low-glycemic-index diet." *American Journal of Clinical Nutrition,* 46:968.

Jenkins, D.J.A. (1982), "Lente carbohydrate: A newer approach to the management of diabetes." *Diabetes Care,* 5:634-639.

Jezova, D., L. Komadel and L. Mikulaj. (1987), "Plasma testosterone response to repeated human chorionic gonadotropin administration is increased in trained athletes." *Endocrinol. Exp.* (Bratisl), 21(2):143-147.

Johnston, D.G. (1985), "Regulation of GH secretion." *Journal of Roy. Soc.* Medicine, 78:319.

Johnston, D.H., P. Thurston and P.J. Ashcroft. (1977), "The Russian Technique of Faradism in the Treatment of Chrondromelacia Patellac." *Physiotherapy Canada,* 29:266-268.

Karlson, J. and B. Saltin. (1971). Diet, muscle glycogen and endurance performance. *Journal of Applied Physiology.* 31(2):203-206.

Kawakami, M., and M. Kuroki. (1993), "Roles of cytokines and growth factors in atherogenesis." *Japanese Journal of Clinical Medicine,* 51(8):2010-5.

Kenyon, A.T., K. Knowlton, G. Lotwin, and I. Sandford. (1942), "Metabolic response of aged men to testosterone propionate." *Journal of Clinical Endocrinology,* 2:690-695.

Kobayashi Matsui, H. (1983), "Analysis of myoelectric signals during dynamic and isometric contraction." *Electromyog Clin Neurophysiol,* 26,147-160.

Komi, P.V. and J.H.T. Viitasalo. (1976), "Signal characteristics of EMG at different levels of muscle tension." *Acta Physiol Scand,* 96:267-276.

Komi, P.V. and E.R. Buskirk. (1972), "Effect of eccentric and concentric muscle conditioning on tension and electrical activity of human muscle." *Ergonomics,* 15:8.

Kowal, M.A. (1983), "Review of the Physiological Effects of Cryotherapy." *The Journal of Orthopaedic and Sports Physical Therapy,* 5(2):66-73.

Kuipers, H. and H.A. Keizer. (1988), "Overtraining in elite athletes: Review and directions for the future." *Sports Medicine,* 6:79-92.

Kupfer, S.R., L.E. Underwood, R.C. Baxter and D.R. Clemmons. (1993), "Enhancement of the anabolic effects of growth hormone and insulin-like growth factor I by use of both agents simultaneously." *Journal of Clinical Investigation,* 91(2):391-6.

Laager, R., R. Ninnis and U. Keller. (1993), "Comparison of the effects of recombinant human insulin-like growth factor-I and insulin on glucose and leucine kinetics in humans." *Journal of Clin. Invest.,* 92(4):1903-1909.

Lahti, E.I., M. Knip and T.J. Laatikainen. (1994), "Plasma insulin-like growth factor I and its binding proteins 1 and 3 in postmenopausal patients with breast cancer receiving long term tamoxifen." *Cancer,* 74(2):618-24.

Lamb, D. (1984). Anabolic steroids in athletics: how do they work and how dangerous are they? *American Journal of Sports Medicine*. 12(1): 31-37.

Lemon, Peter W.R. (1991), "Protein and amino acid needs of the strength athlete." *International Journal of Sport Nutrition*, 1:127-390.

Lima, L., V. Arce, N. Lois, et al. (1989), "Growth hormone responsiveness to GHRH in normal adults is not affected by short-term gonadal blockade." *Acta Endocrinol*, 120(1):31-36.

Lindstrom, L., R. Magnusson, I. Peterson. (1970), "Muscle fatigue and action potential conduction velocity changes studied with frequency analysis of EMG signals." *Journal of Physiology* (Lond), 230:371-390.

Lohman, T.G., M.L. Pollock, M.H. Slaughter, L.J. Brandon, and R.A. Boileau. (1984), "Methodological factors and the prediction of body fat in female athletes." *Medicine and Science in Sports and Exercise*, 16:92-96.

Loucks, A.B. and R. Callister. (1993), "Induction and prevention of low-T3 syndrome in exercising women." *American Journal of Physiology*, 264(5 Pt.2): R924-30.

Low, J. and A. Reed. (1990), *Electrotherapy Explained: Principles and Practice*, London, Boston: Butterworth-Heinemann Ltd.

Lukaski, H.C., P.E. Johnson, W.W. Bolonchuk, and G.I. Lykken. (1985), "Assessment of fat-free mass using bioelectrical impedance measurement of the human body." *American Journal of Clinical Nutrition*, 41:810-817.

Lukaski, H.C. (1985), "Use of tetra polar bioelectrical impedance method to assess human body composition." In N.G. Norgan (Ed.), *Human Body Composition and Fat Distribution* (pp. 143-158). Wageningen, Netherlands: Euronut.

Marsden, C.D., J.C. Meadows and P.A. Merton. (1971). Isolated single motor units in human muscle and their rate of discharge during maximum voluntary effort. *Journal of Physiology*. (London). 217: 12P.

Martikainen, H., M. Alen, P. Rahkila and R. Vihko. (1986), "Testicular responsiveness to human chorionic gonadotrophin during transient hypogonadotrophic hypogonadism induced by androgenic/anabolic steroids in power athletes." *Journal Steroid Biochem.*, 25(1):109-112.

Massey, B.H., R.C. Nelson., B.C. Sharkey., et al. (1965), "Effects of High Frequency Electrical Stimulation on the Size and Strength of Skeletal Muscle." *Journal of Sports Medicine and Physical Fitness,* 5:136-144.

Masuda, A., T. Shibasaki, M. Hotta, et al. (1990), "Insulin-induced hypoglycemia, L-dopa and arginine stimulate GH secretions through different mechanisms in man." *Regul Pept*, 31(1):53-64.

Matsuda, J.J., R.F. Zernicke, A.C. Vailus, V.A. Pedrini, A. Pedrini-Mille and J.A. Maynard. (1986). Structural and mechanical adaptation of immature bone to strenuous exercise. *Journal of Applied Physiology*. 60(6): 2028-2034.

Mauras, N. and B. Beaufrere. (1995), "Recombinant human insulin-like growth factor-I enhances whole body protein anabolism and significantly diminishes the protein catabolic effects of prednisone in humans without a diabetogenic effect." *Journal of Clin. Endocrinol. Metab.*, 80(3):869-74.

May, M.E. and M.G. Buse. (1989), "Effects of branched-chain amino acids on protein turnover." *Diabetes Metab. Rev.*, 5(3):227-245.

McDonagh, M.J.N. and C.T.M. Davis. (1984). Adaptive response of mammalian skeletal muscle to exercise with high loads. *European Journal of Applied Physiology.* 52:139-155.

Melo, G.L. and E. Cafarelli. (1994-95), *Exercise Physiology Laboratory Manual*, 25.

Melzack, R. and P.D. Wall. (1965). Pain mechanisms: a new theory. *Science.* 150: 971-979.

Messing, E.M. and N. Murphy-Brooks. (1994), "Recovery of epidermal growth factor in voided urine of patients with bladder cancer." *Urology*, 44(4):502-6.

Miller, M.F., H.R. Cross, J.J. Wilson and S.B. Smith. (1989), "Acute and long-term lipogenic response to insulin and clenbuterol in bovine intramuscular and subcutaneous adipose tissues." *Journal of Anim. Sci.*, 67(4):928-33.

Moller, A., L.M. Rasmussen, L. Thuesen and J.S. Christansen. (1989), "Impact of human GH on plasma lipoprotein concentrations." *Horm. Metab. Res.*, 21(4):207-9.

Moore, K.L. (1980), *Clinically Oriented Anatomy.* Baltimore: Williams and Wilkins.

Moore, M.A. and R.S. Hutton. (1980). Electromyographic investigation of muscle stretching techniques. *Medicine and Science in Sports and Exercise.* 12: 322-329.

Morgan, R.E. and G.T. Adamson. (1959), *Circuit Weight Training.* London: G. Bell and Sons.

Moritani, T., M. Muro, A. Kijima, F.A. Gaffney, and D. Parsons (1985), "Electro-mechanical changes during electrically induced and maximal voluntary con-tractions: Surface and intramuscular EMG responses during sustained maximal voluntary contractions." *American Journal of Physiological Medicine*, 58:115-130.

Moritani, T. and H.A. deVries. (1987), "Re-examination of the relationship between the surface integrated electromyogram (IEMG) and force of isometric contraction." *American Journal of Physiological Medicine*, 57:263-277.

Moritani, T., M. Muro, and A. Nagata. (1986), "Intramuscular and surface electromyogram changes during muscle fatigue." *Journal of Applied Physiology*, 60:1179-1185.

Moritani, T., A. Nagata, and M. Muro. (1982), "Electromyographic manifesta-tions of muscular fatigue." *Medicine and Science in Sports Exercise*, 14:198-202.

Muller, M.J. and H.J. Seitz. (1984), "Thyroid hormone action on intermediary metabolism. Part III. Protein metabolism in hyper- and hypothyroidism." *Klin Wochenschr*, 62(3):97-102.

Munro, H.N. (1951), "Carbohydrate and fat as factors in protein utilization and metabolism." *Physiol. Rev.*, 31:449-488.

Odell, W.D. and J. Griffin. (1987), "Pulsatile secretion of human chorionic gonadotropin in normal adults." *N. Engl. Journal of Medicine*, 317(27):1688-1691.

Oshida, Y., K. Yamanouchi, S. Hayamizu and Y. Sato. (1989), "Long-term mild jogging increases insulin action despite no influence on body mass index or VO₂max." *Journal of Applied Physiology*, 66(5):2206-2210.

Pakarinen, A., K. Hakkinen and M. Alen. (1991), "Serum thyroid hormones, thyrotropin and thyroxine binding globulin in elite athletes during very intense strength training of one week." *Journal of Sports Medicine & Physical Fitness*, 31(2):142-6.

Petrofsky, J.S. and A.R. Lind (1980), "The influence of temperature on the amplitude and frequency components of the EMG during brief and sustained isometric contractions," *European Journal of Applied Physiology*, 44:189-200.

Petrofsky, J.S. and A.R. Lind. (1980), "Frequency analysis of the surface elctromyogram during sustained isometric contractions." *European Journal of Applied Physiology*, 43:173-182.

Piehl, K. (1974). Time course for refilling of glycogen stores in human muscle fibers following exercise-induced glycogen depletion. *Acta Physiologica Scandinavica*. 90:297-302.

Prentice, W.J. (1990). Rehabilitation techniques in sports medicine. Toronto: *Times Mirror/Mosby College Publishing*.

Reeds, P.J., S.M. Hay, P.M. Dorwood and R.M. Palmer. (1988), "The effect of beta-agonists and antagonists on muscle growth and body composition of young rats." *Comp. Biochem. Physiol.*, 89(2):337-41.

Repcekova, D. and L. Mikulaj. (1977), "Plasma testosterone response to HCG in normal men without and after administration of anabolic drug." *Endokrinologie*, 69(1):115-18.

Richter, E.A., K.J. Mikines, H. Galbo and B. Keins. (1989), "Effect of exercise on insulin action in humans skeletal muscle." *Journal of Applied Physiology*, 66:876-885.

Riondino, G. and F. Strollo. (1981), "Age-dependent changes in epitestosterone urinary excretion in man." *Boll Soc Ital Biol Sper*, 57(22):2215-2221.

Rodriguez, D.O.L., M.C. Valeron, D.A. Carrillo, et al. (1984), "Evaluation of GH stimulation tests using clonidine, glucagon, propanolol, hypoglycemia, arginine and L-dopa in 267 children of short stature." *Rev. Clinc. Esp.*, 173(2):113-6.

Rowlands, R.P. and G.W. Nicholson (1929), "Growth of left testicle with precocious sexual and bodily development (macro-genitosomania)." *Guy's Hosp. Rep.*, 79:401-408.

Sacchi, E. (1895), "A case of infantile gigantism (pedomacrosomia) with a tumor of the testicle." *Riv Sper Freniat*, 21:149-161.

Sadayama, T., T. Masuda, and H. Miyano. (1983), "Relationships between muscle fibre conduction and velocity and frequency parameters of surface EMG during sustained contraction." *European Journal of Applied Physiology*, 51:247-256.

Sahlin, K. (1986). Metabolic changes limiting muscular performance. *Biochemistry of Exercise*. Vol. 16:22-31, 42-53.

Sale, D. (1986), "Neural adaptation in strength and power training." In L. Jones, N. McCartney, and A. McComas (eds.). *Human Muscle Power*, pp. 289-304/ Human Kinetics, Champaign, Illinois.

Schmidbleicher, D. (1992), "Training for power events." In Komi, P.V. (ed.). *Strength and Power in Sport*. Oxford: Blackwell Scientific Publications.

Sherwood, L. (1993), *Human Physiology From Cells to Systems (Second Edition)*. Minneapolis/St.Paul, West Publishing Company.

Smith, L.L., M. McCammon, S. Smith, M. Chamness, R.G. Israel, and K.F. O'Brien. (1989). White blood cell response to uphill walking and downhill jogging at similar metabolic loads. *Eur J. Appl Physiol*. 58: 833-837.

Staron, R.S., F.C. Hagerman, and P.S. Hikida. (1981), "The effects of detraining on an elite power lifter." *Journal of Neurological Sciences*, 51:247-257.

Stephens, J.A., and A. Taylor. (1972), "Fatigue of maintained voluntary muscle contractions in man." *Journal of Physiology* (Lond), 220:1-18.

Stewart, A.G., G.Grigoriadis, and T. Harris. (1994), "Mitogenic actions of endothelin-1 and epidermal growth factor in cultured airway smooth muscle." *Clinical & Experimental Pharmacology & Physiology*, 21(4):277-85.

Strauss, R.H., J.E. Wright, and G.A.M. Finerman. (1983). Side effects of anabolic steroids in weight trained men. *Physician Sportsmedicine*. 11: 87-96.

Terjung R.L. and D.A. Hood. (1986). Biochemical adaptation in skeletal muscle induced by exercise training.

Tesch, P.A. (1980). Muscle fatigue in man. *Acta Physiologica Scandinavica*. Supplementum,480:3-40.

Tesch, P.A., E.G. Colliander, and P. Kaiser.(1986). Muscle metabolism during intense, heavy-resistance exercise. *European Journal of Applied Physiology and Occupational Therapy*.

Thorstensson, A. (1977), "Observations on strength training and detraining." *Acta Physiologic Scandinavica*, 100:491-493.

U.S. Food and Nutrition Board. *Recommended Dietary Allowances*, vol.10, (1989), Washington, D.C.: National Academy Press, pp. 52-77.

U.S. Food and Nutrition Board. *Recommended Dietary Allowances*, 10th Edition. (1989), Washington, D.C.: National Academy Press.

Umpleby, A.M., F. Shojaee-Moradie, M.J. Thomason, et al. (1994), "Effects of insulin-like growth factor-I (IGF-I), insulin and combined IGF-I insulin infusions on protein metabolism in dogs." *European Journal of Investigation*, 24: 337-344.

Vandersticheleet, H., W. Eechaute, E. Lacroix and I. Leusen. (1989), "Effect of tamoxifen on the activity of enzymes of testicular steroidogenesis." *Steroids*, 53(6):713-726.

Wadsworth, H. and A.P.P. Chanmugan. (1983), *Electrophysical Agents in Physiotherapy*, Second Edition, Marrickville, Australia: Science Press.

Walberg, J.L., M.K. Leidy, D.J. Sturgell, D.E. Hinkle, S.J. Ritchie and D.R. Sebott. (1988), "Macronutrient content of a hypoenergy diet affects nitrogen retention and muscle function in weight lifters." *International Journal of Sports Medicine*, 9:261-266.

Walsh, M. (1986). Hydrotherapy: the use of water as a therapeutic agent. In Michlovits, SL, Editor. *Thermal Agent Rehabilitation*. Philadelphia: F.A. Davis Company.

Wardlaw, Gordon M. and Paul M. Insel. (1990), *Perspectives in Nutrition*. St. Louis, MO: Times Mirror/Mosby College Publishing.

Weissberger, A.J. and K.K. Ho. (1993), "Activation of the somatotropic axis by testosterone in adult males: Evidence in the role of aromatization." *Journal of Clinical Endocrinol. Metab.*, 76(6):1407.12.

Whitsett, T., C.V. Manion and M.F. Wilson. (1981), "Cardiac, pulmonary and neuromuscular effects of clenbuterol and terbutaine compared with placebo." *Br Journal of Clinical Pharmacol.*, 12:195-200.

Williams, J.G.P. and M. Street. (1976), "Sequential Faradism in Quadriceps Rehabilitation." *Physiotherapy*, 62:252-254.

Wilmore, J.H. (1986), "Body composition: A roundtable." *The Physician and Sports Medicine*, 14:144-162.

Wilmore, J.H., and D.L. Costill. (1988), Training for Sport and Activity: The Physiological Basis of the Conditioning Process. Dubuque, Iowa: Wm. C. Brown Publishers.

Windsor, R., and D. Dumitru (1989), "Prevalence of anabolic steroid use by male and female adolescents." *Medicine and Science in Sports Exercise*, 21(5):494-497.

Wolf, R.F., M.J. Heslin, E. Newman, et al. (1992), "Growth hormone and insulin combine to improve whole-body and skeletal muscle protein kinetics." *Surgery*, 112(2):284-92.

Wolf, R.F., D.B. Pearlstone, E. Newman, et al. (1992), "Growth hormone and insulin reverse net whole body and skeletal muscle protein catabolism in cancer patients." *Annals of Surgery*, 216(3):280-90.

Wolf, R.F., D.B. Pearlstone, E. Newman, et al. (1992), "Growth hormone and insulin reverse net whole body and skeletal muscle protein catabolism in cancer patients." *Ann.Surgery*, 216(3):280-290.

Wong, J. and L. Rapson. (1983), *L. TENS - Manual of Transutaneous Electrical Nerve Stimulation Therapy.*

Wright, E.J., C. Dahlf and K. Sveningson. (1995). Your hands-on guide to massage. *Muscle & Fitness*. August: 160-166.

Yakovlev, N.N. (1967)

Yang, Y.T. and M.A. McElligott. (1989), "Multiple actions of ?-adrenergic agonists on skeletal muscle and adipose tissue." *Biochemical Journal*, 261:1-10.

Yarasheski, K.E., J.J. Zachweija, T.J. Angelopoulos and D.M. Bier. (1993), "Short-term growth hormone treatment does not increase muscle protein synthesis in experienced weight lifters." *Journal of Applied Physiology*, 74(6):3073-6.

Yessis, M. (1990). *Soviet training methods*. New York: Barnes and Noble Publishing.

Zeman, R.J., R. Ludemann, T.G. Easton and J.D. Etlinger. (1988), "Slow to fast alterations in skeletal muscle fibres caused by clenbuterol, a beta 2-receptor agonist." *American Journal of Physiology*, 254(6):E726-32.

Zuniga, E.N. and D.G. Simons (1969), "Nonlinear relationship between averaged electromyogram potential and muscle tension in normal subjects." *Journal of Physiology* (Lond), 220:1-18.

INDEX

ABOUT THE AUTHORS

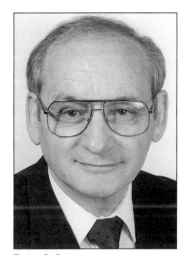

Tudor O. Bompa

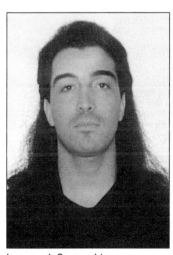

Lorenzo J. Cornacchia

Tudor O. Bompa, PhD, revolutionized western training methods when he introduced his groundbreaking theory of Periodization in Romania in 1963. After adopting his training system, the Eastern Bloc countries dominated international sports through the 1970s and 1980s. In 1988, Dr. Bompa applied his principle of Periodization to the sport of bodybuilding. He has personally trained 11 Olympic Games medalists (including four gold medalists) and has served as a consultant to coaches and athletes worldwide.

Dr. Bompa's books on training methods, including *Theory and Methodology of Training: The Key to Athletic Performance,* have been translated into eight languages. His training programs have been used in coaching certification programs around the world, and he's received certificates of honor and appreciation from such prestigious organizations as the Argentinean Ministry of Culture, the Australian Sports Council, the Spanish Olympic Committee, and the International Olympic Committee.

A member of the Canadian Olympic Association and the Romanian National Council of Sports, Dr. Bompa is full professor at York University in Toronto, Ontario, where he has taught training theories for 25 years. He and his wife, Tamara, live in Sharon, Ontario, where he enjoys walking his dog, gardening, and watching old movies. He is a citizen of both Canada and Romania.

As a personal trainer, kinesiologist, and former bodybuilder, **Lorenzo J. Cornacchia** has conducted extensive electromyography (EMG) research to identify which exercises cause the greatest muscle stimulation and which could potentially cause harm. He publishes a regular column in *Ironman* magazine based on his research.

Cornacchia received his bachelor of arts in physical education and health from York University in Toronto, Ontario. A member of the Association of Kinesiologists of Canada and a resident of Toronto, he enjoys attending wrestling events and playing volleyball and tennis.

MORE BOOKS TO HELP YOU BUILD MUSCLE

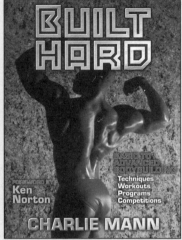

Built Hard shows serious fitness enthusiasts how to enter the sport of body-building and helps veteran bodybuilders make the gains necessary to win in competitions. It features

- important initial steps for beginners;
- comprehensive exercise routines for every part of the body;
- detailed lifting descriptions with more than 200 photographs;
- separate programs for beginner, intermediate, and advanced bodybuilders; and
- special inside tricks that promote faster progress.

1998 • Paper • 280 pp • Item PMAN0696
ISBN 0-88011-696-X • $19.95 ($29.95 Canadian)

Building muscle takes more than just long hours in the gym—what you eat, how much you eat, and when you eat has a big impact on how strong, lean, and powerful you can be. *Power Eating* provides

- detailed advice on 36 supplements, herbs, and hormones, including a powerful technique to boost creatine absorption by 60 percent;
- optimal protein intake formulas for your body type and training goals;
- smart choices for fast food restaurants and vegetarian eating;
- healthy alternatives to steroids; and
- eight complete eating plans to add muscle, cut weight, taper for competition, and maintain muscle gains.

1998 • Paper • 240 pp • Item PKLE0702
ISBN 0-88011-702-8 • $15.95 ($23.95 Canadian)

The best in sports conditioning now combines plyometric, resistance, and sprint training. *Explosive Power and Strength* not only offers these three training methods in one, but also shows you how to create individualized, sports-specific programs. The book features 33 resistance and 45 plyometric exercises with 115 detailed illustrations, plus three ready-to-use workouts for each of 11 sports.

1996 • Paper • 200 pp • Item PCHU0643
ISBN 0-87322-643-7 • $15.95 ($23.95 Canadian)

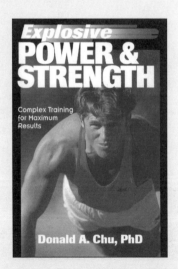

To request more information or to place your order,
U.S. customers call **TOLL FREE 1-800-747-4457**. Customers outside the U.S. place your order using the appropriate telephone number/address shown in the front of this book.

HUMAN KINETICS
The Premier Publisher for Sports & Fitness
http://www.humankinetics.com/